PULMONARY FUNCTION TESTING GUIDELINES AND CONTROVERSIES

Equipment, Methods, and Normal Values

Contributors

Joan F. Abramson, M.S., RCPT
Homer A. Boushey, Jr., M.D.
Wilbur Brandt, M.S., RCPT
Jack L. Clausen, M.D.
Clarence R. Collier, M.D.
Arthur Dawson, M.D.
Robert J. Fallat, M.D.
Catherine Fonzi, RCPT
Philip M. Gold, M.D.
James E. Hansen, M.D.
Darrell Hauer, B.S.
Alfredo A. Jalowayski, Ph.D.
James K. Larson, P.E.
Norman J. Lewiston, M.D.
John C. McQuitty, M.D.
John G. Mohler, M.D.
Frederick J. Nachtwey, M.D.
Craig Pederson, RCPT
Joe W. Ramsdell, M.D.
Andrew L. Ries, M.D.
Dennis W. Schwesinger, RCPT
Michael Snow, RCPT
Antonius L. Van Kessel, B.S., RCPT
Gerda Verkaik, RCPT
Steven Yates, RCPT
L. Powell Zarins, RCPT

PULMONARY FUNCTION TESTING GUIDELINES AND CONTROVERSIES

Equipment, Methods, and Normal Values

A Project of the California Thoracic Society

Edited by

JACK L. CLAUSEN, M.D.
University of California School of Medicine
and
University of California Medical Center
San Diego, California

Assistant Technical Editing by

L. POWELL ZARINS, RCPT
University of California Medical Center
San Diego, California

G&S

GRUNE & STRATTON, INC.
(Harcourt Brace Jovanovich, Publishers)
Orlando San Diego San Francisco New York
London Toronto Montreal Sydney Tokyo São Paulo

Library of Congress Cataloging in Publication Data
Main entry under title:

Pulmonary function testing guidelines and controversies.

"A project of the California Thoracic Society."
Bibliography: p.
Includes index.
1. Pulmonary function tests—Handbooks, manuals, etc.
I. Clausen, Jack L.
RC734.P84P83 1984 616.2'4'075 83-20146
ISBN 0-8089-1647-5 (pbk.)

Printing history: original edition by Academic Press, Inc., © 1982.
Reprinted 1982, 1983 by Academic Press, Inc.
Paperback edition published 1984 by Grune & Stratton, Inc.

Distributed in the United Kingdom by
Grune & Stratton, Inc. (London) Ltd.
24/28 Oval Road, London NW 1

Library of Congress Catalog Number 83-20146
International Standard Book Number 0-8089-1647-5

Printed in the United States of America.

Contents

3 Pulmonary Laboratory Infection Control and Safety

Philip M. Gold, M.D., and Dennis W. Schwesinger, RCPT

4 Measurement: Theory and Practice

John G. Mohler, M.D.

5 Instrumentation

Michael Snow, RCPT

6 Prediction of Normal Values

Jack L. Clausen, M.D.

7 Spirometry and Flow–Volume Curves

Homer A. Boushey, Jr., M.D., and Arthur Dawson, M.D.

8 Microprocessor-Assisted Spirometry

Arthur Dawson, M.D., and John G. Mohler, M.D.

9 Pneumotachography

Arthur Dawson, M.D.

10 Low-Density Gas Spirometry

Arthur Dawson, M.D.

11 Single Breath Nitrogen Test: Closing Volume and Distribution of Ventilation

Philip M. Gold, M.D.

12 Measurement of Lung Volume: The Multiple Breath Nitrogen Method

Alfredo A. Jalowayski, Ph.D., and Arthur Dawson, M.D.

13 Closed Circuit Helium Dilution Method of Lung Volume Measurement

L. Powell Zarins, RCPT

14 Body Plethysmography

L. Powell Zarins, RCPT, and Jack L. Clausen, M.D.

15 Estimation of Lung Volumes from Chest Radiographs

Jack L. Clausen, M.D., and L. Powell Zarins, RCPT

16 Pulmonary Diffusing Capacity for Carbon Monoxide

Antonius L. Van Kessel, B.S., RCPT

17 Maximal Inspiratory and Expiratory Pressures

Jack L. Clausen, M.D.

18 Elastic Recoil and Compliance

Arthur Dawson, M.D.

19 Bronchial Provocation Testing

Joe W. Ramsdell, M.D., Darrell Hauer, B.S., and Frederick J. Nachtwey, M.D.

20 Response to Bronchodilators

Andrew L. Ries, M.D.

21 Blood Gases

John G. Mohler, M.D., Clarence R. Collier, M.D., Wilbur Brandt, M.S., RCPT, Joan F. Abramson, M.S., RCPT, Gerda Verkaik, RCPT, and Steven Yates, RCPT

22 Exercise Testing

James E. Hansen, M.D.

23 Regulation of Ventilation

James E. Hansen, M.D.

24 Bedside Testing and Intensive Care Monitoring of Pulmonary Function

Robert J. Fallat, M.D., and John C. McQuitty, M.D.

25 Hemodynamic Monitoring

Robert J. Fallat, M.D.

Contributors

Numbers in parentheses indicate the pages on which the authors' contributions begin.

Joan F. Abramson, M.S., RCPT (7, 223), Pulmonary Diagnostic Services, White Memorial Medical Center, Los Angeles, California 90033

Homer A. Boushey, Jr., M.D. (61), Department of Medicine and Cardiovascular Research Institute, University of California, San Francisco, California 94143

Wilbur Brandt, M.S., RCPT (223), Pulmonary Laboratory, Los Angeles County/University of Southern California Medical Center, Los Angeles, California 90033

Jack L. Clausen, M.D. (1, 49, 141, 155, 187), Pulmonary Division, University of California Medical Center, San Diego, California 92103

Clarence R. Collier, M.D. (223), University of Southern California School of Medicine, Los Angeles, California 90033

Arthur Dawson, M.D. (61, 83, 91, 99, 115, 193), Division of Chest Medicine, Scripps Clinic and Research Foundation, La Jolla, California 92037

Robert J. Fallat, M.D. (293, 311), Department of Pulmonary Medicine, Pacific Medical Center, San Francisco, California 94120

Catherine Fonzi, RCPT (343), Pulmonary Division, University of California Medical Center, San Diego, California 92103

Philip M. Gold, M.D. (15, 105), Pulmonary Division, Veterans Administration Hospital, Loma Linda, California 92357

James E. Hansen, M.D. (259, 281), Division of Respiratory Physiology and Medicine, Department of Medicine, Harbor/UCLA Medical Center, Torrance, California 90509

Darrell Hauer, B.S. (205), Pulmonary Division, University of California Medical Center, San Diego, California 92103

Alfredo A. Jalowayski, Ph.D. (115), Pediatric Respiratory Unit, University of California Medical Center, San Diego, California 92103

James K. Larson, P.E. (331), Pulmonary Division, University of California Medical Center, San Diego, California 92103

Norman J. Lewiston, M.D. (321), Pediatric Allergy and Pulmonary Disease Division, Children's Hospital, Stanford University, Stanford, California 94303

John C. McQuitty, M.D. (293, 321), Children's Hospital Oakland, Oakland, California 94609

John G. Mohler, M.D. (23, 83, 223), Pulmonary Physiology Laboratories, Los Angeles County/University of Southern California Medical Center, Los Angeles, California 90033

Frederick J. Nachtwey, M.D. (205), Pulmonary Division, University of California Medical Center, San Diego, California 92103

Craig Pederson, RCPT (343), Pulmonary Function Laboratory, University of California Medical Center, San Diego, California 92103

Joe W. Ramsdell, M.D. (205), Pulmonary Division, University of California Medical Center, San Diego, California 92103

Andrew L. Ries, M.D. (215), Pulmonary Division, University of California Medical Center, San Diego, California 92103

Dennis W. Schwesinger, RCPT (15), Cardiopulmonary Department, Century City Hospital, Los Angeles, California 90067

Michael Snow, RCPT (27), Pulmonary Laboratory, Pacific Medical Center, San Francisco, California 94510

Antonius L. Van Kessel, B.S., RCPT (7, 165), Pulmonary Physiology Laboratory, Stanford University Hospital, Stanford, California 94305

Gerda Verkaik, RCPT (223), Pulmonary Physiology Laboratory, Los Angeles County/University of Southern California Medical Center, Los Angeles, California 90033

Steven Yates, RCPT (223), Pulmonary Physiology Laboratories, Los Angeles County/University of Southern California Medical Center, Los Angeles, California 90033

L. Powell Zarins, RCPT (129, 141, 155), Pulmonary Division, University of California Medical Center, San Diego, California 92103

Preface

This volume originated in an ad hoc subcommittee of the California Thoracic Society (CTS) formed to advise the California State Department of Health Services regarding qualifications of laboratory personnel and quality assurance of blood-gas analyses. The combined resources of both technical and medical expertise within the committee were employed to develop recommendations for CTS members concerning methodologies for the various tests performed in pulmonary function laboratories.

The significant differences in test results between laboratories using different equipment, techniques, or normal values led to the conclusion that the more basic technical aspects of testing must first be addressed prior to undertaking meaningful dialogues on the important issues of clinical usefulness, indications for testing, and interpretation of results. (The latter issues will be addressed in another volume, which is currently being developed.)

Chapters in this book were first critically reviewed in a series of committee meetings, revised to reflect committee input, and then subjected to more widespread review when used as the syllabus for a 3-day CTS postgraduate course held in 1980. The guest faculty for this course was selected with the intent of gaining fresh critiques of the recommendations presented in the syllabus. This guest faculty was a rich resource of expertise. We are very appreciative for their helpful comments and suggestions. The faculty included Sonia A. Buist, M.D., Benjamin Burrows, M.D., Edward A. Gaensler, M.D., Reed M. Gardner, Ph.D., Norman L. Jones, M.D., Richard J. Leman, M.D., David A. Mathison, M.D., Alan H. Morris, M.D., Kenneth M. Moser, M.D., Richard M. Peters, M.D., Anton Renzetti, M.D., Joseph R. Rodarte, M.D., John W. Severinghaus, M.D., Gennaro M. Tisi, M.D., Karlman Wasserman, M.D., Ph.D., and Brian Whipp, Ph.D.

Course participants included physicians, technologists, therapists, and representatives of manufacturers of pulmonary laboratory equipment. Although many topics sparked considerable differences of opinion, the course was perceived by most participants as an effective and productive interchange of ideas on the technical aspects of testing. The input from the course was then used by each author in preparing the final versions of the chapters.

One of the most heated controversies that developed during the course concerned the appropriateness of including tests that are not established as clinically useful. It was decided that the primary criterion for inclusion of a test in this text was whether or not the test was then being done in a significant number of clinical laboratories. Questions of clinical usefulness will be addressed in the second volume of this project.

This text does not represent an official policy statement of the CTS, nor does every statement represent the unanimous consensus of the committee. As accurately as possible, the material in each chapter represents the authors' synthesis of their own recommendations with those of the committee and course participants. We view this text as the best body of recommendations that can be made based on the current state of the art.

The primary purpose of this book is to maximize the accuracy and precision of pulmonary function testing, and thereby, increase its clinical utility. We hope that the recommendations in this text will help some laboratories improve efficiency, thereby reducing costs, mainly by eliminating unnecessary quality control procedures and unnecessary steps during testing, reducing the need for repeat testing, and decreasing the likelihood of purchasing inappropriate testing equipment and quality control materials.

This text is also intended to give manufacturers guidelines for the development of equipment in accordance with current needs of pulmonary laboratories, as perceived by both laboratory and clinical personnel. As instruments become more automated, it becomes increasingly important that technical and clinical personnel have both a clear understanding of what their instruments do, and input into the design of future instruments. One purpose of the conference was to stimulate increased dialogue between industry and the medical community involved with pulmonary function testing. Thus, conference invitations were sent to all companies we could identify as being involved with pulmonary function testing. In some instances, draft versions of specific chapters were sent to appropriate industrial personnel for their input.

This book is directed primarily at technologists, physiologists, engineers, and physicians who are responsible for clinical application of pulmonary function testing. It should also be of interest to those doing related clinical, physiological, or epidemiological research, and for students and postgraduate trainees in fields involving pulmonary function testing. It may also be of interest to physicians who must interpret pulmonary function tests and therefore wish to better understand the foundations upon which their clinical interpretation of pulmonary function tests must rest. This book was published to meet the need for a single text containing recommended methodologies for the many pulmonary function tests. Although a number of excellent publications on standardized methodologies are available (see references in Chapter 1), some were developed specifically for research or epidemiological applications, and a number are not readily available in medical libraries. We hope this volume will be useful in the development of more uniform pulmonary function testing.

The first six chapters present general overviews of subjects that interrelate to each of the subsequent chapters. The remaining chapters deal with more specific testing procedures and, wherever possible, were organized in the following format:

The *Introduction* includes a brief review of the clinical applications of the test. The summary of indications for each test does not represent a critical assessment of the clinical usefulness, but is intended to give readers a general perspective. Only a brief review of the pathophysiological basis of the test is included. Greater detail is available in numerous physiological texts and articles.

The *Equipment* sections outline what equipment is necessary and, wherever possible, what the minimal performance characteristics should be. Every effort was made to describe equipment in generic terms.

The *Quality Control* sections present the recommended procedures for assuring the accuracy and precision of clinical tests. The selection of optimal quality control procedures is so dependent on instrument characteristics, however, that in many cases quality control procedures different than those recommended may be required.

In the *Procedures* section, we have emphasized the critical aspects of the testing procedures, including those instructions to the patients that are necessary for optimal test results. The necessity for active patient participation is one of the critical differences between tests performed in pulmonary function laboratories and those conducted in clinical pathology laboratories.

The *Calculations* sections, in addition to presenting the formulas used in data calculations, present sample calculations, which were included to prevent problems in the expression of data in the wrong units, the use of incorrect factors, or the erroneous application of algebraic logic.

The recommendations for *Normal Predictive Values* represent the outcome of considerable thought and committee discussion. Although our goal was to recommend a single set of normal reference values for each test, in very few cases was there sufficient evidence to permit the conclusion that a particular study was "the best." One of the most interesting outcomes from the committee was the appreciation of the diversity of normal values that we chose to use in our own laboratories. In almost every chapter, the selection of optimal reference values remains an unresolved controversy. Chapter 6 presents the important general characteristics of studies of normal subjects that must be considered in selecting the most appropriate set of reference values. In most of the chapters dealing with specific tests, we have presented a number of studies of normal values so that laboratories can evaluate and select the study most appropriate for their particular instrumentation and patient population. When specific sets of normal values were recommended, they usually reflected the opinion of the chapter authors rather than the unanimous consensus of the committee. Clearly one of the more challenging future tasks is the identification or development of prediction equations for normal values that are of maximal clinical usefulness. As greater uniformity in testing procedures is achieved, this task will be easier.

We presented data on *Expected Reproducibility* because we believe that this information is useful for confirming that the precision of a laboratory's own testing methods is adequate. This information is also of obvious importance in interpreting the clinical significance of measurements that differ from those predicted for or previously obtained from the same patient. For comparison with normal values, the within-day reproducibility is most pertinent; for serial measurements, the between-day variability is more appropriate.

In the *Troubleshooting* sections we present what we feel would be the most useful information on sources of error. No attempt was made to include all possibilities. For further information, readers are encouraged to review the excellent instrument-specific publications available from most manufacturers of equipment and quality control products.

The *Controversies* sections attempt to identify and sometimes briefly discuss those testing aspects for which we felt there is insufficient scientific evidence on which to base a recommendation. Because these are issues that usually need further investigation, studies related to these issues will be of obvious interest in the future. Resolution of these controversies will be a key step toward achieving more uniform testing procedures.

Acknowledgments

The financial and administrative support of the California Thoracic Society (CTS) and the California Chapter of the American Lung Association was essential to the development of this text. The considerable administrative support of Elma Plappert, Executive Secretary of the CTS, is particularly appreciated. Dr. Philip Gold was the committee chairman when this project was initiated and later served as president of the CTS. He was a key factor in the development and continued support of this project.

Numerous people contributed very helpful suggestions and corrections to the original course syllabus. They include associates at the various institutions represented by the authors of this text, colleagues within the CTS and other participants in the 1980 postgraduate course. Most useful and appreciated were the detailed suggestions given to us by the guest faculty, as well as the detailed reviews by Barbara Corbett and Paul Koenig. Jan Evans made essential contributions in the typing and communications between myself, the authors, and the publishers. Her cheerful input into this project is gratefully acknowledged. The contributions of Linda Zarins as assistant editor extended well beyond her careful technical documentation and are greatly appreciated.

I enjoyed the privilege of editing this text and assume responsibility for any errors or omissions. Suggestions and corrections will be received with interest and gratitude.

Terms and Abbreviations

The variety of abbreviations used in clinical pulmonary function reports (e.g., MEF 50%, FEF 50%, $\dot{V}$max 50%, and $\dot{V}$ 50%) often leads to considerable confusion, especially for physicians without specific training in pulmonary medicine. Although not perfect, the terminology and abbreviations suggested by an American College of Chest Physicians/American Thoracic Society (ACCP/ATS) joint committee are the best available and should be used whenever possible. Those most relevant to subsequent chapters are given below. Abbreviations marked with an asterisk were not cited by the ACCP/ATS joint committee, but are used in this book.

A	Alveolar
a	Arterial
an	Anatomic
ATPD	Ambient temperature and pressure, dry
ATPS	Ambient temperature and pressure, saturated with water vapor at these conditions
B	Barometric
BTPS	Body conditions: Body temperature, ambient pressure, and saturated with water vapor at these conditions
C	A general symbol for compliance, volume change per unit of applied pressure
c	Capillary
C/V_L	Specific compliance
CD*	Cumulative inhalation dose. The total dose of an agent inhaled during bronchial challenge testing; it is the sum of the products of concentration multiplied by the number of breaths at that concentration
C_{dyn}	Dynamic compliance, compliance measured at point of zero gas

	flow at the mouth during active breathing. The respiratory frequency should be designated; e.g., $C_{dyn}40$
C_{st}	Static compliance, compliance determined from measurements made during conditions of prolonged interruption of air flow
D	Dead space or wasted ventilation (qualifying symbol, e.g., V_D)
D/V_A	Diffusion per unit of alveolar volume
D_k	Diffusion coefficient or permeability constant as described by Krogh; it equals $D \cdot (P_B - P_{H_2O})/V_A$
D_m	Diffusing capacity of the alveolar capillary membrane (STPD)
D_x (or DL_{CO})	Diffusing capacity of the lung expressed as volume (STPD) of gas (x) uptake per unit alveolar-capillary pressure difference for the gas used. Unless otherwise stated, carbon monoxide is assumed to be the test gas, i.e., D is D_{co}. A modifier can be used to designate the technique, e.g., D_{SB} is single breath carbon monoxide diffusing capacity and D_{SS} is steady state CO diffusing capacity. (Editor's note: This recommendation has not widely been accepted. DL_{CO}, $DL_{CO}SB$, and $DL_{CO}SS$ are still the most commonly used abbreviations.)
E	Expired
ERV	Expiratory reserve volume; the maximal volume of air exhaled from the end-expiratory level
est	Estimated
f	Respiratory frequency per minute
F	Fractional concentration of a gas
FEF_{max}	The maximal forced expiratory flow achieved during an FVC
$FEF_{25-75\%}$	Mean forced expiratory flow during the middle half of the FVC (formerly called the maximum mid-expiratory flow rate)
$FEF_{75\%}$	Instantaneous forced expiratory flow after 75% of the FVC has been exhaled
$FEF_{200-1200}$	Mean forced expiratory flow between 200 ml and 1200 ml of the FVC (formerly called the maximum expiratory flow rate)
FEF_x	Forced expiratory flow, related to some portion of the FVC curve. Modifiers refer to the amount of the FVC already *exhaled* when the measurement is made
FET_x	The forced expiratory time for a specified portion of the FVC; e.g., $FET_{95\%}$ is the time required to deliver the first 95% of the FVC and $FET_{25-75\%}$ is the time required to deliver the $FEF_{25-75\%}$
$FEV_t/FVC\%$	Forced expiratory volume (timed) to forced vital capacity ratio, expressed as a percentage
FIF_x	Forced inspiratory flow. As in the case of the FEF, the appropriate modifiers must be used to designate the volume at which flow is

being measured. Unless otherwise specified, the volume qualifiers indicate the volume inspired from RV at the point of the measurement

FRC — Functional residual capacity; the sum of RV and ERV (the volume of air remaining in the lungs at the end-expiratory position). The method of measurement should be indicated as with RV

G_{aw} — Airway conductance, the reciprocal of R_{aw}

G_{aw}/V_L — Specific conductance, expressed per liter of lung volume at which G is measured (also referred to as SG_{aw})

I — Inspired

IRV — Inspiratory reserve volume; the maximal volume of air inhaled from the end-inspiratory level

IC — Inspiratory capacity; the sum of IRV and V_T

L — Lung

max — Maximal

MIP* — Maximal inspiratory pressure

MEP* — Maximal expiratory pressure

MVV_x — Maximal voluntary ventilation. The volume of air expired in a specified period during repetitive maximal respiratory effort. The respiratory frequency is indicated by a numerical qualifier; e.g., MVV_{60} is MVV performed at 60 breaths per minute. If no qualifier is given, an unrestricted frequency is assumed

p — Physiological

P — Pressure, blood or gas

PA* — Pulmonary artery

PD* — Provocative dose; the dose of an agent used in bronchial challenge testing which results in a defined change in a specific physiologic parameter. The parameter tested and the percent change in this parameter is expressed in cumulative dose units over the time following exposure that the positive response occurred. For example, $PD_{35}SG_{aw}$ = x units/y minutes, where x is the cumulative inhalation dose and y the time at which a 35% fall in SG_{aw} was noted

PEF — The highest forced expiratory flow measured with a peak flow meter

P_{st} — Static transpulmonary pressure at a specified lung volume; e.g., $P_{st}TLC$ is static recoil pressure measured at TLC (maximal recoil pressure)

Q_c — Capillary blood volume (usually expressed as V_c in the literature, a symbol inconsistent with those recommended for blood volumes). When determined from the following equation, Q_c represents the effective pulmonary capillary blood volume, i.e., capillary blood volume in intimate association with alveolar gas:

$$1/D = 1/D_m + 1/(\Theta \cdot Q_c)$$

R — A general symbol for resistance, pressure per unit flow

R_{aw} — Airway resistance

rb — Rebreathing

RQ* — Respiratory quotient

R_{us} — Resistance of the airways on the alveolar side (upstream) of the point in the airways where intraluminal pressure equals Ppl, measured under conditions of maximum expiratory flow

RV — Residual volume; that volume of air remaining in the lungs after maximal exhalation. The method of measurement should be indicated in the text or, when necessary, by appropriate qualifying symbols

SBN* — Single breath nitrogen test; a test in which plots of expired N_2 concentration versus expired volume after inspiration of 100% O_2 are recorded. The closing volume and slope of Phase III are two parameters measured by this test

STPD — Standard conditions: temperature 0° C, pressure 760 mm Hg, and dry (0 water vapor)

t — Time

T — Tidal

TGV* — Thoracic gas volume; the volume of gas within the thoracic cage as measured by body plethysmography

TLC — Total lung capacity; the sum of all volume compartments or the volume of air in the lungs after maximal inspiration. The method of measurement should be indicated, as with RV

V — Gas volume. The particular gas as well as its pressure, water vapor conditions, and other special conditions must be specified in text or indicated by appropriate qualifying symbols

v — Venous

$\bar{v}$ — Mixed venous

$\dot{V}_A$ — Alveolar ventilation per minute (BTPS)

$\dot{V}_{CO_2}$ — Carbon dioxide production per minute (STPD)

$\dot{V}_D$ — Ventilation per minute of the physiologic dead space (wasted ventilation), BTPS, defined by the following equation:

$$\dot{V}_D = \dot{V}_E(PaCO_2 - P_ECO_2/(PaCO_2 - P_ICO_2)$$

V_D — The physiologic dead-space volume defined as $\dot{V}_D/f$

$V_D$an — Volume of the anatomic dead space (BTPS)

$\dot{V}_E$ — Expired volume per minute (BTPS)

$\dot{V}_I$ — Inspired volume per minute (BTPS)

Viso$\dot{V}$* — Volume of isoflow; the volume when the expiratory flow rates become identical when flow-volume loops performed after breathing room air and helium-oxygen mixtures are compared

$\dot{V}_{O_2}$ Oxygen consumption per minute (STPD)

$\dot{V}_{max}X$ Forced expiratory flow, related to the total lung capacity or the actual volume of the lung at which the measurement is made. *Modifiers refer to the amount of lung volume remaining when the measurement is made.* For example: $\dot{V}_{max}$ 75% is instantaneous forced expiratory flow when the lung is at 75% of its TLC. $\dot{V}_{max}3.0$ is instantaneous forced expiratory flow when the lung volume is 3.0 liters. [Editor's note: It is still common to find reports in which modifiers refer to the amount of VC remaining.]

V_T Tidal volume; TV is also commonly used

XA or Xa A small capital letter or lowercase letter on the same line following a primary symbol is a qualifier to further define the primary symbol. When small capital letters are not available on typewriters or to printers, large capital letters may be used as subscripts, e.g., X_A = XA

Blood-Gas Measurements

Abbreviations for these values are readily composed by combining the general symbols recommended earlier. The following are examples:

$PaCO_2$ Arterial carbon dioxide tension

$C(a-v)O_2$ Arteriovenous oxygen content difference

CcO_2 Oxygen content of pulmonary end-capillary blood

F_ECO* Fractional concentration of CO in expired gas

$P(A-a)O_2$ Alveolar-arterial oxygen pressure difference; the previously used symbol, $A\text{-}aDO_2$ is not recommended

SaO_2 Arterial oxygen saturation of hemoglobin

Q_{SP} Physiologic shunt flow (total venous admixture) defined by the following equation when gas and blood data are collected during ambient air breathing:

$$Qsp = \frac{CcO_2 - CaO_2}{CcO_2 - CvO_2} \cdot Q$$

$P_{ET}O_2$ PO_2 of end tidal expired gas

$TCPO_2$ Transcutaneous PO_2

CHAPTER 1

Standardization of Clinical Testing Procedures: Pros and Cons

JACK L. CLAUSEN, M.D.

There are a number of publications available that represent efforts to develop standardized or uniform testing procedures for pulmonary function tests (1–16). These resources were reviewed and the recommendations incorporated into this volume whenever appropriate. The advantages and disadvantages of standardization of clinical testing procedures were the focus of much thought and discussion during the development of this book. Some of the issues that arose from those discussions are presented in this chapter.

ARGUMENTS IN FAVOR OF STANDARDIZATION

Widespread standardization of the methodology of pulmonary function testing offers a number of attractive potential benefits. If methodology were uniform, clinicians would find it easier to interpret and compare test results from different laboratories. Standardization would lessen the occasional need for repeat testing when a patient is evaluated at a second facility and increase the usefulness of earlier test results as baseline data.

Standardization might also facilitate dialogues that seek to answer questions regarding the physiological basis or clinical applications of the test. All too often such discussions are stalemated by the conclusion that an opinion based on test methodologies that differ from those utilized by the majority of labs should not be seriously considered.

Standardization could also benefit the product development efforts of manufacturers by spelling out very clearly the capabilities required of future instruments. In addition, if equipment were standardized, the process of training both technical and medical specialists involved with physiological testing would be simplified.

PULMONARY FUNCTION TESTING
GUIDELINES AND CONTROVERSIES

ISBN 0-12-788125-5

A final argument in favor of test standardization is related to the cost. The modification or purchase of new equipment, the development of new normal reference values, and the reinvestigation of the abnormalities observed in specific disease processes all contribute to the costs of adopting significant changes in testing methodology, which are later reflected by increased costs of health care. When projected to a nationwide scale, the magnitude of these costs may be considerable. If the impartial body of expertise responsible for recommending changes in the standardized test procedures incorporated questions related to cost-benefits in their decision-making process, some observers feel that a standardization program would be a potentially effective mechanism for addressing cost-benefit issues before new technology is adopted for widespread use. Some would argue that these are inappropriate issues for a body chosen because of physiological and clinical expertise. Others argue that in the absence of effective consumer feedback, this would be the best, albeit imperfect, decision-making body.

ARGUMENTS AGAINST STANDARDIZATION

The most commonly cited argument against standardization of clinical pulmonary function tests is that for too many tests there is disagreement among the experts as to what the standard method should be, and therefore standardization is currently impossible. If standards were not based on valid and accepted scientific evidence, they would likely be counterproductive. Also, it would be difficult and time-consuming to incorporate valid improvements once a method is standardized. Experience has shown that governmental or national professional task forces can indeed be very slow to officially change established policies or recommendations. Standardization might also encourage the intrusion of big government (or big professional societies) into the practice of medicine and may limit the ability of physicians to select what they consider to be the best diagnostic procedure for each patient under their responsibility.

Another criticism is that standardization may result in mediocrity, stifling creativity and improvements in testing methodology. Also, testing procedures designed for large numbers of screening exams may not be appropriate for a tertiary medical center, which seeks precise measurements for purposes of diagnosis of subtle disease processes.

Standardization initially may be very costly if significant modifications or replacement of existing equipment are required. Seemingly inconsequential specific details, such as the duration of continuously recorded time during the forced expiratory maneuver or the definition of breath-holding time in the single-breath carbon monoxide diffusing capacity ($D_{L_{CO}}$) test may have a profound impact on whether or not specific equipment can be used for testing.

THE SPECTRUM OF STANDARDIZATION

Standardization of testing procedures means that certain aspects of equipment performance and test methodologies would need to be in accord with written standards. Depending upon the specificity of the standards, the tests may or may not be done identically in different laboratories. As it applies to clinical testing, standardization can encompass a number of different forms. At one end of the spectrum is the formulation of exact specifications encompassing all aspects of the testing, so that all equipment, methods, and normal values would be identical in all labs. This approach is the easiest to develop (e.g., use spirometer x and the methods and normal (reference) values used in hospital A) and is the most likely to result in uniformity of testing measurements in the shortest period of time. This approach, however, may be in conflict with the creative forces of industry and medical research labs, which are continually tempting laboratories with improvements (either real or perceived) in equipment, testing methodologies, and normal values. It also may require the replacement of currently functional equipment. This approach is usually applicable only to an organization with a small number of laboratories, all of which have a vested interest in cooperative interactions.

The other end of the spectrum is based on the premise: ''we don't care how you get the results, but they must be comparable to the results obtained by a specific reference method.'' An example would be recommendations consistent with the use of a wide variety of different devices (cylinders floating on water, pistons, bellows, screen, and Pitot-type pneumotachographs, turbines, thermistors, or ultrasonic generators and detectors) for measuring expiratory flow rates. If the new procedure or device results in normal subject and patient values comparable to the results obtained by the specific reference method, then the new method is judged acceptable. This approach is more likely to gain widespread acceptance from the many laboratory personnel who need the freedom to pursue identification of tests and equipment of maximal clinical usefulness and efficiency. Such an approach is the most difficult to develop, however, as it requires consensus on the choice of reference methods, and may require considerable expenditure of time and resources for research that adequately compares each method or piece of equipment with the reference method. Establishing reference values by research of normal subjects is a minor undertaking in comparison with the effort required to study adequate numbers of patients in various stages of disease who have the diversity of defects which the test may be used to detect.

Standards could be established by any of a number of different groups, including manufacturers, hospital associations, technologists, physiologists, medical directors, third-party insurance carriers, or governmental regulatory agencies.

The term ''standardization'' carries the connotation that compliance is mandatory, but participation could be voluntary. However, there are in existence powerful economic and legal forces, which may result in de facto mandatory compliance. For instance, if manufacturers adopt standardization, purchasers of equipment will have fewer options. Also, the pressure from hospitals for laboratory compliance with regulations of the Joint Commission for Accreditation of Hospitals (JCAH), the risk of malpractice liability if diagnostic tests are done contrary to published recommendations and prevailing medical practice, the denial of reimbursement for "nonstandardized" tests from private and governmental insurance carriers, as well as the need to comply with existing state and federal laws and regulations applicable to clinical laboratories and hospitals all tend to encourage standardization.

THE ROLE OF REGULATORY AGENCIES

Standardization can be achieved by a variety of approaches. One possibility is the development of state and federal regulations that require specific aspects of a test to be done in a prescribed manner as a condition for licensing of the laboratories. Examples already in existence are the regulations of the California State Department of Health Services that pertain to blood-gas laboratories. According to these regulations, blood-gas laboratories in California must be licensed if any analyses are done for clinical purposes. The only exception to the need for licensing is a laboratory that makes clinical tests exclusively on patients under the direct care of the physician who is the lab director. Specific examples of minimum requirements for licensing include the following (17):

1. A two-point calibration shall be performed each eight-hour shift when tests are done.
2. A one-point calibration shall be performed before or after each specimen or run.
3. Instrument readings shall be recorded for each calibration.

Laboratories that fail to meet these and other very specific minimal requirements may be required by the state regulatory agency to refer all clinical tests to another licensed lab until licensing requirements are met. Compliance with regulations is evaluated during annual visits to each laboratory by state inspectors. In the past, specialty laboratories, such as blood-gas laboratories, have often not been monitored by the state regulatory agency. In the past few years, however, increasing attention is being directed toward blood-gas laboratories not only by state agencies but also by JCAH inspection teams.

The emotional response to the regulations and inspection visits may sometimes obscure the fact that these activities were established in response to many legislators' perception that clinical testing results are sometimes so erroneous as to be clinically misleading, and from the good intentions of wanting to assure minimal standards of medical care. There is controversy regarding the benefit of such regulatory activities, but it is generally agreed that such agencies rarely have the resources and expertise required to develop satisfactory standards for a field as complicated as physiological testing of patients. Many regulatory agencies recognize these limitations and actively seek input from practicing health professionals for the formulation of reasonable minimal standards.

CONCLUSIONS

Although there are strong disagreements regarding the desirability of any organization's imposition of rigid standards for clinical testing, there is general agreement that it would take many years to achieve effective standardization of clinical pulmonary function tests. For example, the standards for spirometry, the most basic of pulmonary function tests, developed by the American Thoracic Society (1), required a considerable effort by many people extending over many, many months. It was the feeling of a number of participants of the discussions on which this text is based that many of the benefits of rigid standardization could be achieved by voluntary compliance with well-established uniform procedures, and that this approach would be more likely to result in widespread acceptance than attempts at rigid standardization.

The guidelines for testing methods presented in this book can be viewed as current state-of-the-art recommendations, which, combined with future opinions and recommendations from other groups, can be used in a "distillation" process to ultimately yield uniform testing methodologies which are voluntarily and widely accepted.

Although the regulatory activities of the government and JCAH are based upon concerns about the quality of clinical diagnostic testing procedures, there is currently a paucity of objective data regarding the validity of these concerns. Nevertheless, the most appropriate group to develop and establish minimal standards or uniform testing procedures would be a coalition of pulmonary technologists, physicians, and physiologists working with representatives of industry and regulatory agencies.

REFERENCES

1. Gardner RM, Baker CD, Broennle AM Jr, et al: ATS statement—Snowbird workshop on standardization of spirometry. *Am Rev Respir Dis* 119:831-838, 1979.
2. Ferris BG (principal investigator): Epidemiology standardization project. *Am Rev Respir Dis* 118(no.6,2), 1978.
3. Taussig LM, Chernick V, Wood R, et al: Standardization of lung function testing in children. Proceedings and recommendations of the GAP conference committee, Cystic Fibrosis Foundation. *J Pediatr* 97:668-678, 1980.

4. Kanner RE, Morris AH (eds): *Clinical Pulmonary Function Testing. A Manual of Uniform Laboratory Procedures for the Intermountain Area.* Salt Lake City, Utah; Intermountain Thoracic Society, 1975.
5. *Suggested Standardized Procedures for Closing Volume Determinations (Nitrogen Method).* National Heart and Lung Institute, Division of Lung Diseases, 1973.
6. Leith DE, Mead J: *Principles of Body Plethysmography.* National Heart and Lung Institute, Division of Lung Diseases Publication, November 1974.
7. Macklem PT: *Procedures for Standardized Measurements of Lung Mechanics.* National Heart and Lung Institute, Division of Lung Diseases Publication, November 1974.
8. Severinghaus J (ed): Proceedings of the workshop on methodological aspects of transcutaneous blood gas analyses. *Acta Anaesthesiol Scand.,* suppl. 68, 1978, pp. 76–82.
9. Guidelines for bronchial inhalation challenges with pharmacologic and antigenic agents. *Am Thor Soc News,* Spring 1980, pp 11–19.
10. Chai H, Farr RS, Froehlich LA, et al: Standardization of bronchial inhalation challenge procedures. *J Allergy Clin Immunol* 56:323–327, 1975.
11. Assessment of respiratory control in humans; editorial and workshop reports. *Am Rev Respir Dis* 115:1–5, 177–181, 363–365, 541–544, 713, 715–716, 883–887, 1977.
12. Severinghaus JW: Proposed standard determination of ventilatory responses to hypoxia and hypercapnia in man. *Chest,* suppl 70, 1976, pp 129–131.
13. Comroe JH Jr (ed): *Methods in Medical Research; Pulmonary Function Tests.* Chicago, Year Book Publishers Inc, 1950.
14. Bartels H, Bucherl E, Hertz CW et al: *Methods in Pulmonary Physiology.* Workman JM (trans). New York, Hafner Publishing Co, 1963.
15. Pulmonary terms and symbols. A report of the ACCP-ATS joint committee on pulmonary nomenclature.
16. *Definitions of Quantities and Conventions Related to Blood pH and Gas Analysis.* Pennsylvania, National Committee for Clinical Laboratory Standards, 1979.
17. *Quality Control for Blood Gas Analyses, Guidelines to Laboratory Management.* No. C-8 (revised) October 1980. California State Department of Health Services, 1980.

CHAPTER 2

Laboratory Management: Qualifications of Personnel

JOAN F. ABRAMSON, M.S., RCPT
ANTONIUS L. VAN KESSEL, B.S., RCPT

It is difficult, if not impossible, to specify qualifications for lab personnel that will be applicable to all laboratories. Some laboratory medical directors in smaller hospitals employ only a single technician whose responsibilities include the purchase, maintenance, and quality control of instrumentation; development and documentation of testing procedures; performance of all the standard pulmonary function tests, including blood-gas analyses and exercise testing; and the calculation of data and quality-control review of the report. In other hospitals, the medical director may assume many of these administrative responsibilities. Some large laboratories employ numerous personnel whose function is restricted to the performance of large numbers of a single test, such as blood gases or spirometry; this is done in the interest of maximizing quality control, reducing costs, and improving efficiency. In order to provide jobs with more varied daily routines as well as broad experience for optimizing future employment opportunities, other large labs prefer to rotate personnel through all aspects of testing functions.

Despite the difficulties in meaningfully defining qualifications for lab personnel, there are a number of reasons why it is important to do so. For testing which requires active patient participation, the abilities of the person who instructs the patient and performs the test often have much more impact on test results than the performance characteristics of the equipment, the methodology used, or the particular reference values selected.

In the past few years increasing attention has been directed by federal and state regulatory agencies to defining personnel standards for laboratories. These standards are an integral part of the agencies' efforts to assure the accuracy of clinical laboratory test results. In addition to other applications, these statements of qualifications may be used when regulatory agencies attempt to define which classification of personnel is qualified to do a particular test. Whether or not these activities are appropriate or effective, attempts to define which personnel are qualified to perform blood-gas analyses (such as those attempts made in

PULMONARY FUNCTION TESTING
GUIDELINES AND CONTROVERSIES

ISBN 0-12-788125-5

California and Florida in 1979 and 1980) indicate that statements of personnel qualifications *can* have a profound impact on the practice of pulmonary laboratory medicine. Development of acceptable standards from within the professional community, rather than originating from regulatory agencies, is an important step toward ensuring that personnel standards will be reasonable if they are required by such agencies.

Statements of minimal standards for personnel are also increasingly used by hospital administrators to define salary levels. Standards that are too low may result in low salary scales and significant problems for laboratory directors in attracting, training, and keeping adequate personnel. Standards that are unnecessarily high may increase the cost of medical care and may limit the abilities of laboratories in rural areas to hire technicians with qualifications defined as minimal.

Definition of personnel qualifications would also be useful for developing the curricula in specialized college training programs in the rapidly growing field of medical technology and would assure graduates of such programs that their training will be in accord with current job requirements. Although such education has commonly been accomplished by on-the-job training programs in the past (this is still the primary route of training in many laboratories), appropriate specialized training programs can relieve technical and medical directors of much of this ongoing responsibility and free them for tasks that more efficiently utilize their skills.

Thus, there are a number of compelling reasons for attempting to define personnel qualifications in clinical medical laboratories. Although it is obviously impossible to derive statements that are appropriate for all laboratories in all states, the following recommendations represent qualifications which we feel are appropriate for the vast majority of labs.

The single most significant factor in the production of high-quality test data is the person conducting the test. In addition to being motivated to work patiently with sick people, this individual must be well trained if the physician is to be provided with dependable test data. He or she should have ingenuity, a reasonable amount of common sense, and a thorough understanding of the underlying principles of the physiological measurements and the diversity of equipment encountered in the pulmonary lab. Also important is the ability to calculate results either by hand or with calculators or computers. A technologist should be trained to assess the validity of the test results, check for internal consistency, and be able to discuss the observations intelligently with the physician. In addition, the person should have a fundamental knowledge of pertinent physiological principles of health and disease. Lack of a familiarity with the rudiments of respiratory physiology is likely to result in poor judgment concerning proper methodology and procedures.

It is important to realize that many pulmonary function studies are partly subjective in nature and require optimum patient cooperation. Test results dependent on voluntary patient effort will be influenced by the technologist's ability to assume the attitude of a team coach to encourage maximum effort when indicated.

MEDICAL DIRECTOR

QUALIFICATIONS*

Training

The director must possess an M.D. degree or its equivalent, must be authorized to practice medicine in the state where the hospital is located, and should be a member of that hospital or clinic staff. The specialized and distinctive activities of the pulmonary function laboratory indicate that it should be under the direction of a physician with expertise in pulmonary physiology. The director should be certified or eligible for certification by the subspecialty board of pulmonary disease. When such a person is not available, the hospital may temporarily appoint the most qualified individual.

Competency

The director should be familiar with all the common pulmonary function equipment, blood-gas analyzers, and pressure-monitoring devices. The director must also be knowledgeable in normal and abnormal cardiopulmonary physiology. This knowledge should be combined with clinical experience in order to evaluate the significance of the laboratory findings in relation to patient care. Clinical skills must include physical diagnostic capability in pulmonary and cardiac evaluation, and knowledge in electrocardiographic interpretation. Other skills that are essential include the following: venipuncture, arterial puncture, and cardiopulmonary resuscitation. Specialized training in medical instrumentation and electronics, computer utilization, and statistics is also useful.

RESPONSIBILITIES

The medical director is in charge of the laboratory space, equipment, and personnel assigned to the performance of pulmonary physiological studies, and directly accountable to the hospital/clinic administration and the professional medical staff of that institution. He or she is responsible for the safety of testing

*Statements in this section are derived from a position paper of the American Thoracic Society Respiratory Care Committee (1) and have been approved by various state thoracic societies.

procedures, and the accuracy, review, and clinical interpretation of test results. Administrative responsibilities include the appointment, supervision, and evaluation of technical staff, record keeping, and fiscal accountability. Other specific responsibilities of the medical director may vary, depending on the nature of the institution, the scope of pulmonary function tests performed, and the qualification of technical personnel.

SUPERVISORY STAFF

The supervisory staff of the pulmonary function laboratory work with the medical director and often directly with the hospital/clinic administration in developing and implementing laboratory policies and procedures which comply with both optimal laboratory standards and the requirements of regulatory and accreditation agencies. The supervisory staff also has the responsibility of seeing that the technical staff carries out its work in accord with these standards.

The number and designation of the supervisory positions depend on the nature of the institution, the degree of active participation by the medical director or other medical personnel, and the scope of pulmonary physiological tests performed. A large laboratory that performs a wide variety of tests, including around-the-clock blood-gas services, should have a technical director and subordinate supervisors, whereas the medical director in a small community hospital that employs one or two technologists can provide direct supervision.

TECHNICAL DIRECTOR

The technical director is responsible to the medical director and the hospital administration. He works with the subordinate supervisors in maintaining the daily operation of the laboratory. The designation of this position is usually appropriate when the laboratory staff consists of 10 or more people.

Qualifications

The technical director should be registered by the National Society for Cardiopulmonary Technology (NSCPT) as a registered cardiopulmonary technologist (RCPT) with a subspecialty in pulmonary technology, or should be registered by the National Board for Respiratory Therapy as a registered therapist. In either case, it is recommended that he or she have 3 years of "hands-on" experience in the field of pulmonary function testing plus 2 years of supervisory experience in a pulmonary or cardiopulmonary laboratory. Ideally, the technical director should be a graduate of an NSCPT-approved program in cardiopulmonary technology or a JRCRTE (Joint Review Committee for Respiratory Therapy Education) approved program in respiratory therapy, or have a college degree in natural or biological sciences or a closely related field.

Supervisors

The supervisor(s) are accountable to the technical director; in laboratories in which the supervisor is the highest technical position, the supervisor is accountable to the medical director and the hospital administration. A supervisor is typically responsible for 4–10 individuals.

Qualifications

The recommended qualifications for supervisors are similar to those for technical director, except that previous supervisory experience is not essential.

Responsibilities

1. The supervisory staff will appoint, educate, supervise, and evaluate the technical staff of the laboratory according to criteria that meet the approval of the medical director, reflect hospital policy, and satisfy the statutes or guidelines of the appropriate state and federal agencies.
2. The supervisory staff is responsible for developing and maintaining detailed procedure manuals, quality control programs, and safety procedures for the laboratory that meet the approval of the medical director and JCAH (Joint Commission for Accreditation of Hospitals), and satisfy federal, state, and hospital or clinic standards.
3. The supervisory staff directs the technical staff in the setup, calibration, performance, calculation, and report preparation of patient tests. It is responsible for ensuring that proper protocols for testing and patient care situations are followed.
4. The supervisory staff is responsible for establishing and maintaining a preventative maintenance program for all laboratory equipment and, in conjunction with the medical director, evaluating and purchasing new equipment and supplies.
5. The supervisory staff works with the medical director in preparing a list of charges for all tests performed in the pulmonary laboratory and ensuring that all tests performed are billed in a timely manner, according to established hospital or clinic procedure.
6. The supervisory staff is responsible for the training, continuing education, and scheduling of the technical staff.
7. The supervisory staff must constantly maintain and improve its own technical and managerial expertise by attending educational programs in the field and

by maintaining affiliations with professional organizations related to cardiopulmonary medicine and technology.

8. The supervisory staff works with the medical director and clerical and technical staffs in organizing laboratory records, statistics, and the budget, in upgrading the quality of service provided by the laboratory, and in providing education in respiratory physiology to interested parties.

TECHNICAL STAFF

The technical staff of the pulmonary laboratory works under the direction of the supervisory staff or, in cases in which a supervisory staff is not warranted, the medical director. The technical staff performs the daily workload of the laboratory.

The number and types of technical positions depend largely on the size of the hospital, the nature of the tests performed, and the degree of independence expected. Technical positions can be divided into three basic categories:

1. Cardiopulmonary or pulmonary technologist. These individuals are trained and can be expected to independently perform a wide range of cardiopulmonary function tests. They may assist in the training of other members of the technical or medical staff. Personnel in this classification should have passed the NSCPT's certification and/or registration examinations. Eligibility criteria for these examinations are quite flexible and are based on a mixture of background education and practical experience under proper medical supervision.
2. Pulmonary technician. This individual has acquired knowledge and expertise in a simple test or limited group of related tests (e.g., spirometry and lung volumes), but lacks education or experience in the broad scope of pulmonary function testing. The pulmonary technician performs tests only under the supervision of a pulmonary technologist or medical director (or his or her designee).
3. Trainee. This category may include many persons who are receiving practical and didactic training in a well-equipped pulmonary function laboratory. Students rotating through the laboratory as part of an agreement with an educational institution for training in pulmonary physiology testing would fall under this category, as well as college science graduates or others with college science backgrounds.

Qualifications

The report of the American Thoracic Society (ATS) Snowbird Workshop on Standardization of Spirometry (2) recognized the critical importance of properly trained pulmonary function laboratory personnel. To accomplish this goal, the report suggested that proper supervision by the medical director is better than certification. However, the report also states, "a related concern is that many physicians supervising pulmonary function laboratories in community hospitals are not adequately prepared." In addition, the workshop participants did not expect that manufacturers of equipment (even as simple as spirometers) would be able to meet the training needs of laboratory personnel.

This illustrates the need for a flexible approach in recommending qualifications of technical personnel. For example, simple spirometry and lung volume measurements can be adequately performed by a person with minimal training and educational background, particularly if the medical director, or his designate, is an active participant in the operation of the laboratory. On the other hand, if one expects the laboratory staff to be proficient in performing laboratory tests described in the other chapters of this book, then obviously more training and educational background are not only desirable but also necessary.

Responsibilities

1. Performance of test procedures according to established policy including:
   a. preparation and calibration of equipment,
   b. preparation and instruction of patients,
   c. performance of the actual testing procedure,
   d. editing (i.e., assessment of validation of test results),
   e. calculation of test data and preparation of reports for interpretations, and
   f. performance of periodic quality control procedures (as required).
2. Performance of preventive maintenance and calibration of laboratory equipment, according to established policy.
3. Other duties as assigned by the supervisory staff and/or medical director of the laboratory.

CONTINUING EDUCATION

Continuing education is required by the JCAH and many state regulatory agencies, and is necessary to ensure that the laboratory staff upgrades and maintains its skills and keeps abreast of new developments in the field of cardiopulmonary physiology, such as new test procedures, equipment changes, and governmental regulations. Continuing education programs should include a combination of the following:

1. hospital inservice classes and rounds,
2. attendance at technical seminars and workshops sponsored by professional organizations and manufacturers of equipment, and

3. easy access to books and medical technical journals pertaining to pulmonary physiology generally and pulmonary technology specifically.

REFERENCES

1. The ATS respiratory care committee position on the director of the pulmonary function laboratory. *Am Thor Soc News* 4:6, 1978.
2. Gardner RM (chairman): ATS statement—Snowbird workshop on standardization of spirometry. *Am Rev Respir Dis* 119:831-837, 1979.

Pulmonary Laboratory Infection Control and Safety

PHILIP M. GOLD, M.D.
DENNIS W. SCHWESINGER, RCPT

The medical and technical directors of pulmonary laboratories must assume the responsibilities for ensuring the safety of patients and staff. It is recommended that each pulmonary function laboratory develop, document, and enforce procedures for control of infectious diseases, handling of hazardous materials, and general and emergency safety measures.

INFECTION CONTROL

The infection control procedures used by different laboratories vary widely. For example, although the majority of laboratories probably change only the mouthpieces between ventilatory testing of different patients, some laboratories routinely also substitute sterilized tubing and manifolds. Despite the impact of infection control procedures on the cost and efficiency of running a laboratory, there are virtually no data documenting the frequency of infections attributable to pulmonary function testing procedures. The Center for Disease Control (CDC) has no record of nosocomial infections attributed to pulmonary function testing (personal communication 1979). A study performed to determine whether CO_2 absorbers inoculated with *Escherichia coli* or *Mycobacterium tuberculosis* were capable of infecting patients indicated that cultures from breathing circuits containing colonized canisters were sterile (1). The major cause of nosocomial pneumonia associated with respiratory therapy equipment is bacterial contamination of large-volume nebulizers and the subsequent administration of infective aerosols (2). Because such equipment is not ordinarily used in the pulmonary function laboratory, it is unlikely that pulmonary function testing constitutes a significant threat in terms of nosocomial infection.

Currently, there is no indication that a significant risk of infection is associated with pulmonary function testing, and therefore stringent infection control mea-

PULMONARY FUNCTION TESTING
GUIDELINES AND CONTROVERSIES

ISBN 0-12-788125-5

sures that may be expensive and impractical cannot be recommended. A clean mouthpiece should be provided for each patient. The need for more extensive decontamination procedures should be determined on an individual basis by each laboratory. For those laboratories wishing to establish more rigorous infection control procedures, the following recommendations constitute an infection control protocol that offers near maximal protection for patients who are tested with volume and flow measuring devices: All mouthpieces, tubing, valves, and connectors from the patient to the measuring device should be disassembled, cleaned with detergent and water, thoroughly rinsed, and dried following each use. Patient circuits should be stored in sealed plastic bags prior to reuse. Water-filled spirometers should be emptied once a week and refilled with distilled water.

When possible, patients with known communicable diseases should be studied with equipment specifically designated for such use. This equipment should be disassembled, cleaned, and sterilized following each patient. If this is not possible, the use of low-impedance bacterial barrier* is recommended; this device is essentially a disposable bag-in-box system, with the box exiting to the spirometer. Alternatively, patients with communicable diseases should be studied at the end of the day or week. Equipment must then be cleaned in the usual manner and the patient circuits sterilized. If contamination of a water-filled spirometer occurs, the spirometer should be emptied and filled with buffered glutaraldehyde for 30 minutes, drained, thoroughly rinsed, and refilled with distilled water. Alternatively, gas sterilization can be used.

STERILIZATION

Sterilization implies the complete elimination of microbial viability. Disinfection refers to the destruction of only certain infectious agents, usually the vegetative forms of pathogenic bacteria. Some stronger disinfecting processes—known as sporocidal—destroy spores as well. The CDC defines two levels of sterilization and three levels of disinfection.

Level	Definition
Sterilization	
A	Most stringent. Fewer than 1 in 1 million highly resistant organisms survive
B	Safe routine working level. Less than 1 in 1000 organisms survive
Disinfection	
A	Sporocidal
B	No vegetative forms resist treatment
C	Active against certain types of organisms but not others

*Available from SMI Laboratories, 11082 Westline Industrial Drive, St. Louis, Missouri 63141.

METHODS OF STERILIZATION AND DISINFECTION

Steam Autoclaving

The use of high-pressure steam at 121° C for 15 minutes constitutes a safe, effective, and inexpensive method of sterilization. Unfortunately, many materials used in the pulmonary laboratory are sensitive to heat and humidity and cannot be autoclaved (3).

Gas Sterilization

Ethylene oxide sterilization allows for prepackaging of equipment, and most materials used in the pulmonary laboratory can be sterilized with this gas. The equipment must be thoroughly cleaned first, and, since ethylene oxide is toxic, extreme care must be taken in its use. Areas where devices are gas sterilized should be well ventilated. The sterilizer itself must be ventilated to the outside, and periodic inspection of the sterilizer must be conducted. Analysis of ambient ethylene oxide concentrations in the sterilizing area should be made periodically. Equipment sterilized by ethylene oxide must be sufficiently aerated prior to use. The aeration period can be shortened with the use of a heated aerator. Gas sterilization is more expensive and more time-consuming than other methods (3).

Chemical Sterilization

Buffered glutaraldehyde will sterilize equipment immersed for 10 hours and disinfect equipment immersed for 30 minutes. Physical contact is required; therefore, equipment must be thoroughly cleaned prior to immersion, and air bubbles must be removed from tubing and valves. Unbuffered glutaraldehyde will sterilize immersed materials in 1 hour if heated to 60° C. Equipment sterilized or disinfected with liquid chemical agents must be thoroughly rinsed, since chemical residues are toxic (3).

Pasteurization

Immersion in water at 77° C for a minimum of 20 minutes provides effective disinfection and requires no rinsing. This method is simple and economical (3), although obviously not applicable to many devices.

Manufacturers' recommendations regarding appropriate techniques for disinfection or sterilization of pulmonary function equipment should be followed meticulously. If a new program of disinfection or sterilization is initiated, systematic microbiologic sampling of equipment is useful for confirming the efficacy of the program. The cooperation of hospital epidemiologists in developing a monitoring program is recommended.

Devices used to nebulize medications or provide inhalation challenge should be disposable or should be sterilized according to the following recommendations, which are consistent with those published by CDC (4) and The American Hospital Association (3). For nebulization, only sterile solutions should be used, although tap water may be used to rinse the residual solutions from reservoir jars prior to refilling them with fresh sterile solutions. If condensation occurs in the tubing between the nebulizer and the patient, it should be drained into a disposable container, never back into the nebulizer jar. Nebulizer equipment should be sterilized or decontaminated daily. The options include: gas sterilization, steam sterilization at 121° C for 15 minutes, pasteurization at 70–75° C for 30 minutes, or immersion in activated glutaraldehyde for 30 minutes. Each patient should, of course, receive a new or decontaminated breathing circuit.

NECESSARY PRECAUTIONS DURING ARTERIAL PUNCTURE AND BLOOD-GAS ANALYSIS

Personnel performing arterial puncture must be well trained in the pertinent anatomy, techniques, and potential complications, and must demonstrate technical skill to the director or his designee. Puncture sites should be prepared with an iodophor or alcohol and contamination of the site and needle avoided. The need to puncture multiple times in order to obtain a specimen because of lack of skill or experience is unacceptable. After analysis of the sample, disposable needles and syringes should be rendered unusable and placed in special waste receptacles for sharp objects. Blood and the waste material from blood-gas analyses must not contaminate the work area; if disposed of in sinks, splatter must be avoided. Reusable glass syringes should be emptied, disassembled, and allowed to soak in sodium hypochlorite (100 ppm) or an aqueous phenolic 1–3% solution prior to sterilization and reuse. Laboratory coats or gowns should be worn by laboratory personnel having frequent contact with blood specimens. Gloves should be worn by those with cuts or breaks in the skin. Eating, drinking, and smoking should be prohibited in the laboratory and frequent, thorough hand washing practiced (5).

If a laboratory worker experiences potential inoculation of hepatitis virus through a break in the skin or by an inadvertent needle puncture, the hepatitis antigen and antibody status of the donor and worker should be determined promptly. If serologic testing results can be obtained within 7 days, administration of the appropriate immune globulin can be delayed. If the serologic results cannot be obtained within a week, the appropriate immune globulin should be administered as soon as possible after exposure. Antigen- and antibody-negative personnel exposed to blood from hepatitis B antigen-positive patients should receive 5 ml of hepatitis B immune globulin, and this dose should be repeated in 1 month. Personnel exposed to blood from antigen-negative patients with clinical hepatitis should receive 5 ml of immune serum globulin as soon as possible after exposure (6).

When an arterial cannula is inserted for pressure monitoring or because of the need for multiple samples, sterile insertion techniques must be used. Sterile pressure tubing and sterile disposable transducer domes must be used for pressure monitoring (7).

HANDLING OF HAZARDOUS MATERIALS

Compressed gas cylinders should not be left unattended unless secured carefully by means of anchored chains, bolts, or cylinder carriers with four-point floor contact. Gas cylinders should not be dragged or rolled across floors, but must be transported by means of appropriate hand trucks with cylinder caps in place. They should be stored in a cool, weather-protected, well-ventilated area away from flammable materials, and must not be allowed to become part of an electrical circuit. Oxidizing and flammable gas mixtures should not be stored in the same area. Valve protection caps should be in place unless cylinders are in use. Cylinder color codes should not be relied upon to identify gases, since color codes are not rigidly enforced; instead, upon arrival in the laboratory, cylinder contents should be checked for accuracy of gas composition and concentration. Appropriate labels should be affixed and used to identify gases. Empty cylinders should be identified and stored separately. Proper regulators with safety system connectors should be used as specified for each gas. "Cheater" adapters must not be used, and cylinders should not be transfilled in the laboratory (8).

Carbon Monoxide

Newly arrived cylinders should be assayed for concentration or compared to previous cylinders. Cylinders containing high concentrations should be labeled clearly and special precautions undertaken to prevent accidental administration to patients or discharge into closed spaces.

Carbon Dioxide

Patient exposure to carbon dioxide in excessive concentration may occur while breathing laboratory gases or endogenous CO_2 in rebreathing circuits not equipped with CO_2 absorbers. When CO_2 absorbers are not used in rebreathing circuits, and ventilation is not monitored, rebreathing should be limited to periods of 30 seconds or less. Spirometers should be flushed thoroughly with fresh air between each 30-second procedure. If soda lime absorbers are used, they should be changed weekly or, if indicating absorbers are used, when color change occurs. Patients performing rebreathing experiments should be watched closely for evidence of hypercapnia, which initially causes a progressive increase in tidal volume.

Oxygen

When performing tests requiring oxygen administration, patients with chronic hypercapnia should be observed closely for evidence of hypoventilation.

Mercury

Rooms in which mercury or mercury compounds are used should be well ventilated and should be monitored periodically with a mercury vapor detector. The National Institute for Occupational Safety and Health has established 0.1 mg of mercury per cubic meter of air as the upper limit of safe exposure (9). Mercury spillage must be picked up immediately and deposited in a sealed vacuum container. Personnel working with mercury should practice careful personal hygiene to ensure that mercury is not deposited on their hands and clothing, and should not wear jewelry (adherence of mercury to jewelry could become a source of low-level chronic contamination).

Other Chemicals

In laboratories in which strong acids and alkaline solutions are used, ventilation hoods must be present immediately above the area of use. Personnel working with such solutions must be aware of the potential dangers involved and appropriate techniques for handling materials. An easily accessible overhead shower and eye wash must be present within 30 feet of the area where caustics are used (10).

ELECTRICAL SAFETY

All electrical equipment and outlets in the pulmonary laboratory must be checked periodically for electrical hazard. Receptacles must be wired properly and grounded. If improper wiring or grounding is detected, receptacles should be repaired immediately or rendered unuseable. Three-wire power cables of high quality with hospital-grade plugs must be used for all equipment. Patient monitoring cables should be checked on a monthly basis for current leakage, with power on and off. Appropriate inspection records should be maintained, and equipment should be labeled with the date and results of the most recent safety check. Patients with indwelling lines and catheters should be considered electrically sensitive. For such patients, transducers, three-way stopcocks, pacing wires, and other metal parts and conductors must be suitably insulated. Isolated amplifiers should be used, and such patients should not come in contact with grounded metal chassis or electrical applicances.

GENERAL SAFETY RULES

Evacuation procedures for fire should be posted in clearly visible areas. Fire exits should be marked clearly, and fire extinguishers in sufficient number should be placed strategically. Work areas should allow free movement of equipment and personnel. Hazardous areas should be marked. Equipment for basic life support should be available in areas where stress testing and inhalation challenge testing is performed, and a defibrillator and emergency cart with drugs for life support and materials for airway maintenance should be available. All personnel with direct patient contact should be trained in cardiopulmonary resuscitation (11).

A system for periodically reviewing and recording contagious illness among personnel should be maintained; yearly skin testing of tuberculin-negative personnel should be performed. Although it is currently not a widespread practice, yearly hepatitis serology testing has been recommended (5, 6). A system for reporting hazards and accidents should be developed. Periodic safety inspections should be scheduled and recorded. Safety policies and procedures should be revised and updated annually, and employees should be required to review policies and procedures. Periodic inservice education should be provided to maintain awareness of safety requirements.

REFERENCES

1. Adriani J, Rovenstine EA: Experimental studies on carbon dioxide absorbers for anesthesia. *Anaesthesiology* 2:1-19, 1941.
2. Pierce AK, Sanford JP, Thomas GD, Leonard JS: Long-term evaluation of decontamination of inhalation-therapy equipment and the occurrence of necrotizing pneumonia. *N Engl J Med* 282:528-531, 1970.
3. *Infection Control in the Hospital,* ed 4. Chicago, American Hospital Association, 1979, pp. 103-122, 159.
4. *Recommendations for the Disinfection and Maintenance of Respiratory Therapy Equipment.* Atlanta, GA, Center for Disease Control, Hospital Infections Branch and Hospital Infections Laboratory Section, Epidemic Investigations Branch, Bacterial Diseases Division, Bureau of Epidemiology, 1977.

5. American Hospital Association: Statement on hepatitis ''B'' antigen carriers. *Hospitals* 48:95–98, 1974.
6. Seeff LB, Hoofnagle JH: Immunoprophylaxis of viral hepatitis. *Gastroenterology* 77:161–182, 1979.
7. Stamm WE, Colella JJ, Anderson RL, et al.: Indwelling arterial catheters as a source of nosocomial bacteremia. *N Engl J Med* 292:1099–1102, 1975.
8. *Characteristics and Safe Handling of Medical Gases,* ed 6. New York, Compressed Gas Association, 1978, pamphlet P-2.
9. *General Industry Standards and Interpretations.* Washington, DC, U.S. Department of Labor Occupational Safety and Health Administration, 1980, 1910.1000.
10. *Sectional Committee on Hospital Laboratories Safety Standard for Laboratories in Health Related Institutions 56C.* Boston, National Fire Protection Association, 1973.
11. Functional safety and sanitation in *Accreditation Manual for Hospitals.* Chicago, Joint Commission on Accreditation of Hospitals, 1981, pp. 35-50, 173–175.

CHAPTER 4

Measurement: Theory and Practice

JOHN G. MOHLER, M.D.

Measurement theory involves a diversity of disciplines, including mathematics, chemistry, physics, biology, statistics, and even philosophy. The interactions of these disciplines have resulted in increasingly complex techniques in error analysis. In this chapter, the primary emphasis is directed toward the basics of measurement theory and the advantages and limitations of their practical application in the pulmonary laboratory. Many of the issues raised are also applicable to a discussion of normal predictive values, which are discussed in Chapter 6.

ACCURACY AND PRECISION

The concept of accuracy implies that there is a ''correct'' value about which repeat measurements scatter in a gaussian manner. The closer the mean of these measurements is to the correct value, the greater the accuracy.

In some cases, physicians are forced to accept inaccurate measurements. For example, estimates of pleural pressures are made from measurements of pressure within a balloon catheter system that is placed in the esophagus adjacent to the pleural space. Although such measurements will not accurately represent the diversity of pressures found in the pleural space, if standardized methodology is followed and the same methods are used both when developing normal predictive values and when developing an understanding of the changes observed in various disease states, then the measurements may be of clinical value. Such measurements are certainly preferable to the more accurate measurements that could only be obtained by inserting a multitude of intrapleural catheters throughout the pleural space.

The assessment of accuracy is an important aspect of quality control in laboratory measurements, but it obviously is not always an easy task. For physiological measurements, we are often tempted to construct mechanical models, such as those that simulate forced expiratory maneuvers. Models offer the advantage that they are more readily dismantled for measurements of internal dimensions than

PULMONARY FUNCTION TESTING
GUIDELINES AND CONTROVERSIES

ISBN 0-12-788125-5

human subjects and yield more reproducible results with repeated trials. Even for measurements as seemingly simple as the vital capacity, however, it is quite difficult to construct a mechanical model that reproduces the complex flow patterns generated during the forced expiratory maneuvers of human subjects. Volume changes are easy to simulate, while changes in the levels of humidity and temperature in the "expired" air are not. The concentrations of O_2 and CO_2 vary during expiration, changing the total viscosity of the expired gas; this phenomenon is almost never simulated in devices designed to test the accuracy of spirometric devices. Although these factors (changing humidity, temperature, and gas concentrations) may not significantly affect the accuracy of volume displacement devices, they may have a profound effect on pneumotachographs or on devices that measure flow from the rate of cooling of a heated wire (see Chapter 9).

A similar discussion is also applicable to the use of commercially available products for assessing the accuracy of blood-gas analyzers. For pH, buffer solutions are clearly superior to blood for quality control. For assessing the accuracy of measurements of oxygen tension (PO_2), however, the complexities of the hemoglobin disassociation curve have yet to be satisfactorily simulated with artificial solutions or suspensions of denatured hemoglobin or red blood cells. Thus, although maximal accuracy is desired, this goal is often difficult to achieve with the use of models or substitutes.

The concept of precision refers to the reproducibility of repeat measurements, regardless of how close the mean value is to the "correct" value. The standard deviation of repeated measurements is commonly used as an estimate of precision; the smaller the standard deviation, the greater the precision.

The assessment of precision is another useful component of quality control programs. It serves to define both the capabilities of the instrument and, when appropriate, the precision of the entire testing procedure. Precision is usually easier to measure than accuracy. Problems sometimes develop however, when models are used to assess precision. Devices such as large syringes for simulating forced expirations clearly offer the advantage that the repeated test "samples" will be more reproducible than the repeated forced expirations of a human subject, whose possible fatigue, airway spasm, and lack of cooperation all have adverse effects on attempts to define the magnitude of the random error of measurements with a specific spirometer. However, a spinning turbine used for measuring flows may perform differently with repeated expirations of relatively dry air at room temperature than with repeated, increasingly moist exhalations of warm saturated air, which may cause condensation of water on the turbine blades.

Thus, it must be recognized that the precision of an instrument, as assessed from measurements using devices or products that substitute for patients or blood, may differ from that obtained in clinical testing conditions, especially when one considers the inherent variability of most physiological measurements in humans.

Systematic and Random Errors

Systematic errors, such as might occur when a number of blood-gas measurements are made on an instrument that is continuously calibrated erroneously, will affect the *accuracy* of these measurements. Although the *precision* of repeat measurements using such an instrument may be optimal, no matter how many measurements are made, the results may still be clinically misleading.

Conversely, when larger than normal *random errors* occur in measurements, the *precision* of repeat measurements will be most severely affected. For example, suppose several aliquots of arterial blood are to be analyzed for PO_2; air is introduced into the first aliquot resulting in elevation of the PO_2, and the measurement of the other aliquots is delayed as they stand at room temperature, which results in a lowering of the PO_2. It is entirely possible that if enough measurements are made under such circumstances, the mean value may be very close to the "correct" value, despite the poor sample handling techniques. If, however, we rely on a single determination, the result is likely to be very misleading. This example also illustrates a point particularly relevant to determinations done in pulmonary labs: Even though the accuracy and precision of a particular instrument may be within acceptable limits, significant problems in accuracy and precision can occur as the result of faulty sampling (or patient instruction) techniques.

Obviously, we would prefer that all instrumentation and testing methodology used in the pulmonary lab result in maximal accuracy and precision. This ideal is seldom achieved, however, because of the constraints of cost and efficiency and also because of the unavoidable variables inherent in direct patient testing. The purpose of quality control programs and defined testing methodology is to give us assurance that our measurements are being made within *acceptable* limits of accuracy and precision (i.e., that random and systematic errors are within acceptable limits).

SELECTION OF DATA FOR CALCULATIONS

When a parameter is measured several times, an understanding of the physiological determinants of the parameter and an understanding of the methodology, accuracy, and precision of the measurement itself all are key elements in selecting the most appropriate measurement for the report. For example, the vital capacity is defined as the largest volume of air that can be expired after a maximal inspiration. From repeated measurements of forced vital capacity (FVC) in a given patient, therefore, the mean value is ignored, and only the maximal value reported. In contrast, with repeated measurements of tidal volume, we usually report the mean value of a number of measurements, after we eliminate any tidal breaths that we can clearly recognize as outlyers (e.g., sighs).

For some parameters, however, despite an exemplary knowledge of the physiological and mechanical determinants of a particular measurement, even a group of experts may not be able to agree on how a measurement should be selected. An example is our attempt to define how to measure the forced expiratory flow at 50% of the FVC ($FEF_{50\%}$). If the maximal value of a series of trials is reported, this value can be spuriously elevated if the patient stops his expiration above his or her normal residual volume during one or more expirations. Spurious elevations might also occur if transient evaluations of flow measurements due to instrumentation problems occur. Such errors can occur if measurements are made by computer directly from the output signal of very responsive pneumotachographs. These errors will also affect the mean value. Conversely, $FEF_{50\%}$ measurements made from expiratory efforts which, though prolonged, are clearly from submaximal efforts, may seriously underestimate the "correct" value for that patient.

Thus, appropriate selection of data for a report is imperative in order to obtain test results of maximal clinical value. Usually, the person making the measurements initially decides whether to accept or reject the data. In order that undesirable bias is not introduced at this stage, it is essential that the technician be trained to recognize problems in patient cooperation or understanding, sample handling, and instrumentation and only reject data when it is appropriate to do so. The next step in the processing of the measurements obtained is to calculate the reported value according to an established procedure. This may involve the calculation of mean values of repeated measurements from a single instrument, or, as is done in some blood-gas laboratories, the mean of single measurements from two different instruments. For some spirometric parameters, maximal values will be reported; for others, measurements are made from the forced expiratory effort with the largest sum of the FVC and FEV_1. In the following chapters, we have always attempted to define how to select the measurements of specific tests, but, as the controversies sections demonstrate, it is not always possible to obtain a consensus on these basic issues.

The final step in transforming the reported measured value into a valid clinical decision is the interpretation of the results. This requires a complex interaction of the knowledge of the physiological basis for the parameters, the methods of measurement, the normal predictive values appropriate for the patient, and the statistical relationship of the test results to disease.

CHAPTER 5

Instrumentation

MICHAEL SNOW, RCPT

A considerable diversity of instrumentation is available for the many test procedures done in diagnostic pulmonary function laboratories. Although obtaining a detailed knowledge of all these instruments is an unrealistic goal, familiarity with general instrumentation principles is recommended, both for ensuring the purchase of appropriate and useful laboratory equipment, and for ensuring the maximum performance of equipment used in testing. This chapter presents an overview of some of the performance characteristics used in evaluating instruments; the basic principles of operation for instruments encountered most frequently in pulmonary laboratories are then reviewed.

INSTRUMENT CHARACTERISTICS

Accuracy

The accuracy of measurements is one of the most important considerations when evaluating laboratory instrumentation. Accuracy is defined as the degree of conformity to a standard or "true" value, i.e., how close a measurement is to the "correct" value. It is obviously important, but commonly overlooked, that evaluations of accuracy be made over the entire range of values encountered in clinical studies. Another important consideration is that the accuracy of an instrument as evaluated using a reference standard (e.g., evaluation of a spirometer with a calibrating syringe) must be differentiated from the accuracy encountered when studying patients.

In choosing instrumentation, acceptable limits of accuracy are based on a number of considerations. These include an understanding of the range of values encountered in a population of subjects free of disease, the magnitude of the changes expected to occur with disease, and what magnitude of changes one wants to detect as a disease improves or worsens.

The term "precision" has a variety of different meanings. As discussed in Chapter 4, when the term is used to describe the characteristics of a particular

PULMONARY FUNCTION TESTING
GUIDELINES AND CONTROVERSIES

ISBN 0-12-788125-5

testing methodology, it describes the reproducibility of repeat measurements. This is the most common meaning of the term. The precision of a test can be described as either the standard deviation (SD) of repeated measurements on a reference standard (e.g., a calibration syringe for a spirometer or a reference buffer solution for a pH meter), or the repeated measurements from patients or blood samples from patients. And, as is the case when considering accuracy, the requirements for precision are defined by the particular clinical application. Deserving emphasis is the obvious but often overlooked fact that both the accuracy and precision of *test results* are as dependent upon patient instruction (or sample handling) and quality control procedures as they are upon the inherent accuracy and precision capabilities of the *instrument* itself. A mass spectrometer may be very precise but grossly inaccurate if calibrated erroneously.

When used to describe the characteristics of an instrument, the term precision is sometimes defined as the degree of significant figures to which a measurement is reported. In this context, a pH meter that reports a pH as 7.446 might be described as capable of greater precision than a unit that reports 7.45. The number of significant figures required is determined by considering clinical needs. For routine clinical determination of the pH of arterial blood, an instrument reporting the pH to the second decimal place is suitable; for measurements to be used for research involving small changes in cerebrospinal fluid (CSF) pH, an instrument capable of reporting values to the third decimal place would obviously be preferred.

Linearity

The term "linearity" is used to describe the response of an instrument to changes in input signals. If equal increments of input result in equal increments of output signal, the instrument is said to be linear. This is most easily visualized with an X–Y plot of input and output signals. As illustrated in Fig. 1, an instrument may be linear over a limited range (inputs B to C) and alinear at the extremes of input signals (inputs A to B and C to D). If the range of clinical measurements is between B and C, the alinearity observed is of no practical consequence. As is the case with accuracy, the linearity of instruments must be tested over the full operating range. Evaluation of a 9-liter piston-displacement spirometer with a 1-liter calibrating syringe when the spirometer piston is in a forward position would miss alinearity that may occur only when the piston binds during the distal excursion of its movement.

Some instruments are inherently alinear. This is not a problem if the alinearity is recognized and appropriate steps are taken. One approach is to precisely define the alinearity by developing a full-range calibration curve; outputs that are outside the limits of linearity are corrected using the calibration curve. Another

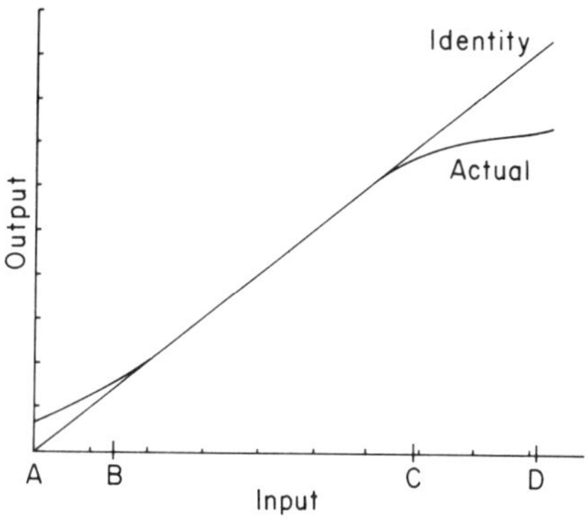

Fig. 1 *Example of alinearity.*

approach used with increasing frequency in recent years is for manufacturers to build circuits or microprocessors directly into the instruments that will automatically linearize the output signal. The presence of such a feature, however, does not obviate the need for regular checks of the linearity as part of the regular quality control program.

Hysteresis

Hysteresis is the phenomenon exhibited when the reaction of a system to change is dependent upon previous reactions to change. This is most easily recognized from a plot of input versus output signals when, after increasing then decreasing the input signal, the plot is not linear, but shows an open loop, as illustrated in Fig. 2. This type of inaccuracy of measurements occurs as a result of the retentivity or memory of the sensor. An example is the hysteresis that may be observed with a Clark electrode system when, following measurements of blood with a high O_2 tension (PO_2), the subsequent analysis of a sample with a low PO_2 may result in measurements erroneously high either due to the "memory effects" of the electrode or the contamination and subsequent release of O_2 from the walls of the tubing and cuvettes.

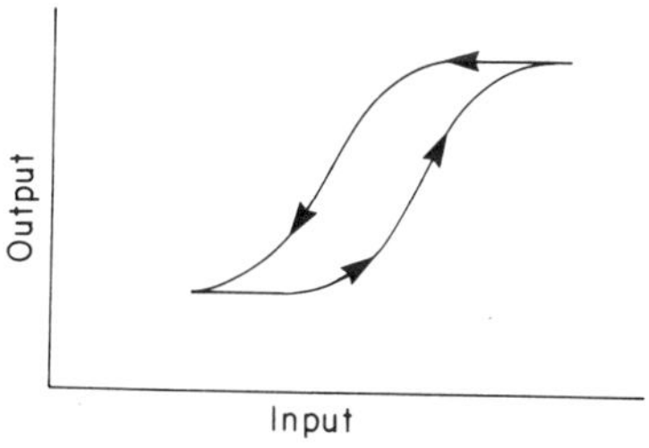

Fig. 2 *Example of hysteresis.*

Frequency Response

Frequency response is a measure of the ability of an instrument to measure the changes of dynamic events within defined levels of accuracy. Specification of frequency response requires defining the amplitude of the input signal, the acceptable limits of accuracy of the output signal, and the maximum (and minimum) frequencies at which the instrument can measure within the acceptable levels of accuracy. For spirometers, this is most commonly assessed using a variable frequency piston pump. Such testing, in conjunction with a knowledge of the frequencies that are expected to occur during testing of patients, is one step in defining acceptable performance characteristics for lab instruments.

In order to meaningfully evaluate the reported frequency response data for a particular instrument, the amplitude of the input signal and the accepted limits of accuracy must be known. A volume displacement spirometer may have a flat (i.e., less than 5% distortion) response to frequencies as high as 12 cycles/sec when tested with oscillations of 50 cc; however, the same instrument may have a flat frequency response to only 0.6 cycles/sec when tested with the more clinically relevant volume of 500 cc.

Damping

Damping is a characteristic that describes the fidelity with which an instrument responds to dynamic changes in input signals. If the output signal temporarily overshoots the input signal in response to a rapid step change, the instrument may be said to be underdamped. This is illustrated in Fig. 3. An example of an underdamped instrument is the chain-compensated, metal bell spirometer, which, due to its inertia, may overshoot during recording of abruptly changing

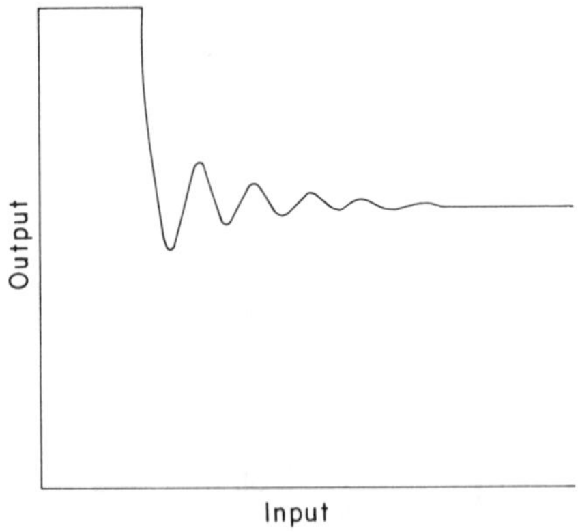

Fig. 3 *Example of underdamping.*

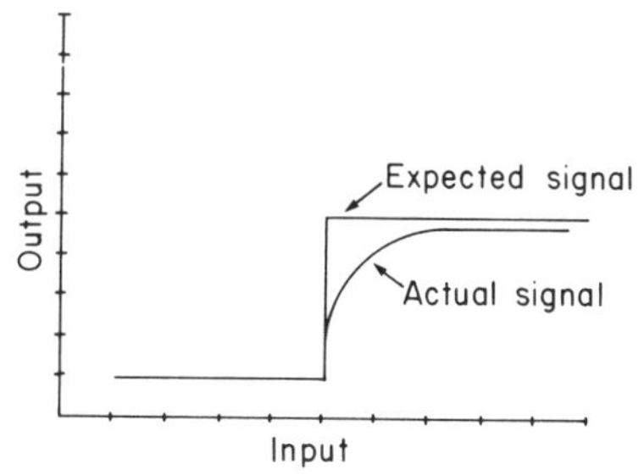

Fig. 4 *Example of overdamping.*

high flow rates. Underdamping is important only if it affects the accuracy of signals within the desired frequencies. Obviously, if damping occurs at frequencies above 30 Hz, this is of little concern for measurements with a spirometer, which need not be accurate at frequencies higher than 10 Hz. Response curves exhibiting an underdamped pattern may be analyzed further to reveal at which frequency damping will occur. The period of the oscillations can be calculated by measuring the time peak to peak. The reciprocal of this period is the damped natural frequency. The damping ratio may be calculated as a quantitative characterization of the degree of underdamping. From this data, the theoretical undamped natural frequency may also be determined.

If the output signal, in response to a rapid step change, approaches the input signal curvilinearly, the instrument is overdamped, as illustrated in Fig. 4. An example of an overdamped instrument is a common PCO_2 electrode with protein contamination. This will slow the response of the electrode significantly, producing a nearly asymptotic response curve. Clearly, a system in this condition cannot faithfully reproduce fast-changing signals.

Testing for damping characteristics need not entail complex equipment. All that is required is the ability to produce a rapid step change in the input signal that is sufficiently faster than the response time of the instrument. For example, the response and damping characteristics of a pressure transducer and recorder can easily be evaluated by attaching a fully inflated toy balloon to the pressure-sensing port of the transducer, so that the transducer records the pressure within the balloon. Piercing the balloon with a sharp pin results in the desired rapid change in input pressure back to atmospheric levels. Obviously, if one then wanted to know the relative contributions of the transducer and the recorder, one would test the response of each separately. The balloon experiment would be repeated, and the output of the transducer would be measured using a different recorder, one with maximal performance characteristics, such as a memory oscilloscope. The fidelity of recording systems can be tested with sudden step changes in input voltage.

Response Time

The response time of an instrument can be characterized by the 90% rise time. This is the time it takes the output to achieve 90% of its final value following a step change in the input, and is indicative of the ability of the instrument to handle rapidly changing signals. Without a sufficiently fast rise time, gas analyzers cannot be used in methodologies of expired gas analyses requiring breath-by-breath analysis. Typically acceptable 90% rise times for such applications are less than 200 msec. Examples of instruments that meet this requirement include mass spectrometers and infrared analyzers; examples of instruments that do not generally meet this requirement include gas chromatographs and paramagnetic oxygen analyzers.

Another component of frequency response that is often confused with rise time is the lag or gas transport time. This is the time it takes the gas sample to reach the analyzer and is a function of the length of sample tubing and the sample flow rate. Knowledge of the magnitude of the lag time may allow correction of the phase shift caused by gas analyses lagging behind volume signals.

Specificity

The specificity with which an instrument makes a measurement is a particularly important characteristic of gas analyzers. Because it makes measurements based on the molecular mass of a particular gas, the mass spectrometer has relatively high specificity. It does not have infinite specificity, however, and cannot, for instance, distinguish carbon monoxide from nitrogen, because both have the same molecular mass.

The commonly used thermal conductivity type of analyzer for measuring helium is an example of an instrument with relatively poor specificity. Although it can usually measure helium concentrations very accurately because of the high thermal conductivity of helium in relation to common respiratory gases, the helium readings may be very erroneous if hydrogen is also in the gas mixture. Elevated concentrations of oxygen also may interfere with the accuracy of measurements of helium concentrations by thermal conductivity methods.

Compatibility

The compatibility of various components of a testing system is an important aspect to be considered both when purchasing instruments and when altering testing protocols. Good compatibility means that when the various components of a system are assembled, there will not be adverse effects on instrument performance because of other components in the system. Poor compatibility can occur, for example, in the utilization of a fuel cell for the analysis of CO in series with a thermal conductivity helium analyzer placed distal to the fuel cell. Water

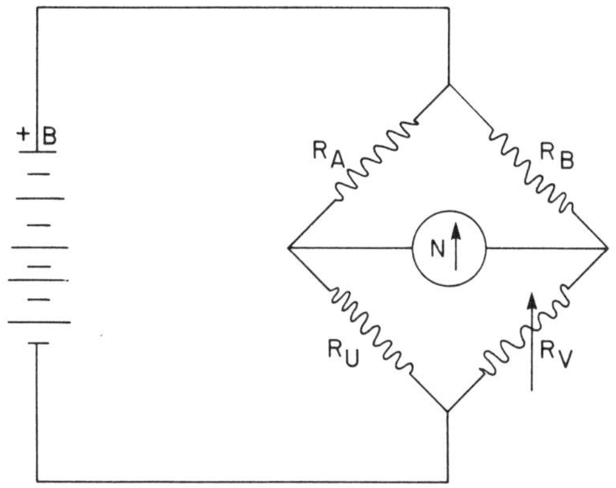

Fig. 5 *Wheatstone bridge.* R_A, R_B = *known resistance;* R_V = *variable known resistance;* R_U = *unknown resistance;* B = *power source;* N = *null meter.*

is an unavoidable end-product of the chemical reaction of the fuel cell; if a dessicant water trap is not inserted between the fuel cell and helium analyzer, the water vapor may seriously interfere with measurements of the thermal conductivity system.

BASIC INSTRUMENTS

Wheatstone Bridge

Although seldom seen as a separate instrument in pulmonary laboratories, the Wheatstone bridge is a basic component of a wide variety of instruments, such as pressure transducers and thermal conductivity detectors. The electronic analogue of a precision laboratory balance, the resistive bridge, as illustrated in Fig. 5, is used to accurately measure the unknown resistance of a detector component (R_U in Fig. 5) using known resistances (R_A and R_B) and a variable but known resistance (R_V). The null meter is used for precise determination of when the resistances are balanced ($R_U/R_V = R_A/R_B$). The sensor resistor is designed so that changes in the input signal (e.g., pressure) are directly related to the measurable changes in the sensor resistance (R_U). Since the main source of error in a Wheatstone bridge is the inaccuracy of the three known resistances, use of precision resistors can make the device extremely accurate.

Volume-Flow Instruments

Devices capable of measuring gas volumes and/or flow generally can be divided into two categories: those based on primary measurements of volume with derived measurements of flow, and devices that measure flow directly with derived measurements of volumes. A number of such devices are discussed in detail in Chapters 7 and 9.

Volume displacement spirometers reflect changes in volume through the physical movement of a collection device, most commonly either an inverted sealed cylinder floating on water, or a moveable piston or bellows. Systems in which the output signal is obtained from the movement of a pen connected to the displaceable collector are simple to operate, usually inexpensive, and need minimal calibration. Attaching potentiometers to the displaceable collectors gives the advantages of greater flexibility for recording data, (e.g., volume versus flow plots), the possibility of on-line computer collection of data, and the potential for direct measurements of both volume and flow. The most important disadvantages are that potentiometers add to the initial cost of the system and require frequent calibration.

Flow-type spirometers utilize a variety of different concepts. These include differential pressure pneumotachographs, heated wire anemometers (which measure flows from rates of cooling), and turbine-blade devices. Turbine-type flow measuring devices may exhibit considerable problems with damping because of their inherent inertia during abrupt changes in flow. One device utilizes a bias flow to keep the turbine constantly in motion, thus reducing the inertia.

All flow-type devices share the common feature that volume measurements are obtained by integration of the flow signals. Such devices may have better frequency responses than volume-measuring devices and hence more accurately measure rapidly changing flow rates. Problems related to appropriate damping of output signals are also less for such devices than for volume displacement instruments. Because they are usually "flow-through" rather than "flow-collection" devices, these flow-measuring devices are more suitable for situations requiring continuous monitoring, e.g., during exercise or in an intensive care unit (ICU). However, their sensitivity to "noise," gas viscosity, humidity, and temperature, which makes accurate integration of flow into volume difficult, as well as their requirements for frequent calibration, are significant disadvantages for some applications.

Transducers

By convention, a transducer is a sensor that converts one kind of energy into another. This definition would include every instrument in a pulmonary laboratory from a counter-balanced, volume displacement spirometer to a mass spectrometer. Discussion is limited here to four types: variable reluctance pressure transducers, strain gauge pressure transducers, variable capacitance pressure transducers, and positional displacement transducers.

A variable reluctance pressure transducer consists of a stainless steel diaphragm

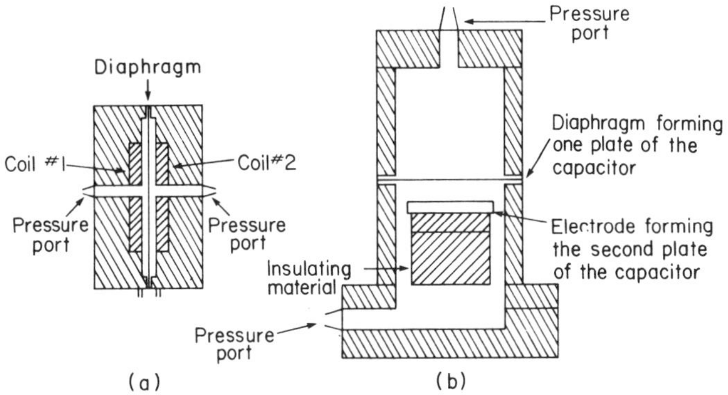

Fig. 6 *Cross sections of (a) variable reluctance and (b) variable capacitance transducers.*

between two coils. This creates equal inductance on both sides, with the diaphragm in an unflexed position. With the application of differential pressure, the diaphragm will flex, creating an imbalance between the two coils. The coils are connected in a bridge circuit that produces an output proportional to the differential pressure. These transducers have a very small internal volume, which results in an excellent frequency response and relative insensitivity to vibration and shock.

Strain gauge pressure transducers use a metal wire or pressure-sensitive semiconductor, which, when elongated due to the application of pressure, increases its electrical resistance. Most commonly, the strain gauges form the active arms of a Wheatstone bridge, with variations in length resulting in a proportional change in resistance and output voltage.

Variable capacitance pressure transducers are very similar in nature to variable reluctance pressure transducers, with notable exceptions in performance. Figure 6 illustrates these similarities. In operation, the diaphragm forms one plate of the capacitor with a stationary electrode forming the other plate. Movement of the diaphragm alters the capacitance, which results in an output voltage proportional to the differential pressure. In general, this technique utilizes relatively large internal volumes which results in an extremely vibration-sensitive system and relatively poor frequency response when compared to the variable reluctance transducer. The transducer's relatively large internal volume also allows considerable warping of the diaphragm as a result of overpressures, which may create a significant zero offset or permanently damage the transducer.

Positional displacement transducers most commonly are potentiometric. Essentially they utilize a variable resistor. Positional displacement varies the resistance and creates a change in voltage proportional to the change in displacement. A typical application is found in a volume displacement spirometer.

Transcutaneous Monitoring Devices

An area of intense interest and current controversy is the subject of transcutaneous monitoring of pO_2 and pCO_2. The capillary bed is vasodilated by heating the skin to 41–45° C, using a heating element. A polarographic electrode with a platinum cathode and a silver anode in combination with a liquid electrolyte is attached to the skin with a heating element and covered by a selectively permeable membrane. This technique has shown significant clinical applicability in infants.

Significant errors may occur if perfusion does not greatly exceed the cellular metabolism, allowing gas depletion, or if the temperature is not closely controlled. Additional difficulties have been experienced with the thickening of the dermis after infancy. Clinical applicability in adults remains controversial. Difficulties relating to electrode placement and maintenance are discussed in more detail in Chapter 24.

Gas Chromatography

Analysis by gas chromatography utilizes two distinct steps. The first step is the separation of the sample into its constituent gases by selective adsorption. The second step involves the quantification of the gases. In the pulmonary laboratory, quantification is generally accomplished using thermal conductivity. During the analysis, a carrier gas is used to carry the sample through the columns. Helium is usually selected, due to its relatively low adsorption and high thermal conductivity. The result of utilizing helium as a carrier gas is that the chromatograph cannot detect the presence of helium in a sample. Diffusion studies generally utilize an inert, insoluble gas such as helium or neon to estimate the alveolar volume. When using gas chromatography, an inert gas different from the carrier gas must, obviously, be selected. The gas usually chosen is neon, which like helium, is relatively insoluble.

The gas sample to be analyzed is injected into a column containing a packing that separates the constituent gases according to their molecular size by selective adsorption. This is illustrated in Fig. 7. Essentially, the column acts as a delay network, releasing the gases into the detector in a predictable, sequential pattern.

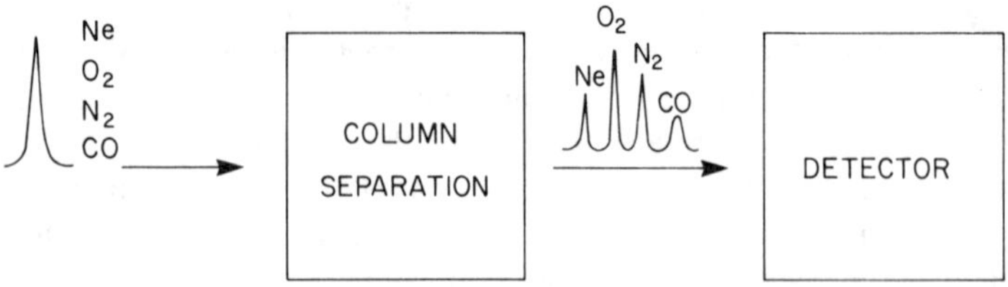

Fig. 7 *Gas separation by chromatography.*

In practice, nearly any of the respiratory gases can be separated. An exception is argon, which has not been successfully separated from oxygen by chromatography.

Certain heat-activated diatomaceous earths, commonly referred to as molecular sieves, are widely used to separate neon, oxygen, nitrogen, and carbon monoxide. Porous polymers, such as chromosorb, separate carbon dioxide and the higher hydrocarbons. Commonly, combinations of columns are utilized to provide a complete analysis of respiratory gases. The molecular sieve column does not elute (or pass) CO_2, which (with time) will gradually cause the column to deteriorate. Water vapor will also eventually contaminate both types of columns, which will necessitate replacing or reconditioning the columns. Columns are reconditioned by baking them at high temperatures, which elutes the CO_2 and removes the accumulated moisture. The problem of water vapor can be minimized by interposing a dessicant between the sample and the column or maintaining the columns at a high temperature during analysis. The utilization of isolated thermal ovens in a chromatograph introduces additional complications and increases the cost of the instrument. Chromatographs currently marketed range from inexpensive room-temperature models to sophisticated models utilizing several distinct thermal regions.

Although a chromatograph is an extremely versatile instrument, its major drawback is that it measures discretely rather than continuously. The instrument cannot be utilized in a dynamic breath-by-breath mode. The analysis time, ranging from 30 seconds to several minutes, depends upon many factors, including carrier gas flow, column length, and temperature and age of the packing material. Currently available models analyze nitrogen, oxygen, and carbon dioxide within 30 seconds. These units can be modified so that expired air continuously passes through the chromatograph and is sampled periodically to provide 30-second averages for expired oxygen and carbon dioxide.

Thermal Conductivity Detectors

Thermal conductivity detectors are widely used as the analyzer in gas chromatography and in the common helium analyzer. The detectors operate on the principle that heat is conducted away from a hot body in a gas at a rate dependent on the nature of the gas. Thermal conductivity detectors usually contain metal filaments with high temperature coefficients of resistance, mounted axially in a space containing the gas. In some cases, a thermistor bead is used in place of the filaments. The sensor is heated by a constant electric current. When the gas to be analyzed is directed over the sensor, heat is conducted away from the sensor at a rate dependent upon the thermal conductivity of the gas. The higher the thermal conductivity of the gas, the greater the conduction of heat away from the sensor.

When used in association with a gas chromatograph to detect the relative concentrations of gases appearing sequentially, the resistance of the sensor will vary according to the relative concentration of each gas. Since the detector measures thermal conductivity sequentially as the gases appear, the specificity of the analyzer is dependent only on the ability of the columns to adequately separate the sample into its constituents.

When used as a helium analyzer, changes in the concentration of helium are measured by the changes in the resistance of the thermistor. If other gases are present, they will impose their own effect and modify the detection of helium to some degree. Since the thermal conductivity of helium is some 8–10 times that of O_2 and CO_2, small variations in the concentrations of the latter gases usually do not create significant problems. However, background gas concentrations must be considered if the system will be utilizing a high concentration of oxygen. Gases with thermal conductivities similar to helium, such as hydrogen, cannot be accurately measured in the same gas sample with helium.

To measure changes in resistance, the sensitive element is inserted in a Wheatstone bridge network. In order to eliminate, as far as possible, effects other than thermal conductivity, the opposing side of the Wheatstone bridge is attached to a second element, which is introduced into a reference gas. When the sensor detects an element not present on the reference side, the bridge is unbalanced. The resultant output voltage is proportional to the concentration of the foreign gas. The output is generally an analog signal appropriate for displaying to a recorder.

As with gas chromatography, the major drawback of thermal conductivity detectors is their relatively slow response time, on the order of 10–20 seconds. Thus, they are practical only for discrete measurements.

Mass Spectrometer

The mass spectrometer is designed to separate charged gas molecules according to their mass. Most commonly, the gas sample to be analyzed is drawn into an ionization chamber, where the gas molecules are ionized by bombardment from an electron source. The positively charged ions are drawn out of the chamber by a negatively charged electrode, with the remaining ions being removed by vacuum. The beam is focused by a powerful magnetic field, which forces the ions into circular trajectories. This is illustrated in Fig. 8.

Each ion will move with a velocity determined by its charge-to-mass ratio. With the magnetic field strength known, it is possible to provide individual collectors for specific gases; each collector is located along the specific trajectory resulting from a specific mass. The current produced by the collector is proportional to the number of ions striking the collector (i.e., the concentration of the gas in the sample). The current is amplified and generally is displayed both as an

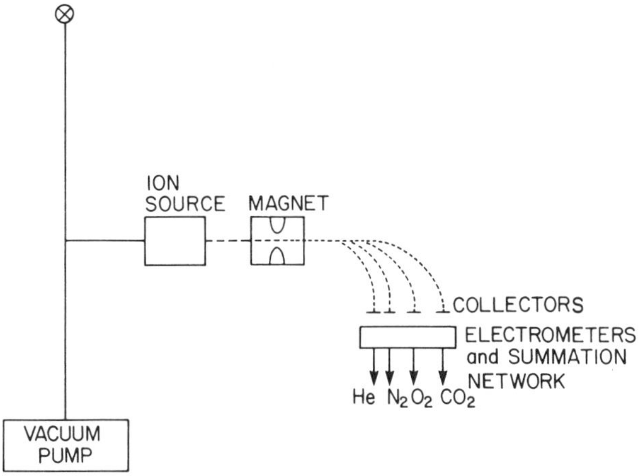

Fig. 8 *Block diagram of a mass spectrometer.*

analog output for interfacing with a microprocessor or recorder and as a digital output for the front panel display.

In theory, the number of gases that may be analyzed simultaneously is limited only by the requirement that their molecular weights differ. In practice, most manufacturers offer machines capable of analyzing three or four standard gases, and optional gases upon request. It is important to note that carbon monoxide and nitrogen have the same molecular weight and, as a result, cannot be differentiated. An expensive solution is utilizing carbon monoxide labeled with the nonradioactive ^{18}O atom, thus giving carbon monoxide a different molecular weight than nitrogen.

The mass spectrometer is an extremely fast responding analyzer suitable for highly specific measurements on an array of respiratory and inert tracer gases. Because of its response time and stability, it lends itself easily to computerized applications. The mass spectrometer may be used in conjunction with most techniques requiring gas analysis.

In vivo determinations of blood-gas tensions have been successfully made with a mass spectrometer. The technique involves gas sampling across a permeable membrane, using an indwelling catheter. No blood is withdrawn, as only dissolved gases pass the membrane to be quantitatively analyzed. The membrane must be sufficiently permeable to achieve the gas density required by the mass spectrometer, but not so permeable that the rate of removal exceeds the rate of replacement from the blood supply. Difficulties have been experienced with thrombosis and degradation of the membrane, necessitating systemic anticoagulation; these difficulties have limited the routine clinical application of this technique.

The most frequently cited drawbacks of mass spectrometry are the cost of the instrument, its complexity, and, for some instruments, the expense of effective maintenance programs. The primary advantages of utilizing a mass spectrometer are its ability to be controlled by microprocessors and its multigas analyzing capability. The cost factor may be minimized when the cost of the separate analyzers necessary to provide the range of analyses available with a mass spectrometer is considered. This is particularly true in the intensive care setting.

Optical Transmission Analyzers

Emission spectroscopy is the most commonly used method to determine nitrogen concentration. Basically, a vacuum pump draws the sample gas through a needle valve into an ionization chamber, where the gas is ionized by the application of a high voltage. The light emitted by this process is filtered; only that within the spectral range of nitrogen is passed and detected by a photocell. This is then amplified and displayed on a meter or as an analog signal.

Emission spectroscopy is affected by the presence of helium, CO_2, and water vapor. The linearity of the instrument is a function of the stability of the vacuum pressure; with higher vacuum pressures, the signal is more linear but also more sensitive to pressure variations caused by pump fluctuations. The instrument is relatively inexpensive, stable, and has a typical response time of approximately 30 msec.

The determination of oxyhemoglobin saturation utilizes monochromatic light. When hemoglobin is saturated with oxygen or carbon monoxide, the transmission of light through the blood or the reflection of light from blood allows the level of saturation to be quantified. The fact that hemoglobin is not a homogenous solution produces alinearity over wide ranges of hematocrit levels. Furthermore, the presence of methemoglobin acts as an optical absorbent. By utilizing several wavelengths and assuming independent and additive absorption by each factor, these factors can be minimized.

Infrared Analyzers

The basis for infrared analysis is the fact that certain gases, such as CO and CO_2, absorb infrared radiation. Infrared analyzers consist of three components, the source, the cell, and the detector, as illustrated in Fig. 9. The source of an infrared analyzer is constructed with a filter network to allow specific wavelengths to pass. Since the wavelength at which a particular gas will absorb infrared radiation is well defined, analyzers can be designed to detect a specific gas.

The cell consists of two parts, a measuring cell and a reference cell. The reference cell contains the environmental atmosphere against which the specific

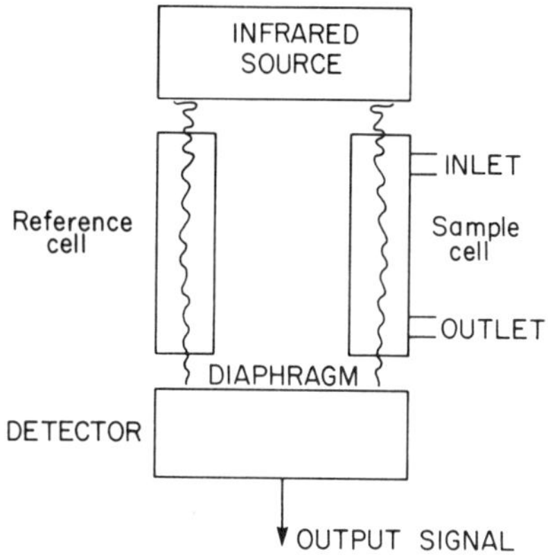

Fig. 9 *Infrared analyzer.*

gas is to be compared. Thus, when the specific gas is present in the measuring cell, a larger amount of radiation is absorbed there than is absorbed in the reference cell. The resulting difference is proportional to the concentration of the analyzed gas

The detector most commonly consists of two chambers separated by a membrane. The amount of radiation emitted from each cell heats and expands the gases in the respective chambers, resulting in movement of the membrane. A perforated metal plate close to the membrane, but electrically isolated from it, creates a condenser. Inclusion of a chopper, which interrupts the radiation at specified intervals (normally about 50 times a minute), causes the condenser to emit a pulsating dc signal proportional to the infrared absorbance of the gas being analyzed. Another method utilizes a photon detector to sense the differences in infrared radiation transmitted.

Paramagnetic Analyzers

Oxygen is an example of a paramagnetic gas, because it tends to distort a magnetic field. Gases such as nitrogen and carbon dioxide are said to be diamagnetic, since they are repelled by a magnetic field. In application, a glass dumbbell filled with a diamagnetic gas is suspended in a strong magnetic field. Introduction of oxygen will cause a displacement of the dumbbell proportional to the concentration of oxygen. The greater the concentration of oxygen, the greater the displacement. This is illustrated in Fig. 10.

Most commonly, the displacement is measured by affixing a mirror to the dumbbell and reflecting light upon a calibrated scale. Another model is based upon a pneumatic analogue of the Wheatstone bridge and utilizes a differential pressure transducer.

The sensitivity of a paramagnetic oxygen analyzer is affected by the magnetic

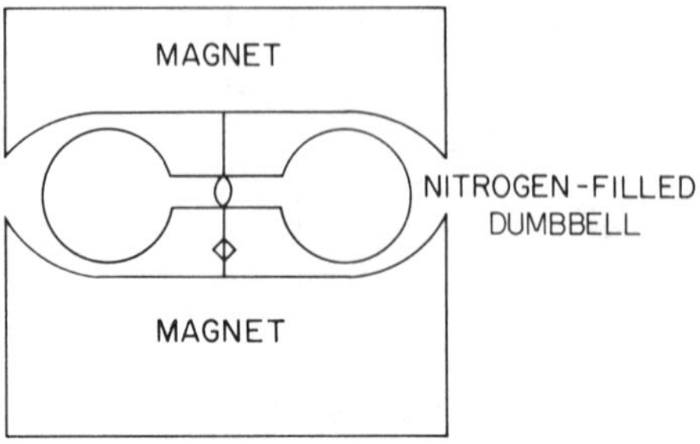

Fig. 10 *Paramagnetic analyzer.*

properties of the background gas, and most gases have magnetic properties proportional to their densities. Thus, accuracy is affected by pressure, which alters density.

Polarographic Electrodes

Miniature polarographic electrodes, similar to the Clark electrode discussed in Chapter 21 have been developed utilizing a variety of cathode-anode combinations. Polarographic electrodes generally require frequent calibration due to drift problems, and have a 90% response time of 30–90 seconds. One commercially available system improves the response time by utilizing internal circuitry to provide an inverse to the sensor's transfer function. By subjecting the input change to the sensor's normal transfer function, then to its inverse, the output will faithfully represent input changes with a response time of 200 msec. This allows the instrument to function as a fast-reacting system appropriate to most monitoring purposes. Without such specialized circuitry, polarographic electrodes will not generally meet the response criteria for monitoring fast-changing signals.

Fuel Cell Analyzers

Fuel cells have been developed for the determination of both oxygen and carbon monoxide concentrations. The fuel cell uses a solid electrolyte of zirconium and calcium oxides, coated with porous platinum. The electrolyte acts as a semipermeable membrane selective for oxygen ions. In practice, the cell is heated to approximately 800° C to improve the conductivity for oxygen ions. The output of the cell is logarithmic, but is generally converted to a linear output. Typical 90% response time is approximately 200 msec. The cell is specific for oxygen and therefore is not affected by other respiratory gases, but it is affected by the presence of hydrogen, hydrocarbons, and other combustibles.

A cell has been developed to electrochemically determine carbon monoxide levels. The carbon monoxide is electro-oxidized to carbon dioxide by a catalytically active electrode, such as platinum in an aqueous electrolyte. The current measured is proportional to the partial pressure of carbon monoxide in the sample. A linearizing network is necessary, and the cell is sensitive to alcohol. In addition to increased concentrations of CO_2, water vapor is also a by-product in the discharge gas stream. The cell exhibits a 90% rise time of approximately 20 sec and requires a relatively large sample of 300–500 ml. The cell has been used successfully in applications not requiring fast response times.

Recorders

Regardless of the instrument used, it is often important to provide a written record of the output. For example, the American Thoracic Society (ATS) Snowbird Report on Standardization of Spirometry recommended that diagnostic spirometry include a copy of the volume–time tracing in addition to the calculation of volume and flow parameters; it is increasingly common to see trend recordings in the intensive care setting.

Recorders are generally categorized by the device that converts the electrical input signal to movement. The basic recorder mechanisms are galvanometric, potentiometric, and optical. Each may be further categorized by the format of the recording, such as curvilinear or rectilinear and as strip chart recorders, X–Y recorders, and continuous recording cameras.

Galvanometric mechanisms utilize a moving coil and magnet assembly, with a stylus attached to the moving coil. The mechanisms normally provide a stylus deflection proportional to the magnitude of input current. The concept of damping, previously discussed, is essential in a galvanometric recorder. Without appropriate damping, the stylus may oscillate around the "true" position. Damping allows the stylus to assume an equilibrium position with minimum delay.

The frequency response of the system is defined by maximum angular acceleration resulting from the finite mass of the stylus and the finite force developed by the galvanometric mechanism. Frequency responses for galvanometric recorders can range up to about 200 Hz.

Potentiometric recorders operate on a servo principle. In this system, the position of the stylus is detected by a contact mechanism attached to the stylus arm and in contact with a fixed slide wire. The servo system will move the stylus until the potential between the slide wire contact and the input voltage is zero. The linearity and accuracy of the system are dependent only on the characteristics of the slide wire and associated electronics. In general, potentiometric recorders provide greater accuracy and better linearity than galvanometric recorders.

Damping in the potentiometric recorder is generally accomplished electronically within the servo amplifier. Due to the inherent speed limitations of moving the stylus and the frictional forces associated with the slide wire, potentiometric recorders rarely achieve a frequency response above 20 Hz. When used in conjunction with most gas analyzers, low frequency response is not a serious limitation. However, for many other applications, the combination of limited frequency response and generally high cost limits the utilization of potentiometric recorders.

Optical coupling between the recorder and the chart allows adequate frequency response for very fast changing signals. Continuous motion recording is achieved by moving photographically sensitive paper past the oscilloscope cathode-ray tube (CRT). This provides the frequency response required by eliminating the need to physically move a stylus with its attendant inertia and friction. This system provides the accuracy associated with potentiometric recorders and a higher frequency response than is possible with galvanometric recorders. Since only the light beam need respond, no damping is necessary. Its primary drawback is the price. Its applications tend to be limited to body plethysmography or specialized applications that require very high frequency response.

A pivoting stylus transcribing an arc with a pen is one of the simplest recording mechanisms, but the format is inconvenient and seldom used. Rectilinear recording is achieved with the galvonmetric mechanism illustrated in Fig. 11. As illustrated, the contact between the stylus and the chart paper moves up and down the stylus arm as the stylus pivots. It is apparent when analyzing the geometry of the setup that the stylus movement will not be directly proportional to the angular deflection of the stylus arm, and will produce alinearity. The alinearity is less than 1% if the total stylus deflection is limited to half the perpendicular distance between the pivot point and the pen tip. This mechanism is most commonly used in electrocardiograph (ECG) recording.

Strip chart recorders are widely used in the pulmonary laboratory, and, as the name implies, they utilize one or more pens and transcribe on a sheet of paper that moves past at pre-set speeds. This allows the option of spreading the signal out for close scrutiny or monitoring trends by slowing the paper speed and compressing the signal.

An X-Y recorder plots one variable against another. Generally these recorders utilize servo mechanisms with slide wires; the two axes may have significantly different frequency response characteristics. The two most important frequency response characteristics are slewing speed and peak acceleration.

Slewing speed refers to the minimum time necessary to move the pen a discrete distance, generally expressed in terms of inches or millimeters per second. Obviously, for recording data such as flow volume loops, higher slewing speeds are preferred. Appropriate ranges for flow volume loops are 20–30 inches/sec. Slewing speed is an important limitation to consider when attempting to expand flow volume loops to larger scales.

Peak acceleration refers to the limits of the response of the recorder output to the acceleration of the input signal. It is an intuitively obvious, but often overlooked fact that the maximum acceleration capabilities of the axis of the pen

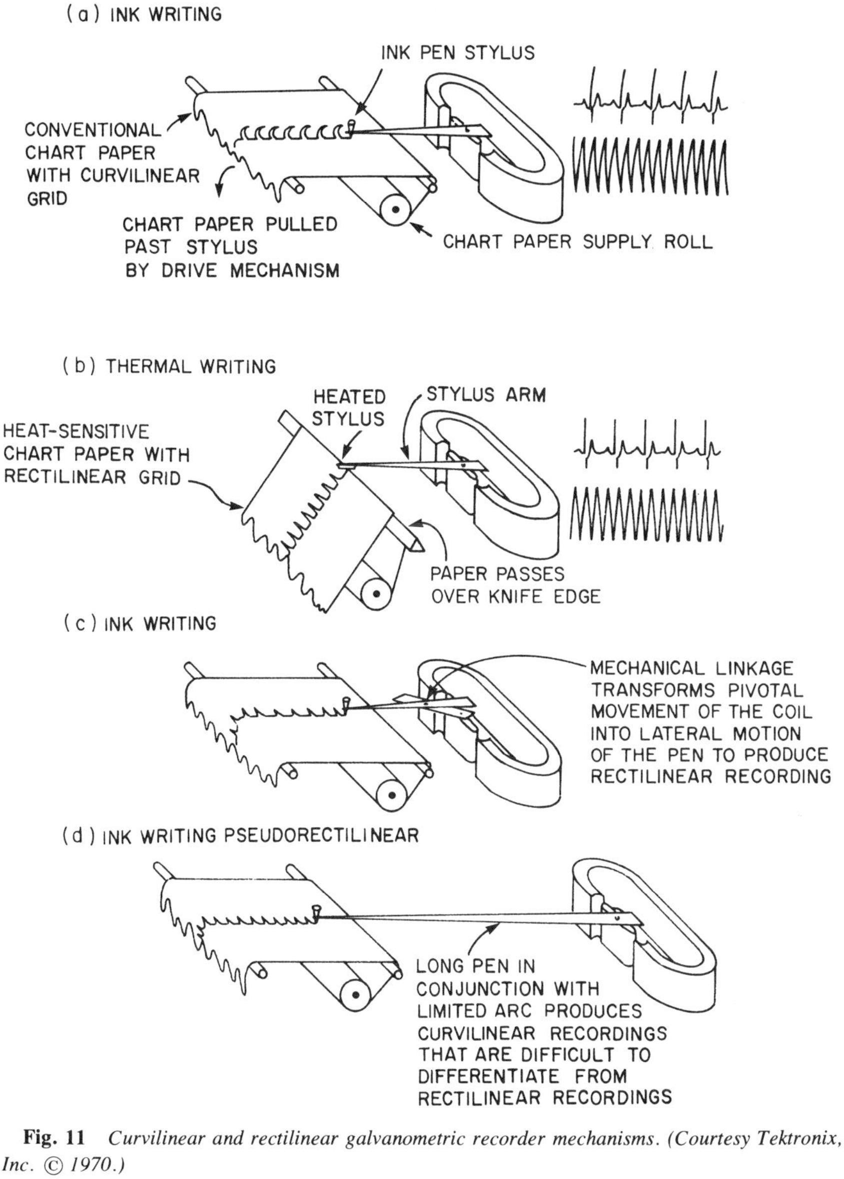

Fig. 11 *Curvilinear and rectilinear galvanometric recorder mechanisms. (Courtesy Tektronix, Inc. © 1970.)*

moving along the slide wire will be superior to the maximum acceleration possible when moving the entire slide wire housing on the other axis. Obviously, the faster changing signal should be placed on the axis with the superior acceleration. Typical peak acceleration specifications for servo-type X–Y recorders are

2000–3000 inches/sec^2. It should, perhaps, be pointed out that an X–Y oscilloscope has very high performance characteristics for both slewing speed and acceleration, and is frequently used for recording flow volume loops and body plethysmography tracings.

CALIBRATION AND QUALITY CONTROL

Calibration of the various instruments discussed depends on the type of analysis performed. For instance, analyses requiring only *relative* concentrations of gases may require only periodic linearity checks, whereas quantitative analyses require calibration with known standards in the appropriate range. Traditionally, known standards are gas cylinders that have been analyzed with a Scholander apparatus, or otherwise certified as a primary standard, traceable to the National Bureau of Standards. It is always advisable to be skeptical of the certified analysis of newly received cylinders, even if precision analysis has been requested. A simple way to check is to compare gas concentrations of the new cylinder with previously accepted cylinders. Because of their higher cost, the primary standard cylinders should be utilized mainly to verify other cylinders used for routine calibration.

Many instruments provide electrical simulations or internal checks not involving the sensor. These should never be accepted as the sole guarantee of operational status. Whenever possible, it is advisable to verify the system as an entity rather than as individual components. This verification should cover the desired operating range and should, when appropriate, simulate the physiological signal.

Quality control should be performed in the context of an established program on a periodic basis. The frequency should be determined by the stability of the analyzer. For instance, a gas chromatograph is quite stable in normal operation and may require quality control on a less frequent basis than a blood-gas analyzer, which is subject to wide fluctuations and varying characteristics. On any analyzer, the quality control program should provide vertification over the entire desired operating range. This verification requires at least three points to assess linearity and accuracy. These points may be achieved by multiple gas cylinders or by careful dilution of a primary standard, using a mixing chamber or calibrated syringe.

GENERAL REFERENCES

1. Brantigan JW, Gott VL, Vestal ML, et al.: A nonthrombogenic diffusion membrane for continuous in vivo measurement of blood gases by mass spectrometry. *J Appl Physiol* 28:375–377, 1970.
2. Fowler KT: The respiratory mass spectrometer. *Phys Med Biol* 14:185–199, 1969.

3. Gardner RM, Baker CD, Broennle AM Jr, et al.: ATS statement—Snowbird workshop on standardization of spirometry. *Am Rev Respir Dis* 119:831-838, 1979.
4. Gardner RM, Hankinson JL, West BJ: Evaluating commercially available spirometers. *Am Rev Respir Dis* 121:73-81, 1980.
5. Lilly JC: Studies on the mixing of gases within the respiratory system with a new type nitrogen meter. *Fed Proc* 5:64, 1946.
6. McCall CB, Hyatt RE, Noble FW, et al.: Harmonic content of certain respiratory flow phenomena of normal individuals. *J Appl Physiol* 10:215-218, 1957.
7. Mitchell RR: Incorporating the gas analyzer response time in gas exchange computations. *J Appl Physiol* 47:1118-1122, 1979.
8. Norton AC: Accuracy in pulmonary measurements. *Respir Care* 24:131-137, 1979.
9. Peabody JL, Gregory GA, Willis MM, et al.: Transcutaneous oxygen tension in sick infants. *Am Rev Respir Dis* 118:83-87, 1978.
10. Saunders NA, Powles ACP, Rebuck AS: Ear oximetry: Accuracy and practicability in the assessment of arterial oxygenation. *Am Rev Respir Dis* 113:745-749, 1976.
11. Stead WS, Wells HS, Gault NL, et al.: Inaccuracy of the conventional water-filled spirometer for recording rapid breathing. *J Appl Physiol* 14:448-450, 1959.
12. Wood EH, Geraaci JE: Photoelectric determinations of the arterial oxygen saturation in man. *J Lab Clin Med* 34:387, 1949.

CHAPTER 6

Prediction of Normal Values

JACK L. CLAUSEN, M.D.

Predictive normal values for pulmonary function parameters are essential for meaningful clinical interpretations of these measurements. Improvements in the accuracy of predictive values will result in increased accuracy of interpretations as well as increased sensitivity of these tests for the detection of early disease. Despite the important role of predictive normal values, for many parameters the currently available normal values are inadequate. A clear understanding of these inadequacies is necessary for meaningful selection and utilization of normal values and for choosing optimal studies of normal values in the future.

A few pulmonary function parameters have a very narrow range of values in normal subjects and are independent of physical characteristics, such as height or age (e.g., the pH of arterial blood; see Fig. 1). Selection of useful upper and lower limits of normal values for such pulmonary function parameters is, therefore, relatively simple. For the vast majority of pulmonary function tests, however, the range of values observed in a population of normal subjects is much broader, making selection of the limits of normal values more difficult. An example is the distribution of normal values of vital capacity (VC) in adults shown in Fig. 2. Since predictive normal values for many of these parameters correlate significantly with selected physical characteristics, regression equations can be developed from studies of large populations of normal subjects and used to predict a narrower range of normal values for subjects with specific physical

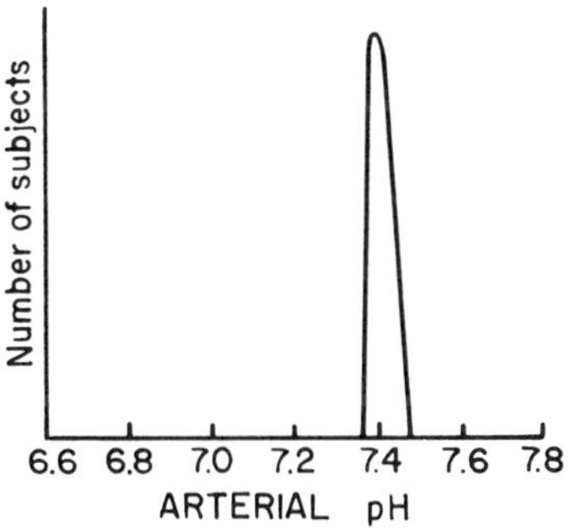

Fig. 1 *Distribution of arterial blood pH in normal subjects.*

PULMONARY FUNCTION TESTING
GUIDELINES AND CONTROVERSIES

ISBN 0-12-788125-5

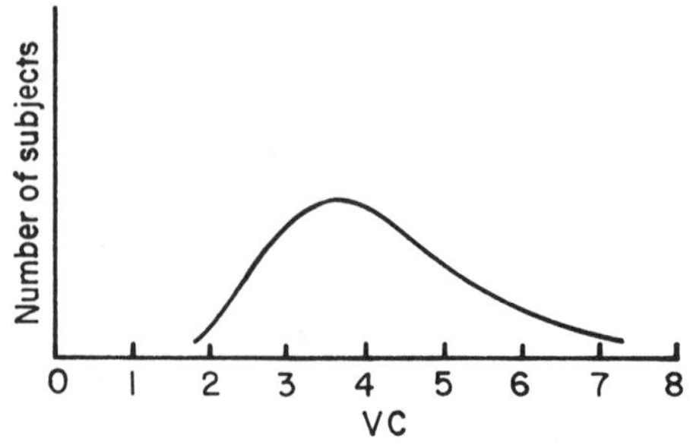

Fig. 2 *Distribution of VC in normal adults.*

characteristics. Figure 3 illustrates the reduction in range of predicted VC that may result from the use of this type of regression equation. Factors of recognized usefulness for the prediction of many pulmonary function parameters include age, height, weight, and sex.

Predictive equations for normal values are usually expressed as linear regression equations, utilizing those physical characteristics that contribute statistically significant reductions in the variability of predictive normal values. However, not all pulmonary function parameters are linearly dependent on physical characteristics; for children and the elderly, curvilinear or power functions may more accurately predict the relationships between pulmonary function parameters and physical characteristics. Although such equations (e.g., in males less than 18 years old, $VC = 4.4 \times 10^{-3}\ Ht^{2.67}$) may be difficult to calculate manually, with calculators or computers these more complex but potentially more accurate equations are simple to use. The recent advent of low-cost microprocessors and time-sharing computer services has significantly increased the feasibility of using those equations. It is important to note, however, that with nonlinear regression

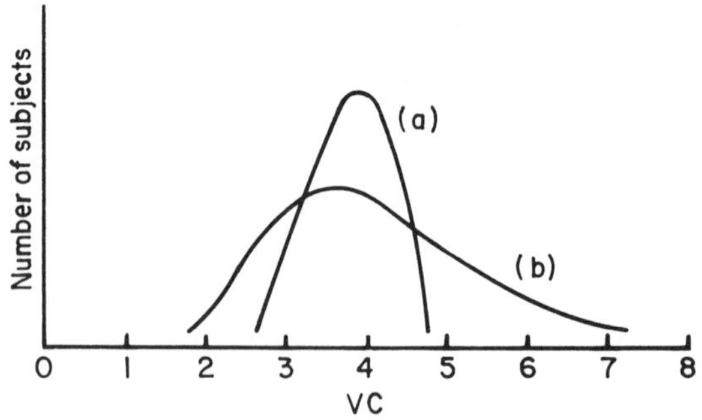

Fig. 3 *Distribution of VC from entire sample of normal adults and the distribution predicted for a specific age, height, and sex. (a) Predicted normal value for a specific age and sex. (b) Distribution of entire sample.*

equations (particularly exponential forms), very substantial errors can result from the application of such equations to subjects with ages, heights, weights (or other factors) that are outside the boundaries within which the equations are appropriate.

A potential disadvantage of many of the currently available normal predictive equations is that the raw data were analyzed only with linear regression equations. The more recent studies of Knudson et al. (1) and Schoenberg et al. (2) both used curvilinear analyses of data; the latter study has a particularly in-depth discussion of sophisticated statistical techniques for analyzing normal predictive data.

RELATIONSHIP TO AGE

Table 1 lists predicted pulmonary function results for two males of different ages and illustrates the very profound significance of aging on certain parameters.

A number of studies (1-3) have noted that VC increases until the ages of 23-27, then shows a steady decrease. If a single best-fit linear regression equation is used to predict the VC from ages 18 and above, the VC will be overestimated in the age range of 18-23; either a curvilinear equation should be used (2) or two different regression equations, as done by Knudson et al. (1), for males less than and more than 25 years old. For parameters other than VC and expiratory flows, the potential uses of curvilinear relationships to aging have not been adequately studied. The precise relationship of aging to decrements in pulmonary function is obscured somewhat by the interactions of height and age. Height reductions associated with increasing age have been attributed to the effects of aging on the width of the intervertebral spaces; however, it has also been observed that older adults were shorter in their youths than the current generation of young adults (presumably due to nutritional effects). The undefined relationship

Table 1 *Significance of Age on Predicted Values for a Subject 176 cm Tall*

	20 (yr)	70 (yr)
PO_2 (mm Hg)	100	79
VC (liters)	5.18	3.93
RV (liters)	1.48	2.33
FEV_1 (liters)	4.26	2.66
$FEF_{25-75\%}$ (liters/sec)	4.76	2.51
$FEF_{75\%}$ (liters/sec)	2.19	0.99
$DL_{CO}SB$ (ml/min/mm Hg)	29	16.5
CV/VC(%)	7.7	25.5

between height and survival may add another potential bias inherent in cross-sectional studies.

RELATIONSHIP TO SEX

For many pulmonary function parameters, there are differences in predictive normal values related to the sex of the subjects and independent of height and weight differences. For such parameters, separate regression equations for each sex are usually defined.

RELATIONSHIP TO HEIGHT AND WEIGHT

In children, many pulmonary function parameters can be better predicted from heights than from ages, and are often best related to curvilinear regression equations. In adults, published regression equations that include height almost always utilize linear relationships. Schoenberg's regression equations included some interactive terms between height and weight that may be similar to the use of body surface area for predictive terms in many older studies (2). An example of the interactions that can be better defined by curvilinear equations is the observation that in adults of the same height, predicted lung volumes first increase as weights increase in the lower range of normal values (''muscularity effect''), then decrease as weights increase further (''obesity effect'') (2).

RELATIONSHIP TO RACE AND ETHNIC BACKGROUND

Differences in predictive values related to racial and ethnic backgrounds are often overlooked in pulmonary function testing and are not adequately documented. A number of studies have shown the VC and TLC of blacks are 13–15% lower than those of whites matched for age, height, and sex (2, 4–6). In one study, the VC, FRC, and TLC of Chinese adults (approximately 20% were light smokers) showed values 20–25% lower than those of height-matched whites (7). Indians in Guyana were noted to have VCs about 5% lower than those of comparable African adults (8). Useful data for Mexican-Americans are unavailable and of obvious importance in California. The changing nutritional conditions in underdeveloped countries and the resultant effects on heights and weights add additional complexity to efforts to define predictive equations for these populations. Differences in normal values between different ethnic groups of white Europeans (e.g., Swedes versus Italians) have been hypothesized but not verified.

RELATIONSHIP TO ALTITUDE

The relationships between normal values and the altitude histories of subjects in a study are also not well defined. They are important both for laboratories at significant elevations above sea level, and for interpreting the results of published normal studies done at higher altitudes [e.g., Goldman and Becklake's study of lung volumes was done at an elevation of 1756 m (5760 feet)]. From an analysis of five published studies, Schoenberg et al. concluded that the mean FVC increase was 100 cc for every 300 m increase in altitude of residence (2). In a comparison of values from spirometry studies of normal subjects residing at 3100 m with published normal values of subjects at sea level, Kryger et al. (9) concluded that there was no significant different in the FVC, but the $FEF_{25-75\%}$ was as much as 30% higher in younger subjects residing at high altitudes. The interpretations of most of these studies on the chronic effects of altitude on pulmonary function parameters are limited by differences in equipment, testing methodologies, and populations studied. Many questions about the effects of altitude remain unanswered.

RELATIONSHIP TO AIR POLLUTION AND OTHER ENVIRONMENTAL FACTORS

Exposure to high levels of "reducing"-type air pollution (usually associated with the combustion of high-sulfur coal) has been shown to have some deleterious effects on pulmonary function. However, chronic exposure to the oxidant-type air pollution that prevails in California has not been associated with demonstrable alterations in pulmonary function (10). The relationship (if any) of normal values of pulmonary tests to fog or extremes of ambient temperatures has not been defined.

LOWER LIMITS OF NORMAL VALUES

Regardless of whether linear or more complex regression equations are used, they predict the mean value expected for a population of normal subjects with specific physical characteristics. Although this mean value is of definite worth when clinicially interpreting the pulmonary function tests, a more useful interpretation often requires knowledge of the limits of normal values (11). If the data from normal values follow a Gaussian (that is, "normal") distribution, one can express an observed value as a multiple of the standard deviation (SD) of the normal population in order to define the probability that an observed value is within normal limits, as illustrated in Fig. 4. In contrast with many statistical analyses, during clinical pulmonary function testing a question that requires

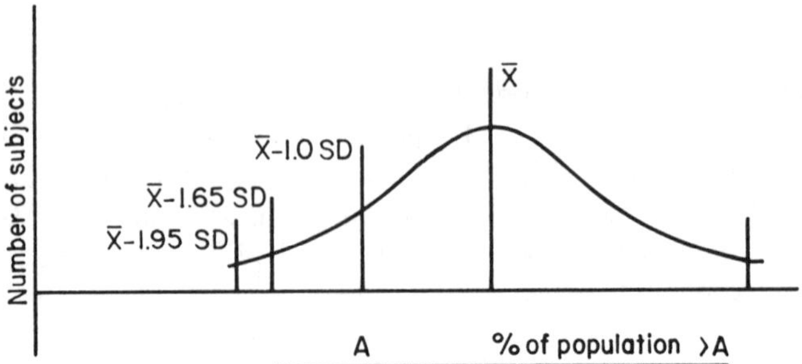

A	% of population >A
X̄-1.95 SD	97.5
X̄-1.65 SD	95.0
X̄-1.0 SD	84.0
X̄	50.0

Fig. 4 *Proportion of a population above various limits of normalcy.*

defining *either* the upper or lower limit of normal values is usually being asked. For these purposes, the one-tailed t-test is the appropriate statistical test; thus, the lower limits of normal values at a confidence level of 95% would be the mean minus 1.65 SD, in contrast with the less sensitive limits of 1.96 SD used for a two-tailed t-test.

The validity of the standard statistical approach is dependent upon the correctness of the assumption that the data from normal subjects are normally distributed for subjects of all ages and heights. In most published studies of normal subjects, this assumption often has not been tested, especially in the older age groups.

Figure 5 shows the distribution of $FEF_{25-75\%}$ measurements that would be predicted to be observed in a population of normal 48-year-old males 170 cm in

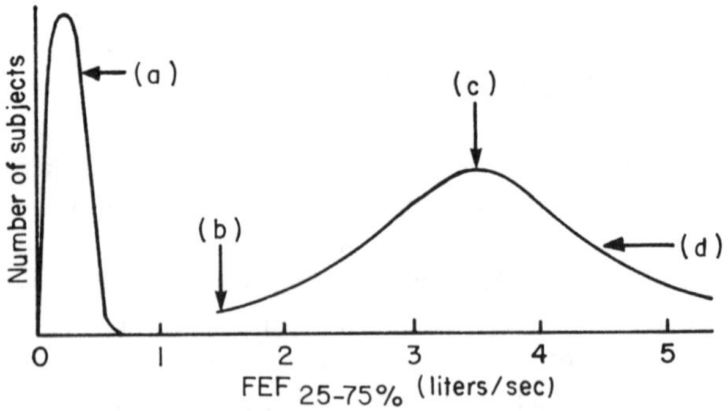

Fig. 5 *Distribution of $FEF_{25-75\%}$ measurements. (a) Patients with severe COPD. (b) Lower limit of predicted normal values ($p < 0.05$). (c) Predicted normal value (mean). (d) Normal.*

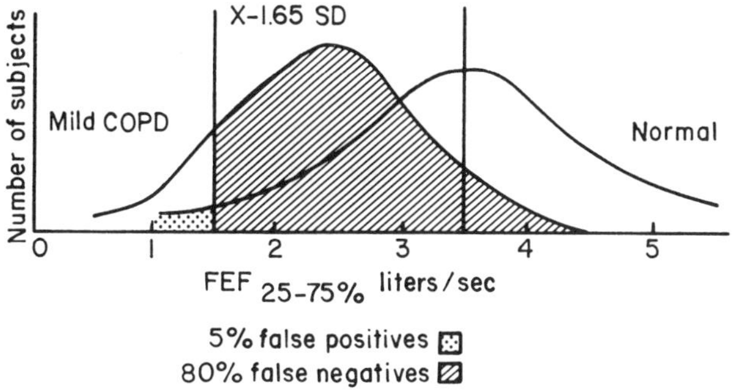

Fig. 6 *Distribution of $FEF_{25-75\%}$ measurements in sample of normal subjects and patients with mild COPD.*

height and in a population of patients with severe obstructive lung disease; this figure illustrates that the lower limit of normal value of the mean minus 1.65 SD would be useful for separating subjects into one of these two populations. In contrast, Fig. 6 illustrates the problems that would arise in attempting to define useful lower limits of normal values if one of the study populations was comprised of patients with "early" mild chronic obstructive pulmonary disease (COPD) in whom there is a considerable overlap of values of $FEF_{25-75\%}$ with those observed in normal subjects. If normalcy is defined as an $FEF_{25-75\%}$ greater than the 95% confidence level ($\bar{x}$ − 1.65 SD), 80% of the patients with early mild disease would be falsely called normal. If 80% of the predicted mean is used as the lower limit of normal values (Fig. 7), one would reduce the false negatives to 40%, but would include 25% of the normal population in the "abnormal" group.

Although somewhat narrower predictive distributions may be available in the future through the use of more sophisticated regression equations, for most

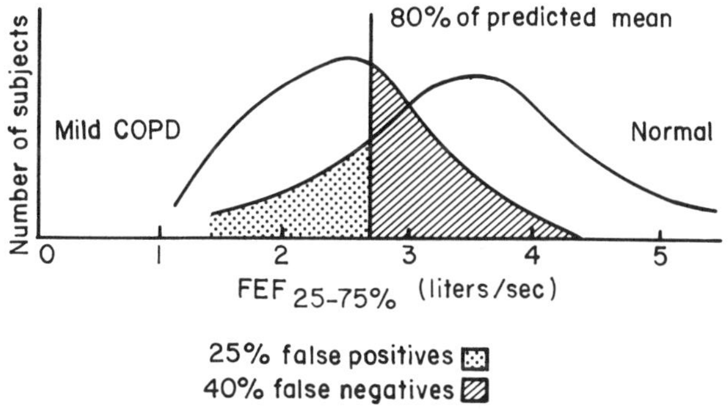

Fig. 7 *Significance of using 80% of predicted mean for defining normalcy.*

pulmonary function parameters the residual "unexplained" intersubject variability will remain, and the large and inherent overlap between normalcy and disease states will persist as a limtation in pulmonary function test interpretations. *Hence, one cannot arbitrarily assign a lower limit of normal values that will be useful for all situations.* If the purpose of testing is to initially screen for *possible* disease, higher limits of normal values would be more useful; if, in contrast, one is testing subjects applying for life insurance, a limit of normal values at the 5% confidence level would assure the physician that there would be a minimal number of false positives.

A more thorough analysis of the clinical applications of the limits of normalcy is more pertinent to a discussion of interpretation of test results. In the context of this chapter, the importance lies in choosing studies of normal subjects in which the lower limits of normal values are meaningfully and accurately defined.

REFERENCING PREDICTIVE VALUES TO OTHER PHYSIOLOGICAL PARAMETERS

Intersubject variability may be reduced for the predictive values of some pulmonary function parameters by relating them to other physiological parameters (e.g., DL_{CO}/V_A, RV/TLC, or FEV_1/FVC). Many other potentially useful interactions remain to be defined. For example, it is well recognized that elevations of residual volume (RV) are commonly associated with decreases in maximal expiratory flow rates in COPD. If a patient has an observed RV of 125% of the predicted value and a $FEF_{25-75\%}$ of 70% of the predicted value, each of these parameters falls within normal limits. What is currently unavailable is the percentile distribution in a normal population of the probability of *both* of these observations occurring in the same subject.

COMPARISONS OF PUBLISHED PREDICTIVE EQUATIONS FOR NORMAL ADULTS

There are many factors that can result in apparently equivalent studies yielding significantly different predictive values in a given patient. Table 2 is an example of differences that might be attributable to performance characteristics of test equipment, in this instance two standard Collins spirometers. More extreme differences in spirometer performance have been well documented in other studies. The considerable efforts of the American Thoracic Society to establish performance standards for spirometers should reduce this problem in the future, but there are a number of unanswered questions about differences in spirometer

Table 2 *Comparison of $FEF_{200-1200}$*[a]

Spirometer	$FEF_{200-1200}$ (liters/sec)
Collins metal bell	9.35
Collins plastic bell (Stead-Wells)	7.27

[a] Measured using two different spirometers in 37 normal subjects (12).

and pneumotachograph performance for studies of normal subjects already published.

A comprehensive comparison of predictive equations for pulmonary function tests is not currently available. To be most useful, such a comparison should include data calculated from the extremes of ages, heights, and weights likely to be encountered in a clinical lab, as it is for these cases that regression equations are most likely to be misleading. That the results of such a comparison can be quite disconcerting is illustrated by the following comparisons of published predictive regression equations for RV and $FEF_{25-75\%}$ using representative ages, heights, and weights that are often encountered in most laboratories (Tables 3 and 4).

With the data available, we do not currently understand the determinants of the differences observed in Tables 3 and 4. Possible factors include differing methodologies for selecting data (e.g., constructing composite curves of highest flow rates versus selecting flow rates from expiratory curves demonstrating the best effort), differences between testing instruments (e.g., pneumotachograph versus volume displacement spirometer), or real physiological differences between the populations studied. Less likely explanations include postures of subjects during testing, differences between the altitudes where the studies were

Table 3 *Comparison of RVs*[a]

Study	RV (liters)
Permutt et al. (13)	1.00
Boren et al. (14)	1.49
Turner et al. (15)	1.66
Grimby and Soderholm (16)	1.70
Goldman and Becklake (17)	1.87
Needham et al. (18)	2.05
Cumming and Semple (19)	2.25

[a] Calculated from published predictive equations for a 30-year-old male, height 178 cm, weight 73 kg.

Table 4 *Comparison of Predicted Normal Values for a 65-Year-Old Male 183 cm Tall*

Study	$FEF_{25-75\%}$ (liters/sec)
Morris et al. (20)	2.97
Knudson et al. (1)	4.35

conducted, or derivation of regression equations that are not applicable to the ages, heights, and weights selected for examples in Table 3 and 4.

SELECTION OF PREDICTIVE VALUES FOR YOUR LABORATORY

The unavoidable conclusion from the previous comparison of published normal values is that, because of these inexplicable differences, there is no one recommended set of prediction equations applicable to all labs and patient populations. The approach that is recommended is as follows: make a preliminary selection of one or more predictive regression equations from studies whose testing equipment, methodologies, and patient populations most clearly resemble those used in your laboratory. Measure each of the pulmonary function parameters used clinically in a small number of normal subjects (n = 10–20) who are representative (race, age, height, etc.) of the patient population normally studied. If more than 3 out of 10 of the presumably normal subjects have observed values that fall outside of the 95% confidence interval for normal limits, then all aspects of your testing procedures should be reviewed. If the study of another 10 subjects again results in 3 or more falling outside the limits, then it is most likely that either the testing is inaccurate or the selected normal values are inappropriate for your instrumentation and patient population.

For each laboratory to establish its own predictive regression equations is a task that should not be embarked upon without due consideration of the considerable work lying ahead. Establishing predictive regression equations that are valid for the wide ranges of heights, weights, and ages encountered in clinical labs is a major undertaking well beyond the resources available to most labs.

REFERENCES

1. Knudson RJ, Slatin RC, Lebowitz MD, et al.: The maximal expiratory flow-volume curve. Normal standards, variability, and effects of age. *Am Rev Respir Dis* 113:587–600, 1976.
2. Schoenberg JB, Beck GJ, Bouhuys A: Growth and decay of pulmonary function in healthy blacks and whites. *Respir Physiol* 33:367–393, 1978.

3. Hutchinson J: On the capacity of the lungs and on the respiratory movements with the view of establishing a precise and easy method of detecting disease by the spirometer. *Trans Med Chir Soc Lond* 29:137-252, 1846.
4. Seltzer C, Siegelaub AB, Freidman GD, et al.: Differences in pulmonary function related to smoking habits and race. *Am Rev Respir Dis* 110:598-608, 1974.
5. Lapp NL, Amandus HE, Hall R, et al.: Lung volumes and flow rates in black and white subjects. *Thorax* 29:185-188, 1974.
6. Abramowitz S, Leiner GC, Lewis WA, et al.: Vital capacity in the negro. *Am Rev Respir Dis* 92:287-292, 1965.
7. Da Costa JL: Pulmonary function studies in healthy Chinese adults in Singapore. *Am Rev Respir Dis* 104:128-131, 1971.
8. Miller GJ, Aschroft MT, Swan AV, et al.: Ethnic variation in FEV and FVC of African and Indian adults in Guyana. *Am Rev Respir Dis* 102:979-981, 1970.
9. Kryger M, Aldrich F, Reeves JT, et al.: Diagnosis of airflow obstruction at high altitude. *Am Rev Respir Dis* 117:1055-1058, 1978.
10. Cohen CA, Hudson AR, Clausen JL, et al.: Respiratory symptoms, spirometry and oxidant air-pollution in nonsmoking adults. *Am Rev Respir Dis* 105:251-261, 1972.
11. Knudson RJ, Lebowitz MD: Maximal mix-expiratory flow (FEF 25-75): Normal limits and assessment of sensitivity. *Am Rev Respir Dis* 117:609-610, 1978.
12. Kory RC, Hamilton LH: Evaluation of spirometers used in pulmonary function studies. *Am Rev Respir Dis* 87:228-238, 1963.
13. Altman PL, Dittmer DS (eds): *Respiration and circulation*. Bethesda, MD, Fed Am Soc Exp Biol, 1971, pp 52-53.
14. Boren HG, Kory RC, Syner JC: The Veterans Administration-Army cooperative study of pulmonary function: II. The lung volume and its subdivisions in normal man. *Am J Med* 41:96-114, 1966.
15. Turner JM, Mead J, Wohl ME: Elasticity of human lungs in relation to age. *J Appl Physiol* 25:644-671, 1968.
16. Grimby G, Soderholm B: Spirometric studies in normal subjects: III. Static lung volumes and maximum voluntary ventilation in adults with a note on physical fitness. *Acta Med Scand* 173:199-206, 1963.
17. Goldman HI, Becklake MR: Respiratory function tests: Normal values at median altitudes and the prediction of normal results. *Am Rev Tuberc* 79:457-467, 1959.
18. Needham CD, Rogan MC, McDonald I: Normal standards for lung volumes, intrapulmonary gas mixing, and maximum breathing capacity. *Thorax* 9:313-325, 1954.
19. Cumming G, Semple SJ: *Disorders of the Respiratory System*. Oxford, Blackwell Scientific Publications, 1973, p 30.
20. Morris JF, Koski A, Johnson LC: Spirometric standards for healthy non-smoking adults. *Am Rev Respir Dis* 103:57-67, 1971.

CHAPTER 7

Spirometry and Flow–Volume Curves

HOMER A. BOUSHEY, JR., M.D.
ARTHUR DAWSON, M.D.

The ultimate purpose of performing spirometry or measuring a patient's flow–volume curve was well summarized in the title of John Hutchinson's 1846 paper: "On the capacity of the lungs and on the respiratory functions with a view of establishing a precise and easy method of detecting disease by a spirometer" (1). A reduction in the volume that can be exhaled from total lung capacity—the vital capacity (VC)—can certainly be detected easily, but it is a relatively nonspecific index of disease, for it may be caused either by a reduction in total lung capacity (due to chest wall, neuromuscular, pleural, or interstitial disease) or by an increase in residual volume (due to airways obstruction or loss of lung recoil). A reduction in the maximal rate at which air is exhaled can also be detected easily by routine spirometry or by measuring the instantaneous expiratory flow at different lung volumes, as from a flow–volume curve. But a reduction in flow does not in itself permit a precise definition of the site or nature of disease, because it may be caused by inadequate expiratory effort, loss of lung recoil, an increase in the resistance of the airways, or abnormal compressibility of the intrathoracic trachea (2–4). However, careful analysis of the pattern of abnormalities in forced vital capacity and maximal expiratory flow and correlation with the data obtained from the history, physical exam, and other laboratory tests permit reasonably secure inferences about the nature of the underlying pulmonary disease and provide a direct, precise estimate of the severity of disease. Measurement of the forced vital capacity or the flow–volume curve has therefore become the most commonly used physiological test for the detection of lung disease. Also, after the nature of the disease has been established, these measurements permit assessment of changes in its severity or its response to treatment. For example, daily measurement of forced expiratory capacity in 1 second (FEV_1) has been advocated as indispensable in following the course of acutely ill, hospitalized asthmatic patients (5).

PULMONARY FUNCTION TESTING
GUIDELINES AND CONTROVERSIES

ISBN 0-12-788125-5

Although the flow–volume curve contains no more information than the spirogram (in fact, the flow–volume curve can be derived from the spirogram), it permits easier recognition of abnormalities confined to either extreme of the respiratory tract. Abnormal narrowing of large, central airways, such as the larynx or trachea, produces a characteristic pattern on the inspiratory and expiratory portion of the flow–volume loop (6, 7). Obstruction of small, peripheral airways may cause a reduction in flow at low lung volumes, which is readily detected from the concave shape of the flow–volume curve (8) but which may be overlooked in standard analysis of the expiratory spirogram. More precise localization of the site of air flow limitation within the respiratory tree may also be possible by comparing the flow–volume curves obtained with the subject breathing air and then a low-density gas, such as "heliox," a mixture of helium (80%) and oxygen (20%) (9). The use of "heliox" flow–volume curves in clinical research has yielded provocative insights into the site and persistence of abnormalities in the airways of patients with asthma and bronchitis (10), but has yet to be shown to have an important role in clinical practice (see Chapter 10).

EQUIPMENT

For measurements obtained with different devices to be comparable, the devices must meet certain minimal standards, so that differences in results are more apt to be due to differences in the performance of the subject, rather than to differences in the behavior of equipment. For static measurements (e.g., vital capacity), the requirements of equipment are that it be stable, linear, and free from hysteresis. Stability implies the absence of drift (change over time) of the zero point and of the endpoint. A device is linear if the ratio of output to input is constant over the entire range of the device. Freedom from hysteresis is present if the output resulting from a certain input is the same whether the input is reached by increasing from a lower value or by decreasing from a higher value.

In general, instruments that measure volume by recording the displacement of a bellows, bell, wedge, or piston meet these criteria. Instruments that obtain volume by integrating flow are accurate only if the flow signal is stable, linear, and free from hysteresis over the entire range of expiratory flows. These instruments often measure volume less accurately and require more frequent calibration (11). The linearity of volume measurements derived from flow-measuring devices should be verified by both slow and rapid injection of known volumes of gas.

The response time of an instrument is seldom important for the measurement of vital capacity and other lung volumes. As long as the instrument is stable and its final output is linear, it is not important if it overshoots or undershoots the input signal. For measurement of dynamic events, however, the rate of response of the equipment becomes critical. The more rapid the rate of change of the event measured, the greater the demands on the equipment. For measurement of forced expiratory maneuvers, spirometers must be able to respond to a rapidly changing input signal, as might be generated by an oscillating pump.

The importance of measuring the response of a spirometer to a sinusoidal test signal (the frequency response) is obvious if one plans to use the instrument for measuring maximal voluntary ventilation, in which case the input signal is cyclical. The importance of measuring a device's frequency response if one plans to use it for measuring maximal expiratory flow becomes apparent when it is recognized that any waveform can be broken down into a collection of sine waves of different amplitudes and frequencies (Fourier analysis). If the instrument magnifies some components of the input signal (for example, those with a frequency of 5–8 Hz) and does not respond to those oscillating at a different frequency (e.g., those with a frequency of greater than 8 Hz)., the resulting net output will distort the shape of the input signal. McCall and co-workers (12) have analyzed the harmonic content of the waveform of forced expiration and have concluded that if the frequency response of an instrument is flat (does not reduce or magnify the input signal) up to 12 Hz, the instrument will not significantly distort any of the waveforms commonly analyzed in respiratory physiology. If an instrument magnifies or diminishes the input signal well below 12 Hz, the output will be most distorted for measurements involving rapid change, such as the peak expiratory flow rate and maximum voluntary ventilation.

In the early 1950s, the spirometers in use for testing pulmonary function had been designed for calculating oxygen uptake during measurement of the basic metabolic rate. Stead and his coworkers (13) recognized the importance of the dynamic response of the equipment used to measure rapid spirometric maneuvers. Their analysis of the 13.5-liter Collins metal-bell spirometer showed that when the input was varied at more than 0.6 Hz, the output no longer followed. With simulated fast breaths, the overshoot of the instrument was as much as 24%. Their suggestions for improvement led to the construction of the Stead–Wells spirometer; its lighter weight and diminished dead space enable it to record accurately inputs of up to 6 Hz (13). The Stead-Wells spirometer was subsequently used in a number of epidemiological studies and became the device against which other spirometers were compared until the American Thoracic Society (ATS) defined standards for spirometers (14) in 1979.

It should be recognized that these recommendations of the ATS apply not just to the spirometer itself but also to the spirometer and its recording device as a unit. This is particularly important if, as if often the case, a spirometer and an X–Y recorder are purchased separately to assemble a system for recording flow-volume curves. If the pen on the X–Y recorder cannot follow a rapidly changing signal, the tracing provided will distort the input signal just as much as if the spirometer itself were sluggish.

The performance standards proposed by the ATS incorporate the principles of instrumentation, as just reviewed, and define the range of values over which the instruments must be accurate to include at least 95% of the American population (14). Spirometers need not meet the standards for all tests, but they should meet the standards for each of the tests for which they are to be used. Unless it is demonstrated that a CO_2 absorber in a specific system does not significantly affect spirometry results from both normals and subjects with lung disease and prolonged expirations, CO_2 absorbers should be removed or bypassed during spirometry (see Controversies).

Performance Standards for Spirometers and Recommended Test Signals

The performance standards suggested are essentially those recommended by the ATS task force at the Snowbird Workshop (14).

1. Vital capacity (VC) The spirometer should have a volume range of at least 7.0 liters, and its output should be within 3% or 50 ml of the input, whichever is greater, when gas is injected into the system at any rate between 0.2 and 12 liters/sec. It should be able to accumulate volume for at least 30 seconds. The test signal will be a calibrated syringe with a volume of at least 3 liters.

2. Forced vital capacity (FVC) The standards for performance are identical, except that the instrument must be capable of accumulating volume for only 10 seconds.

3. Forced expiratory volume, timed (FEV_t) The standards for volume range, linearity, and time of accumulating air are identical to those for the FVC. In addition, the resistance to airflow should be less than 1.5 cm H_2O/liter/sec at a flow rate of 12.0 liters/sec. Although the ATS task force proposed that the test signals should be simulated "exponential" volume-time curves, one with an FVC of 5 liters and a time constant of 0.4 second, and one with an FVC of 3.5 liters and a time constant of 2.4 seconds, devices that generate these curves are not widely available. An acceptable alternate test is to measure the frequency response of the spirometer to a sinusoidally varying input of more than 1 liter. If it is flat to 4 Hz. then the spirometer is adequate for measuring timed forced expiratory volumes. Flow generators capable of delivering 12.0 liter/sec and sinusoidal pumps are not available in most community hospitals. Until calibration devices are available at reasonable cost, most laboratories will have to rely on the manufacturer's test results or on those of independent agencies for the comprehensive evaluation of dynamic performance.

4. Mean forced expiratory flow during the middle half of the FVC ($FEF_{25-75\%}$) and instantaneous forced expiratory flow (e.g., $FEF_{50\%}$) may be measured electronically or graphically. Flow should be measured to within $\pm 5\%$ or ± 0.2 liter/sec (whichever is greater) of reference calibrating flow rates over the range

from 0 to 12 liter/sec. Instruments that measure volume as the primary signal can be tested by drawing air from the spirometer at a constant rate, using a negative pressure source (e.g., a vacuum cleaner), and displaying the change in volume over time simultaneously with the signal for flow. The flow calculated from the volume-time curve should correspond to the amplitude of the flow signal. Alternatively, flows can be generated through a rotameter using a positive pressure source or using a syringe that delivers flows at known rates. In devices that integrate the signal from a flow transducer to measure volume, the system can be tested by injecting air from a calibrated syringe at different rates (e.g., over 0.5, 3, and 10 seconds). The volume signal produced by the integrator should be accurate to within 3% or 50 ml, whichever is greater.

5. Maximum voluntary ventilation (MVV) The MVV may be measured by an open circuit method or by a spirometer that has low resistance and inertance. The open circuit method and the requirements for its performance are described in the Epidemiology Standardization Project (15). The closed circuit method employs a spirometer that should be accurate to within 5% when driven by a sinusoidal pump at up to 250 liters/min with a maximum stroke volume of 2 liters (14). The resistance and inertance of the system should be low enough so that pressure within the spirometer is less than 10 cm H_2O at a stroke volume of 2 liter at 2 Hz (14). These standards will be met by most spirometers that meet the standards for measurement of timed forced expiratory volume.

For diagnostic spirometry, flow-volume curves, and maximal voluntary ventilation, a graphic record is required. A permanent tracing is not required if spirometry is done for screening purposes only or for follow-up studies in patients who have already had diagnostic spirometry. If a paper record is made, the paper speed should be at least 2 cm/sec. Volume sensitivity should be at least 10 mm of chart per liter of volume. Flow sensitivity should be at least 4 mm/liter/sec of flow (14).

QUALITY CONTROL

In the initial evaluation of equipment, its response to the test signals already described should be measured for each of the tests for which the device is to be used. Volume calibration by injection of a known quantity of air from a 3.0-liter syringe over the entire range for which measurements are made clinically should be performed at least once a week, but preferably daily. An electrical calibration signal may be used for daily calibration, but its use does not eliminate the need for periodically calibrating with a known volume of air. Flow calibration (previously described as the test signal for measuring flow) should be done (at a minimum) quarterly.

Recording paper speed should be tested periodically (e.g., quarterly or whenever measurement errors are suspected). Paper speed can be tested by closing a half-filled spirometer and pressing slightly on the bell at a 10-second interval timed with a stop watch (15). For practical purposes, this test should detect problems with paper speed, although it is possible to miss compensating fluctuations in paper speed during the 10-second interval.

As a simple means of confirming the accuracy of equipment initially, many laboratories perform tests in 10 or 20 healthy individuals, checking that the measured values fall within the predicted ranges. After this initial validation, some laboratories find it useful to measure the forced vital capacity and maximal expiratory flow in the same healthy individuals every morning before diagnostic studies are performed. The values for FEV_1 and FVC in normal subjects should vary by less than 5% from day to day (16).

PROCEDURE

After the procedure has been explained in simple terms, the subject should be instructed to loosen any tight clothing (especially collar, necktie, or brassiere). For adults, the test may be performed with the subject seated or standing; children should be studied while standing. The mouthpiece should be positioned, so that the subject's chin is slightly elevated and the neck extended. Noseclips should be applied and are required if tidal respirations and the maximal inspiratory effort are to be recorded on a closed circuit system immediately before the FVC maneuver is performed. After the mouthpiece is inserted, a check should be made to ensure that no leaks are present (it may be necessary to remove dentures). The subject then takes a full inspiration from a normal breathing pattern and exhales as rapidly, forcefully, and completely as possible. The recording paper should be turned to its appropriate speed 1 or 2 seconds prior to the beginning of forced expiration, so that it has reached a constant speed before recording the maneuver.

The performance of the maneuver should be evaluated by inspecting the graphic output, and the patient should be re-instructed, if necessary. Three acceptable tracings should be obtained in which the effort appears maximal, starts without hesitation, is sustained for 6 seconds, and is free of cough. In nonobstructed subjects who exert a maximal effort, the volume–time tracing will approach the horizontal asymptotically. In many patients with severe obstructive lung disease, however, the volume–time tracing does not plateau, and expiration can continue for 20 seconds or longer. In such cases, there is no consensus as to how long the FVC maneuver should be. Prolonged FVC efforts run the risk of syncopal episodes. It seems reasonable to stop the FVC maneuver after 10 seconds, unless terminated earlier because of dsypnea or lightheadedness of the subject, or observation of flow rates less than 0.05 liter/sec over at least a 0.5-second interval.

If measurements of tidal volume, expiratory reserve volume, and inspiratory vital capacity are desired, the subject should be seated and the mouthpiece inserted as just described. A period of quiet breathing is maintained until a constant end-tidal point is reached for three consecutive breaths. The subject is then instructed to exhale slowly and maximally. When expiration is maximal, that is, when residual volume (RV) has been reached, the subject is told to breathe in as deeply as possible [to total lung capacity (TLC)]. Forced expiration can be initiated from this point.

In the procedure for the flow-volume curve, the instructions to the subject, his posture, and the performance of the test are similar to those for the forced vital capacity. After a brief period of quiet breathing, the subject is instructed to inhale as rapidly and as forcefully as possible to TLC, to hold the inspiratory effort at TLC for 1 or 2 seconds, then to exhale as rapidly, forcefully, and completely as possible. As RV is reached (shown by the gradual decrease in expiratory flow rates toward zero), the subject is again instructed to inhale rapidly to TLC and to repeat the maneuver. If the instrument provides a continuous record, the reproducibility of the efforts can be verified by showing that the points of maximal inspiration (TLC) and maximal expiration (RV) are identical in the two efforts, and the expiratory portions of the curve are superimposable. Submaximal effort is suggested by reduction of flow rates at high lung volumes, flattening of the expiratory portion of the curve, and poor reproducibility. In such cases, maximal expiratory flow may be estimated by having the subject initiate a series of coughs from TLC (6).

To measure maximum voluntary ventilation, the subject is instructed to breathe the maximal possible amount of air over a 15- to 20-second interval, choosing his or her own rate. The observer should demonstrate the maneuver, and the subject should be permitted to perform practice runs for a brief period, in order to become familiar with the procedure. The respiratory frequency used in performing the MVV should be noted and the value recorded in a subscript, e.g., MVV_{90} or MVV_{110}. Most subjects achieve maximum levels at between 70 and 120 breaths/min; the choice of respiratory frequency does not greatly affect the result (15). The maximum ventilation over any 12 consecutive seconds of the maneuver is converted to BTPS and is expressed in liter/min. The highest value achieved in at least two runs, separated by a brief rest period, is reported.

CALCULATIONS

A consensus has not yet been reached on the issue of how to select spirometric data for report. It appears acceptable to report the largest FEV_1 and largest FVC from three acceptable tracings, even if the values do not come from the same curve ("maximal" data) (14, 15, 17, 18). It was the intent of the ATS Snowbird workshop, however, to recommend that all other parameters such as $FEF_{25-75\%}$ and $V_{max50\%}$ be measured from the "best test" FVC, defined as the maneuver that generated the largest sum of FVC and FEV_1 (14, and personal communication, Reed Gardner, June 1981). Recently, Sorensen et al. reexamined data obtained from 1101 subjects, 675 of whom showed varying degrees of expiratory obstruction, and found that the differences between "maximal" and "best test" values for FVC and FEV_1 were clinically insignificant (18). Therefore, in the interests of convenience and consistency, we recommend that when the FEV_1 is available, all flow measurements be made from the maneuver that meets the ATS "best test" criteria. Unfortunately, with many of the currently available flow-volume systems, FEV_1 is difficult, if not impossible, to obtain. Until this issue is resolved, in those cases in which FEV_1 is not obtainable, we recommend:

1. The FVCs of the curves considered for selection must be within 5% of the maximal FVC observed.
2. The maximal inspiratory volumes should be assumed to be identical, and the flow-volume loops should be considered to be superimposed at TLC; the volume intervals for maximal flow points (e.g., $FEF_{50\%}$) should be taken from the largest observed FVC (15, 41).
3. All data should be reported from the curve with the largest sum of FVC (in liters) and $FEF_{50\%}$ (in liter/sec), or from the curve with the largest FVC that appears to have been made with maximal effort.

Additional discussion is found in Controversies.

Calculations of flow are performed according to the recommendations of the American Thoracic Society (14). For timed maneuvers, the point at which exhalation is assumed to have begun (zero time) is determined by drawing a tangent to the steep, initial portion of the tracing and extrapolating it backward to the point of intersection with the maximal inspiratory line (Fig. 1). To achieve accurate zero time, the extrapolated volume should be less than 10% of the FVC or 100 ml, whichever is greater. Computer-determined extrapolation gives similar values for timed expired volumes. Other methods of estimating zero time, used primarily by electronic spirometers, include determining the point at which 30 ml have been expired, expiratory flow exceeds 0.1 liter/sec, or 200 ml have been expired. All methods give values significantly different from the extrapolation technique, but only the final method—using zero time as the moment when 200 ml are expired—gives values so different as to be of clinical importance (19).

Forced vital capacity, timed forced expiratory volume, and mean forced expiratory flow during the middle half of the vital capacity ($FEF_{25-75\%}$) are calculated as defined by the ATS Snowbird Workshop (14). All volumes should be corrected to BTPS. In expressing maximal flow, it should be remembered that

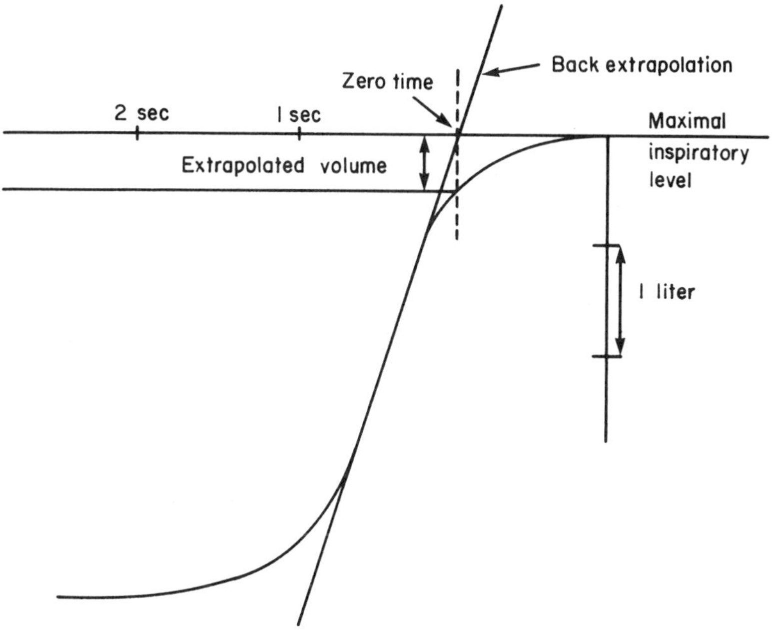

Fig. 1 *Backward extrapolation method for determining zero time for calculation of forced expiratory volume, one second (FEV_1). Zero time is determined by the intersection of a straight line drawn tangentially to the steepest portion of the spirogram and of a line drawn horizontally from the maximum inspiratory level. (Used with permission from ATS Statement, Snowbird Workshop on Standardization of Spirometry,* Amer Rev Respir Dis *119:831–838, 1979.)*

the subscript for FEF_x refers to the amount of the *vital capacity* that has already been exhaled, whereas the subscript for $\dot{V}_{max}$ refers to the percentage of total lung capacity *remaining* when the measurement is made (20).

Measurements made from the flow-volume curve include vital capacity, maximum expiratory flow rate (FEF_{max}), and flow at particular lung volumes (e.g., $FEF_{50\%}$). Failure of the subject to exhale completely to RV will spuriously elevate the flows measured at fixed percentages of the vital capacity. If the apparatus is equipped with a timing device, the volume expired is 1 second can also be determined.

NORMAL VALUES

Normal values for forced expiratory flow and spirometric measurements, related to the subject's age, height, and sex have been provided by studies of large numbers of subjects without symptoms of lung disease (21–34). The considerable differences between some of the reported normal values may partly reflect technical differences in the equipment and methods of measurement but may also be due to real differences in the study of populations. In the absence of any generally accepted prediction standards, each laboratory must review the published data and regression equations, selecting those that appear most applicable to its methodology and patient population.

Many of the older studies of normal spirometry made only limited efforts to exclude subjects with mild chronic respiratory disease and included smokers in the "healthy population." Several more recent investigations have studied only nonsmokers who have been carefully screened by questionnaire, physical examination, and chest radiograph. The exclusion of smokers from the normal population makes good medical sense because of the well-documented adverse effects of cigarette smoking on the spirometric indices, but it does have the unfortunate statistical effect of introducing a major bias into the selection of the normal study population. Apart from the theoretical considerations of whether those who have abstained from smoking may differ from the general population in other important biological characteristics, the nonsmoking group is clearly deficient in older males. Thus, men over 35 years made up only 133 (4.4%) of the 3046 subjects studied by Schoenberg and co-workers (21) and men over 39 only 72 (9.7%) of the 746 subjects of Knudson and associates (22). The nonsmokers studied by Morris and his colleagues (23) show a more balanced age distribution but still include only 26 men over age 64 out of a total of 517 adult males.

It has clearly been shown that regression equations derived from persons of European origin do not accurately predict the average spirometric indices of blacks (21) or of Asiatics (24). Of the recent studies summarized here, only that of Schoenberg and co-workers (21) give separate prediction equations for blacks and for whites, and it is unknown which set of equations would better predict the normal spirometric indices of Americans of Asiatic or native American extraction. The whole question is further complicated by the fact that many Americans who are classified as "black" may be genetically of predominantly European extraction. Nevertheless, the different prediction equations for blacks and for whites do seem to reflect real biological differences in the relationship between height and lung size, and their use, therefore, does seem justifiable.

Differences in methodology may also contribute to some of the reported differences between studies of normal spirometric values. The Snowbird Workshop reported that, in general, flow-measuring devices performed less accurately than volume-measuring devices, and, therefore, laboratories that use conventional water-filled or wedge spirometers might give careful consideration before using normal data derived from pneumotachography (25).

None of the published normal series has conformed to the recommendations of the Snowbird Workshop for selection of the best trials in reporting spirometric values (14). If values such as the $FEF_{50\%}$ or the $FEF_{25-75\%}$ are taken from expirations with a low FVC because of incomplete expirations, the value obtained will be falsely elevated. Knudson and associates (26) have suggested that this phenomenon may account for their failure to demonstrate an increase in concavity of the descending limb of the flow-volume loop in older normal subjects in their study of the normal maximal expiratory flow-volume curve (22). It is not clear in the studies that analyzed data from the best of two or three trials whether they took the value of FVC, FEV_1, and $FEF_{25-75\%}$ from the best single trial, or whether they took each value from the expiration showing the highest value for the spirometric index. Those laboratories changing their procedure to conform to the recent recommendations of the Snowbird Workshop must remember that the predicted values they are using may not be strictly applicable.

Another important difference between the currently recommended standards and the methods used in some studies of normal subjects has to do with the calculation of zero time on the spirographic tracing. The Veterans Administration-Army cooperative study (27) and the study conducted by Morris and co-workers (23) both defined zero time as the moment at which 200 ml had been exhaled. This method provided significantly different values for FEV_1 and FVC than the extrapolation technique recommended by the ATS (14).

Most of the published studies give prediction equations only for the mean values of the spirometric indices. They may report standard deviation or some other estimate of the population variance, but this is of limited use in predicting the lower limit of normal values, which is the number most often desired for clinical purposes. A single value for the standard deviation of the whole population will tend to give too low an estimate of the lower limit of normal values for small subjects whose predicted mean values are below the average. A more serious objection is that spirometric indices tend to have a nonnormal distribution skewed toward high values. If the population is asymmetrically distributed about the mean value, too low an estimate of the lower limit of normal values is given if 1.65 SD is subtracted from the predicted mean. Three of the cited studies (21, 22, 35) have addressed this problem and provide estimates of the lower limit of normal values in addition to the predicted mean values.

Finally, in order to simplify calculations, most of the published studies give multiple linear regression equations relating spirometric indices to sex, age, and height, though it is recognized that the regressions may actually be curvilinear. As computers are increasingly acquired, more laboratories will be easily able to use nonlinear regression formulas, and it will become practical to include other variables, such as body weight, in the equations. Of the recent studies cited, only that of Schoenberg and co-workers (21) provides nonlinear regression equations.

Recommended Equations

At present, there are no universally accepted prediction equations for spirometric indices, and all of the published studies suffer from at least some shortcomings. No study, for example, has provided equations for all of the

Table 1 *Comparison of Some Recent Studies of Normal Spirometric Values*

	Morris et al. (23,34)	Schmidt et al. (31)	Dickman et al. (32)	Bass (28)	Cherniak and Raber (29)	Knudson et al. (22)	Schoenberg et al. (21)
Age range	20–84	55–94	18+	21–71+	15–79	8–90	7–65+
Number of subjects							
adult male	471	295	604	149	782	128	256
adult female	517	237	134	98	382	321	569
male, <20 yr	0	0	0	0	88	163	1073
female, <20 yr	0	0	0	0	70	134	1148
Smokers included?	No	Yes	Yes	No	No	No	No[a]
Equipment	SWS[b]	CS[c]	CS[c]	WS[d]	WS[e]	PT[f]	PT[f]
Number of trials	best of 2	best of 2	best of 3	best of 2	best of 3	avg. best 2 of 5	avg. best 2 of 5
Separate predictions for blacks?	No	No	No	No	No	No	Yes
Nonlinear regression equations?	No	No	No	No	No	No	Yes

Estimate of lower limit of normal values?	No	No	No	No	No	Yes	Yes
Spirometric Indices Reported							
FVC	X	X	X	X	X	X	X
FEV_1	X	X	X		X	X	X
FEV_1/FVC	X	X				X	X
FEV_2						X	
FEV_3						X	
PEF				X	X	X	X
$FEF_{25\%}$				X	X	X	
$FEF_{50\%}$				X	X	X	X
$FEF_{75\%}$				X	X	X	X
$FEF_{25-75\%}$	X	X	X		X	X	
$FEF_{0.2-1.2}$	X	X	X				

[a] Except for black males.
[b] Stead-Wells spirometer.
[c] Online data acquisition, using a 13.5-liter Collins spirometer.
[d] Wedge spirometer.
[e] Online data acquisition, using a wedge spirometer.
[f] Online data acquisition, using a pneumotachograph.

Table 2 *Prediction Equations*

Parameter	Sex	Equations (adults)				Reference
FVC	M	0.0583H[a]	− 0.025A[b]	− 4.241		23
	F	0.0453H	− 0.024A	− 2.852		23
FEV_1	M	0.0362H	− 0.032A	− 1.26		23
	F	0.035H	− 0.025A	− 1.932		23
$FEV_1/FVC\%$	M	−0.123H	− 0.242A	+ 107.1		34
	F		− 0.179A	+ 84.23		34
FEF_{max}	M	0.094H	− 0.035A	− 5.993		22
	F	0.049H	− 0.025A	− 0.735		22
$FEF_{50\%}$	M	−0.042H	− 0.038A	+ 2.35S[c]	+ 9.45	28
	F		− 0.029A		+ 5.37	28
$FEF_{75\%}$	M		− 0.024A	+ 0.613S	+ 1.61	28
	F		− 0.023A		+ 2.59	28
$FEF_{25-75\%}$	M	0.0185H	− 0.045A	+ 2.513		23
	F	0.0236H	− 0.030A	+ 0.551		23
$FIF_{50\%}$	M	−0.026A	+ 6.28			28
	F	−0.020A	+ 1.07S	+ 2.78		28
MVV	M	−1.42A	+ 0.79H	+ 76		33
	F	−0.77A	+ 138			33
		Equations (children)				
FVC	M (<25 yr)	0.078A	+ 0.05H	− 5.508		22
	F (<20 yr)	0.092A	+ 0.033H	− 3.469		22
FEV_1	M	0.045A	+ 0.046H	− 4.808		22
	F	0.085A	+ 0.027H	− 2.703		22
FEV_1/FVC		Same equation as adults				22
PEF	M	0.166A	+ 0.078H	− 8.060		22
	F	0.157A	+ 0.049H	− 3.916		22
$FEF_{50\%}$	M	0.081A	+ 0.051H	− 4.975		22
	F	0.120A	+ 0.034H	− 2.531		22
$FEF_{75\%}$	M		+ 0.032H	− 2.455		22
	F	0.139A		+ 0.692		22
$FEF_{25-75\%}$	M		+ 0.059H	− 5.334		22
	F	0.121A	+ 0.025H	− 1.893		22

[a] H is height in centimeters.
[b] A is age in years.
[c] Body surface area in square meters.

commonly used spirometric values (see Table 1). The following recommendations must therefore be considered tentative, but they are offered with the hope that they may be useful to laboratory directors purchasing new equipment or considering a change of the equations they are currently using.

For those with computers capable of performing the calculations, the equations of Schoenberg and co-workers (21) probably provide the most satisfactory predictions for the mean and lower limits of normal values for FVC, FEV_1, FEV_1/FVC, FEF_{max}, $FEF_{50\%}$, and $FEF_{25\%}$. Separate equations are given for adults and children, for males and females, and for blacks and whites.

For those preferring linear equations, several formulas are acceptable (see Table 2). For adults, the data of Morris and co-workers (23) are the most generally used in this country, but there are several other satisfactory studies. The equations of Knudson and associates (22) are suggested for FEF_{max}, but not for $FEF_{50\%}$ or $FEF_{75\%}$ since evaluation in a number of laboratories has suggested that the Knudson predicted values for $FEF_{50\%}$ and $FEF_{75\%}$ are higher than those seen in most normal subjects. For these parameters, the equations of Bass (28) are suggested, in spite of the relatively small number of subjects in that study. For children, the prediction equations of Polgar and Promadhat (30) are probably the most generally used; these equations were derived from data pooled from several different studies. While this might be a good way to determine average predicted values, especially if the number of subjects in the individual studies is small, the estimate of variance of the pooled data will necessarily be biased by the variance of the study with the highest experimental error. The large coefficients of variation (the coefficient of variation equals the standard deviation divided by the mean) probably reflect the difficulty in getting good cooperation from younger subjects, as Polgar and Promadhat (30) point out in their interesting monograph. Since an overestimate of the variance will give too low an estimate of the lower limit of normal values, the equations of Knudson and associates (22) may be preferable.

EXPECTED REPRODUCIBILITY

Small changes in FVC, FEV_1, or maximal expiratory flow may be found in the same subject studied repeatedly on the same day or on consecutive days. When multiple measurements are made, the variability of the data can be expressed as the coefficient of variation. The variability of tests obtained at the same time of day on several consecutive days is no less than that of tests obtained throughout a day (22), suggesting that diurnal variation in maximal flow does not occur. In a direct study of diurnal variation, Hruby and Butler found no significant pattern of change in vital capacity or FEV_1 from 8 AM to 6 PM (16). The maximal range of values for vital capacity and FEV_1 in normal subjects was from 6% above to 4% below and from 11% above to 10% below their respective means. Patients with obstructive lung disease showed greater variability than normal subjects.

Using a Fleisch pneumotachograph system and online computerized data acquisition, Nickerson et al. studied the variability of spirometric measurements in 15 normal subjects, ages 8–34 years, and 15 subjects with cystic fibrosis, ages

7-36 years, who underwent a 10-minute period of "extensive training" in the art of spirometric performance (36). The within-subject coefficients of variations (SD/mean × 100) were as follows:

	VC	FEV_1	FEF_{max}	$FEF_{25-75\%}$	$FEF_{50\%}$	$FEF_{75\%}$
Normals	3.5	3.6	5.8	5.5	6.1	8.4
Patients	6.0	5.3	6.6	9.3	10.1	11.3

TROUBLESHOOTING

The most common source of error in tests of maximal expiratory flow is inadequate patient cooperation, as evidenced by the poor reproducibility of forced vital capacity. It is easily recognized by analyzing consecutive flow-volume curves. In normal subjects, the flow-volume envelope should be highly reproducibile, so that consecutive curves are superimposable. In patients with hyperreactive airways, however, inhalation to TLC may trigger bronchoconstriction, so that maximal flow on the first effort may be greater than on all subsequent efforts (37).

Spuriously low values may be caused by leakage at the mouthpiece (especially in patients wearing dentures) or at any point in the tubing or apparatus. Leaks are easily detected on consecutive flow-volume curves, because the TLC point shifts to progressively smaller (inspiratory leak) or larger (expiratory leak) values.

Other causes of erroneous values vary with the particular device being used. With conventional water spirometers, errors may result from insufficient water, a cracked or perforated bell, leaks in the tubing or the thermometer, or a malfunction of the motor driving the kymograph. If apparently erroneous results cannot be explained by improper patient performance, the system should be checked with a calibrated syringe, or the test should be performed on one of the laboratory personnel whose values are known.

CONTROVERSIAL ISSUES

Selection of FVC Effort for Calculation of Volume-Related Maximal Expiratory Flow Rates

The Epidemiology Standardization Project (15) recommended that if flow rates are measured from a single curve, the curve selected should be that with the largest sum of FVC and FEV_1; if multiple curves are used, "it is assumed that the maximal inspiratory volume will be identical and the *largest* $\dot{V}_{max}$ values will be measured at volumes corresponding to 50 and 75% of the largest FVC." The first recommendation presents obvious problems for flow-volume systems that plot volume versus flow and from which FEV_1 cannot be measured. The problems inherent in the second recommendation were discussed by Knudson et al. (38), whose normal values were originally selected from a "composite" flow-volume curve that may yield larger values for maximal flow (39); they later redefined their normal population and adopted the ATS Snowbird Workshop criteria. This is consistent with the Intermountain manual recommendation that "it is more practical to choose one spirogram representing the patient's best effort and perform all calculations on that tracing, rather than mix computations made from different tracings. The best spirogram will be chosen from three reproducible recordings on the basis of a single tracing with the largest sum of FVC and FEV_1" (40).

None of the currently available published studies on normal values for spirometry have used the FVC + FEV_1 sum criteria for measurement; although it is unlikely that this would change the predicted values significantly, this issue awaits resolution. Another problem with these criteria is that none of the currently available computerized spirometer or flow-volume systems are programed to meet these criteria. Also, for laboratories utilizing manual systems, these calculations add to the time required for measurements.

Validity of BTPS Corrections

Almost all standardization reports and studies of normal values have utilized a BTPS correction of volumes and flows. However, there are theoretical reasons to question whether this is justifiable. Recent studies presented as abstracts have suggested that the BTPS correction may, indeed, not be valid (41, 42).

Reasons for Differences among Predicted Values for Maximal Flow Rates

Attempts to analyze flow at low lung volumes as a means for early detection of chronic airflow obstruction have been frustrated by the large variability of values obtained in normal subjects within a given population sample. The problem is compounded by the large differences between the *mean* values of the maximal expiratory flows at low lung volumes published by different groups (and differences between predicted values using regression equations derived from the data). These differences might be attributed to variations in equipment performance, small but crucial differences in calculation methods, or inherent differences between the populations sampled.

SIGNIFICANCE OF "NEGATIVE EFFORT DEPENDENCE"

In some patients, greater expiratory efforts result in a decrease in expired volume or, more commonly, in maximal expiratory flows. There are a number of unanswered questions related to this phenomenon: does a difference between the forced vital capacity and the vital capacity obtained with a relaxed effort imply effort-related closure of airways? If the difference is great, will reporting the FEV_1 as a percentage of the smaller, forced vital capacity underestimate the severity of obstructive lung disease, and should, therefore, a "slow" vital capacity always be measured before the forced vital capacity is obtained? Does maximal expiratory flow refer to the highest flow observed with any effort, or to the flow observed with maximal effort?

SHOULD INSPIRATORY VITAL CAPACITY BE MEASURED?

A related controversy has to do with the use of an inspiratory vital capacity (IVC). Some workers believe that problems caused by the forced vital capacity being smaller than the slow vital capacity can be avoided by recording flow and volume on an X-Y recorder while the patient first exhales to residual volume and then inhales to TLC, thereby providing the inspiratory vital capacity. The subsequent maximal expiratory effort need be maintained only until 80% of the vital capacity has been exhaled for the $FEF_{75\%}$, $FEF_{50\%}$, and $FEF_{25\%}$ to be determined. This method of performing the forced expiratory maneuver offers the advantage of simplified computer calculations of volume-specific flow rates (only the IVC needs to be stored in the memory rather than the entire expiratory curve). It also would eliminate the need for prolonged forced expiratory vital capacity maneuvers in patients with markedly reduced flow rates during the expiration of the last 20% of the vital capacity. However, it is not a methodology recommended by any of the standardization efforts (14, 15, 39) or followed by any of the commonly used studies of normal values (21–24, 27–29).

DURATION OF EXPIRATORY EFFORT

There also appears to be disagreement over the duration of the maximal expiratory effort, which the ATS statement (14) did not specify. It did, however, specify that for the measurement of the FVC, the spirometer should be capable of accumulating volume for 10 seconds. The "end of test" is said to occur when the average flow over 0.5 second is less than 25 ml. This recommendation was based on the observation that in 205 miners with FEV_1/FVC less than 70%, these end of test criteria (flow less than 0.05 liter/sec) were met by 94% of the subjects. In the Epidemiology Standardization Project, however, it was noted that in 100 consecutive spirograms of *patients* with chronic obstructive lung disease (COPD) referred to a hospital laboratory, 18% did not meet the ATS end-of-test criteria within 10 seconds. It was concluded that although the 10-second minimum time may be appropriate for field studies, it may not be adequate for clinical laboratories (15). Prolongation of forced expiratory efforts beyond 10 seconds, however, runs the risk of syncopal episodes during testing.

Performance Standards for Spirometers

Although some have argued that spirometers used for screening, monitoring of therapy, or "office spirometry" need not meet the same stringent requirements as recommended by the Snowbird Workshop for "clinical, diagnostic, or epidemiologic purposes" (14), compelling arguments can be made that the former applications deserve the same standards of accuracy. Other unresolved questions include the following: What are the practical consequences of using a 13.5 liter water-sealed bell spirometer with a flat frequency response to only 2–4 cps? What are the consequences of using spirometers that do not continuously record volume versus time tracings for at least 10 seconds during a FVC maneuver? How does one decide if the errors caused by substandard equipment are severe enough to warrant the purchase of new and often costly equipment? What is required of devices used for bedside studies or for measuring tidal volume and vital capacity in an intubated patient who is being weaned from a respirator?

Impact of CO_2 Absorbers on Spirometry Results

Since a number of spirometers that are also used for helium dilution procedures have CO_2 absorbers built into the spirometry circuit, the absorbers cannot be easily bypassed during measurements of forced expiratory flow rates. In most studies that defined normal reference values, CO_2 absorbers were removed during spirometry. Neither the Snowbird Workshop (14) nor the Epidemiology Standardization Project (15) specifically made recommendations regarding CO_2 absorbers. The Intermountain manual recommends that unidirectional valves and CO_2 absorbers be removed during spirometry (39). It is important to emphasize that equipment must meet the performance standards defined by the ATS task force (14) in the configuration in which it is to be used in testing patients. It is also important to recognize that although the testing of spirometry with room air using syringes, sine wave pumps, or forced expiration simulators may effectively evaluate the impact of the added resistance of a CO_2 absorber, it will not detect the volume loss due to CO_2 absorption from the expired gas during clinical spirometry.

Accuracy Required when Flow Is the Primary Input

The ATS Snowbird Workshop recommended that a flow measuring device be capable of recording flow within ±0.2 liter/sec (or ±5% of the true reading, whichever is greater) over a range of 0–12 liters/sec. Some patients with severe obstructive lung disease may show expiratory flow rates of 0.2 liter/sec or less through most of their forced expiration; in such patients if volumes were derived by integration of the flow signal from a device which barely met the flow standards, the calculated measurements of volumes could be grossly inaccurate. The Snowbird standard for the accuracy of vital capacity measurements states that "the instrument should be capable of measuring volumes of at least 7 liters (BTPS) independent of flow rate for flows between 0 and 12 liters/sec. Accuracy required is at least ±3 percent of reading or ±50 ml., whichever is greater" (14). Although this recommendation implies that the assessment of accuracy of VC measurements should include evaluation at low flow rates, recommendations for testing at specific low flow rates were not made. For accurate measurements of VC in patients with severe obstruction using devices which integrate the flow signal, it is clear that much greater accuracy than ±0.2 liters/sec for flow rates may be required in order to meet the standards for volume measurements.

REFERENCES

1. Hutchinson J: On the capacity of the lungs and on the respiratory functions, with a view of establishing a precise and easy method of detecting disease by the spirometer. *Trans Med Chir Soc Lond* 29:137–252, 1846.
2. Mead J. Turner JM, Macklem PT, et al.: Significance of the relationship between lung recoil and maximal expiratory flow. *J Appl Physiol* 22:95–108, 1967.
3. Jones JG, Fraser RB, Nadel JA: Prediction of maximum expiratory flow rate from area-transmural pressure curve of compressed airway. *J Appl Physiol* 38:1002–1011, 1975.
4. Jones JG, Fraser RB, Nadel JA: Effect of changing airway mechanics on maximum expiratory flow. *J Appl Physiol* 38:1012–1021, 1975.
5. Gold WM: Asthma. *Basics RD* 4(3), 1976.
6. Hyatt RE, Black LF: The flow-volume curve; a current perspective *Am Rev Respir Dis* 107:191–199, 1973.
7. Miller RD, Hyatt RE: Evaluation of obstructing lesions of the trachea and larynx by flow-volume loops. *Am Rev Respir Dis* 108:475–481, 1973.
8. Gelb, AF, Zamel N: Simplified diagnosis of small airway obstruction. *N Engl J Med* 288:395–398, 1973.
9. Despas PJ, Leroux M, Macklem PT: Site of airway obstruction in asthma as determined by measuring maximal expiratory flow breathing air and a helium-oxygen mixture. *J Clin Invest* 51:3235–3243, 1972.
10. Gelb AF, Molony PA, Klein E, et al.: Sensitivity of volume of isoflow in the detection of mild airway obstruction. *Am Rev Respir Dis* 112:401–405, 1975.

11. Fitzgerald MX, Smith AA, Gaensler EA: Evaluation of "electronic" spirometers. *N Engl J Med* 289:1283-1288, 1973.
12. McCall CB, Hyatt RE, Nobel FW, et al.: Harmonic content of certain respiratory flow phenomena of normal individuals. *J Appl Physiol* 10:215-218, 1957.
13. Stead WS, Wells, HS, Gault NL, et al.: Inaccuracy of the conventional water-filled spirometer for recording rapid breathing. *J Appl Physiol;* 14:448-450, 1959.
14. Gardner, RM, Baker CD, Broennle AM Jr, et al.: ATS statement—Snowbird workshop on standardization of spirometry. *Am Rev Respir Dis* 119:831-838, 1979.
15. Ferris BG: Epidemiology standardization project. *Am Rev Respir Dis* 118:1-120, 1978.
16. Hruby J, Butler J: Variability of routine pulmonary function tests. *Thorax* 30:548-553, 1975.
17. Nathan SP, Lebowitz MD, Knudson RJ: Spirometric testing* number of tests required and selection of data. *Chest* 76:384-388, 1979.
18. Sorensen JB, Morris AH, Crapo RO, et al.: Selection of the best spirometric values for interpretation. *Am Rev Respir Dis* 122:802-805, 1980.
19. Smith AA, Gaensler EA: Timing of forced expiratory volume in one second. *Am Rev Respir Dis* 112:882-885, 1975.
20. Pulmonary terms and symbols. Report of the ACCP-ATS Joint Committee on Pulmonary Nomenclature. *Chest* 67:583-593, 1975.
21. Schoenberg JB, Beck GJ, Bouhuys A: Growth and decay of pulmonary function in healthy blacks and whites. *Respir Physiol* 33:367-393, 1978.
22. Knudson RJ, Slatin RC, Lebowitz MD, et al.: The maximal expiratory flow-volume curve: Normal standards, variability and effects of age. *Am Rev Respir Dis* 113:587-600, 1976.
23. Morris JF, Koski A, Johnson LC: Spirometric standards for healthy nonsmoking adults. *Am Rev Respir Dis* 103:57-67, 1971.
24. DaCosta JL: Pulmonary function studies in healthy Chinese adults in Singapore. *Am Rev Respir Dis* 104:128-131, 1971.
25. Gardner RM, Hankinson JL, West BJ: Testing spirometers—ATS standards. *ATS News* 3:24-25, 1977.
26. Knudson RJ, Clark DF, Kennedy TC, et al.: Effect of aging alone on mechanical properties of the normal adult human lung. *J Appl Physiol* 43:1054-1062, 1977.
27. Kory RC, Callahan R, Boren H, et al.: The Veterans Administration-Army cooperative study of pulmonary function. I. Clinical spirometry in normal man. *Am J Med* 30:243-258, 1961.
28. Bass H: The flow volume loop: Normal standards and abnormalities in chronic obstructive pulmonary disease. *Chest* 63:171-176, 1973.
29. Cherniack RM, Raber MB: Normal standards for ventilatory function using an automated wedge spirometer. *Am Rev Respir Dis* 106:38-46, 1972.
30. Polgar G, Promadhat V: *Pulmonary Function Testing in Children; Techniques and Standards.* Philadelphia, WB Saunders Co, 1971.
31. Schmidt CD, Dickman ML, Gardner RM, et al.: Spirometric standards for healthy elderly men and women. *Am Rev Respir Dis* 108:933-939, 1973.
32. Dickman ML, Schmidt CD, Gardner RM, et al.: On-line computerized spirometry in 738 normal adults. *Am Rev Respir Dis* 100:780-790, 1969.
33. Grimby G, Soderholm B: Spirometric studies in normal subjects: III. Static lung volumes and maximum voluntary ventilation in adults with a note on physical fitness. *Acta Med Scand* 173:199-206, 1963.
34. Morris JF, Temple WP, Koski A: Normal values for the ratio of one-second forced expiratory volume to forced vital capacity. *Am Rev Respir Dis* 108:1000-1003, 1973.
35. Knudson RJ, Lebowitz MD: Maximal mid-expiratory flow ($FEF_{25-75\%}$): Normal limits and assessment of sensitivity. *Am Rev Respir Dis* 117:609-610, 1978.

36. Nickerson BG, Lemen RJ, Gerdes CB, et al.: Within-subject variability and percent change for significance of spirometry in normal subjects and in patients with cystic fibrosis. *Am Rev Respir Dis* 122:859–866, 1980.
37. Gayrard P, Orehek J, Grimaud C, et al.: Bronchoconstrictor effects of a deep inspiration in patients with asthma. *Am Rev Respir Dis* 111:433–439, 1975.
38. Knudson RJ, Slatin RC, Lebowitz MD, et al.: Response to letter of RB Douglas. The maximal expiratory flow-volume curve, normal standards, variability, and effects of age. *Am Rev Respir Dis* 122:990–991, 1980.
39. Peslin R, Bohadana A, Hannhart B, et al.: Comparison of various methods for reading maximal expiratory flow-volume curves. *Am Rev Respir Dis* 119:271–277, 1979.
40. Kanner RE, Morris AH (ed); *Clinical Pulmonary Function Testing.* Salt Lake City, Utah, Intermountain Thoracic Society, 1975.
41. Tashkin D, Patel A, Calvarese B, et al.: Over-estimation of forced expiratory volumes and flow rates measured by volumetric spirometry when ATPS to BTPS correction is applied. *Am Rev Respir Dis* 123:83, (abstract) 1981.
42. Perks WH, Sopwith T, Brown D, et al.: The effect of temperature on the vitalograph spirometer. (Abstract), *Am Rev Respir Dis* 123:124, 1981.

CHAPTER 8

Microprocessor-Assisted Spirometry

ARTHUR DAWSON, M.D.
JOHN G. MOHLER, M.D.

In the past few years, a number of computer-assisted spirometry systems have appeared on the market. They are already used in many small hospital laboratories, and their price is decreasing to the point where pulmonary physicians may begin to use them in office practice. Therefore, although it is difficult to do justice to this rapidly evolving field, we feel it would be unrealistic in a manual on technical aspects of lung function testing not to discuss special problems of standardization and quality in computerized systems. Most users of computers in the pulmonary laboratory will not wish to do their own programing or to modify the packaged software they receive with their system, but it is important for those performing and interpreting the tests to have sufficient understanding of their equipment to recognize its limitations.

Regardless of the specific hardware used, the computer performs two basic tasks. The first task is the input of a series of data points from the spirometer to the computer memory. This input represents instantaneous flow or volume at each discrete small interval of time after the point recognized as the beginning of test. The second task is "number crunching"—i.e., calculation of the various spirometric indices, determination of predicted values from regression equations, and output of the final report, according to the format determined by the program. Most of the problems peculiar to computerized spirometry occur in connection with the input portion of this process. In the pages that follow, we shall review some of the standards recommended by the Snowbird Workshop (1) and consider how they relate to the performance of computer-based systems.

RANGE AND ACCURACY

Obviously, no computer-based spirometry system can be more accurate than the spirometer on which it is based, but there are additional requirements so that no unacceptable loss of accuracy occurs in the course of data acquisition and processing. If a volume signal is the input, it should have a range of 7 liters and

PULMONARY FUNCTION TESTING
GUIDELINES AND CONTROVERSIES

ISBN 0-12-788125-5

an accuracy of ±50 ml. If each data point is converted by an analog-to-digital converter (ADC) to an 8-bit binary "word" and 7 liters is equivalent to the maximum output of the ADC ($2^8 - 1$ or 255), then the resolution of the ADC is 7000/255 or about 27 ml. If the output voltage of the spirometer and the voltage range of the ADC are not optimally matched, the resolution will be correspondingly poorer. For a flow signal the recommended range is 12 liters/sec and the accuracy 0.2 liter/sec. If an 8-bit ADC has an output of 255 for a flow input of 12 liters/sec, then its resolution will be 12/255 or about 0.05 liter/sec. If both positive and negative flows are to be sensed and the maximum positive output of +127 is given for a flow of +12 liters/sec, then the resolution will be 12/127 or about 0.09 liter/sec. The resolution should be sufficient to detect a change of half the recommended accuracy, and, therefore, the performance of an optimally matched spirometer and 8-bit ADC would be adequate, but barely adequate, to meet the Snowbird standard. The accuracy would be improved by using an ADC with greater resolution (e.g., a 10-bit or a 12-bit ADC) (2).

The accuracy of a computerized spirometry test is also affected by the sampling rate of the ADC. If a series of instantaneous flow measurements is integrated to calculate volume, the instantaneous value is assumed to be the average flow over the time interval between conversions. If the cost of the system were no consideration, one would simply accumulate data at the maximum conversion rate of the ADC and store the information in memory, so that the calculations would be done after completion of the forced expiration or other respiratory maneuver. If each conversion required 2 bytes of memory and conversions were made at 100 Hz for a 15-second test, then a single forced expiration would occupy 3000 (3K) bytes. This would present no difficulty for systems with 8K or more of memory but might add excessively to the cost of a small dedicated system. If the sampling rate can be reduced without unacceptable loss of accuracy, there is not only the advantage of reduced memory requirements, but there may also be time for the microprocessor to perform additional tasks between data-point conversions. For example, the accumulated expired volume could be displayed to tell the operator whether expiratory effort should be continued, or a flow–volume trace could be shown on the cathode-ray tube (CRT) as it is generated. A compromise solution is to accumulate data rapidly during the initial part of a forced expiration while flow is changing rapidly, and then to slow the sampling rate for the remainder of the test. For example, if each conversion requires 2 bytes of memory and data are accumulated at 100 Hz for 1 second and at 20 Hz for the remaining 14 seconds, the memory requirement would decrease from 3000 to 760 bytes, and the 50 msec between conversions would allow ample time for the microprocessor to calculate and display results in "real time."

A word of caution is appropriate concerning measurements of the $FEF_{25-75\%}$. If the sampling rate is slowed during the terminal portion of the forced expiration in order to save memory, the resolution may be inadequate, since the slope of the line drawn from 25% to 75% of the forced vital capacity (FVC) is affected by the value of each point. A similar problem exists if measurements of instantaneous flow during the terminal part of the expiration are reported. If computerized spirometry is to be used to detect small airways disease, the sampling rate must be adequate during the entire expiration.

DURATION OF EXPIRATION

The Snowbird Workshop recommended that a spirometer be capable of accumulating volume for at least 30 seconds for measurement of vital capacity and 10 seconds for forced vital capacity (1). This should present no problem for a computerized spirometry system, except for the amount of memory required to store individual flow data points if volume is obtained by integration after completion of the expiratory maneuver. The user should be sure that his system meets this standard.

IDENTIFICATION OF START OF TEST

It is recommended that the "start of test" (the point from which zero time is measured) be determined by back-extrapolation of the volume versus time curve, or by a method shown to be equivalent (1). This implies that all data points from the initial part of the forced expiration must be stored until the completion of the breath, in order that the back-extrapolation can be done. In most published descriptions of the back-extrapolation method, an "eyeball" or pattern-recognition approach is used by the operator to fit a tangent to the steepest portion of the curve. One method that has been proposed for computer analysis is to store the volume expired at 100-msec intervals. The slope of the interval with the greatest volume change is extrapolated back to zero volume expired. Results from this method have been found to be almost identical to results obtained by manual back-extrapolation (3).

IDENTIFICATION OF END OF TEST

The Snowbird Workshop recommended that the accumulation of expiratory volume or flow data be terminated when the average flow over an interval of 0.5 second is less than 50 ml/sec or when the volume change in a 0.5-second interval is less than 25 ml. The computer can accomplish this in two ways. It can store all data points until recognition of a critical inspiratory flow value indicates that expiration certainly is completed, then calculate back point by point until it identifies a 0.5-second interval with less than the critical average flow or volume change. Alternatively, it can hold a half-second "window" (string of data points) and note the average flow or volume change, subtracting the "oldest" point in the window as each new data point is accumulated. The data accumulation is automatically terminated when the half-second score falls below a critical level. It might seem much simpler merely to terminate the test at the point at which the flow or volume signal changes sign. However, this will often result in premature shutoff of the test, especially in patients with severe airways obstruction. In the terminal portion of the forced expiration, very low flows may be maintained for several seconds, and there is considerable noise in the signal, which may result in a number of flow zero-crossings before the true end of expiration.

NEED FOR A GRAPHIC OUTPUT

If the computer system includes a printer with graphic capability, a "hard copy" report can be generated in either a volume–time or flow–volume format. Printers may be slow and noisy, however, and for purposes of quality control it is much preferable if a display can be provided on a CRT screen. It is often difficult to judge the adequacy of tbe patient's performance if the calculated data can only be viewed at the completion of each trial of the forced expiratory maneuver. If the computer system does not allow a convenient immediate display, we would recommend that the spirometer should be provided with an analog recording device (strip chart recorder, X–Y recorder, or oscilloscope), so that the results of each spirometric maneuver can be evaluated by the technician. Also, unless a hard copy report is to be printed after each trial, the computer should be able to store the data from all trials until completion of the test, in order that the best trial can be used in the final report.

NUMBER OF TRIALS

The Snowbird recommendations state that a minimum of three acceptable forced vital capacity maneuvers should be performed and that the best two should agree within 5% of reading or 100 ml, whichever is greater. If the computer can store the results of all trials, it can easily select the best trial (see the following) and cue the operator whether more trials are needed. Preferably, there should be capacity to store more than three trials. The final report should include a tabulation of the results of all trials, in order that the interpreter can be assured that an adequate number of trials has been done and can make some assessment of the patient's consistency of performance.

SELECTION OF THE FORCED EXPIRATION FROM WHICH TO CALCULATE DATA

Concerning which forced expiration to use for the calculation of flow parameters, the Snowbird Workshop suggested that "if the $FEF_{25-75\%}$ and/or instantaneous maximum expiratory flows ($\dot{V}$) are obtained from a single test, the test used will be the one with the largest sum of the FVC and $FEV_{1.0}$" (1). The FVC and FEV_1 should be taken from the trial giving the highest value, even if the two values do not come from the same curve. For the most part, currently available computerized spirometry packages do not satisfy this requirement. Appropriate changes in the software should be made in systems that can be altered.

MAXIMUM INSPIRATORY FLOW RATE

If inspiration is to be recorded as a continuation of the preceding forced expiration, additional storage capacity will be required in the computer memory. If the rate of sampling has been decreased during the latter part of the expiration, it should again be increased at the beginning of inspiration to equal the rate during the first part of expiration. If limitation of memory makes this impossible, slower rates are acceptable, because the pattern of the inspirogram is much less variable than the expirogram. The maximum forced inspiratory flow (FIF_{max}) can be computed from the steepest portion of the inspirogram. Rather than storing all data points, the computer can store a window of 10 data points, dropping the oldest as the next is sampled. The maximum value of the average slope over 10 points (100 msec) can be stored as the FIF_{max}. This has been shown to agree within acceptable error with other methods of calculation.

COMPUTERIZED INTERPRETATION OF SPIROMETRY

Using the calculated values, the computer can rapidly analyze the spirogram and generate a report concerning the presence and severity of expiratory obstruction, inspiratory obstruction, and restriction of the vital capacity while the patient is still present in the laboratory. First, the computer must be provided with a set of objective criteria for data analysis. It can then select a coherent interpretation from a library of sentences and paragraphs. This is much more useful to the clinician than a sentence statement referring to each reported value without regard to their overall meaning.

A BUYER'S CHECKLIST

Those considering the purchase of a computerized spirometry system may find it helpful to ask the following questions of the sales representative. Probably none of the currently available systems will meet all of these requirements, although they should do so in order to conform to the recommendations of the Snowbird Workshop.

1. What is the maximum value of volume or flow that can be accepted by the ADC? (They should be at least 7 liters and 12 liters/sec, respectively.)
2. What is the resolution of the ADC? (Divide the maximum accepted value by the largest positive number the ADC can output. Half of that value should be, at most, 50 ml for a volume signal and 0.2 liter/sec for a flow signal.)
3. What is the sampling rate of the ADC? (It should be at least 50 Hz for the first 1 second of the forced expiration if FEF_{max} is to be reported, and at least 15 Hz through the rest of the test.)
4. Can the computer accumulate data for at least 10 seconds for a forced expiration and 30 seconds for measurement of the vital capacity?
5. How is "start of test" identified? Is an acceptable method of back-extrapolation used?
6. How is "end of test" identified? Is flow or volume averaged over an interval of 0.5 seconds?
7. Is there a graphic output of volume versus time or flow versus volume, providing a hard copy for the permanent record?
8. Can the graphic tracing and numerical data be viewed after each trial in order to judge patient cooperation and consistency of performance?
9. Is there a means of cueing the operator that more trials are needed if the best two trials fail to agree within 5%?
10. Are the best trials selected according to the Snowbird recommendations? That is, are FVC and FEV_1 taken from the trial giving the highest value for those spirometric indices? Are the $FEF_{25-75\%}$ and $FEF_{50\%}$ taken from the trial with the best sum of FVC and FEV_1?

There are other questions not specifically related to the Snowbird recommendations which may be of importance to the individual user.

11. What is the input device? Is its accuracy acceptable? Can the system accept an input signal from a spirometer other than the one provided in the "package"?

12. What predicted values are used? Can they be changed if the user prefers another set of regression equations or if newly reported regression equations prove to be preferable to those in current use?

13. Can the software be changed if necessary? Is it possible to add new spirometric calculations to those included in the original package?

14. Are listing and documentation of the programs available? (Even carefully developed programs sometimes contain undetected bugs.)

One can confidently predict that over the next few years we shall be able to buy more computer power for fewer dollars. Perhaps we will see more systems in which the software can be readily changed to accommodate new developments and improvements in the clinical applications of spirometry. Much more complex and extensive predicted data will be included in the calculations, and statistical confidence limits will be reported routinely. Nonlinear regression equations may be used—including exponential and logarithmic terms and multiple input variables—in addition to the usual parameters of sex, age, and height. It will be possible to calculate more elaborate spirometric indices, such as moment analysis of the expired volume versus time curve or the area under the flow-volume curve. It remains to be demonstrated whether computerization will increase the clinical usefulness of spirometry, but it certainly can greatly speed up the calculations and, if properly used, improve the accuracy of the test.

REFERENCES

1. Gardner, RM, Baker CD, Broennle AM Jr, et al.: ATS statement—Snowbird workshop on standardization of spirometry. *Am Rev Respir Dis* 119:831-838, 1979.
2. Black KH, Petusevsky ML, Gaensler EA: A general purpose microprocessor for spirometry. *Chest* 78:605-612, 1980.
3. Smith AA, Gaensler EA: Timing of forced expiratory volume in one second. *Am Rev Respir Dis* 112:882-885, 1975.

CHAPTER 9

Pneumotachography

ARTHUR DAWSON, M.D.

A pneumotachograph is a device that measures instantaneous respiratory air flow. Pneumotachographs—such as the ultrasonic flowmeter and the hot wire anemometer—have been developed based on several different physical principles. By far the most commonly used type is the differential pressure flow transducer, in which a sensitive manometer detects the pressure drop across a slight resistance placed in the airstream.

Each type of pneumotachograph has its own technical problems that must be overcome if the output of the transducer is to reflect accurately the instantaneous flow of gas through it. The present discussion will be confined to the Fleisch pneumotachograph, which is widely used in clinical lung function testing. This device is simple in principle, but there are a number of factors, some of which are difficult to analyze, that can significantly affect its linearity and accuracy. These are discussed in some detail, because the information cannot readily be found in the standard works on clinical lung physiology.

PRINCIPLES OF OPERATION

In the Fleisch pneumotachograph, a small resistance to the airflow is provided by a bundle of parallel capillary tubes. The pressure drop across the resistance is measured by a sensitive differential manometer. The parallel small-diameter tubes tend to maintain laminar flow in the gas passing through the pneumotachograph. An electrical heating element keeps the temperature at 37°–38° C, to prevent condensation of expired water vapor in the capillary tubes which would change their resistance.

The pressure drop (ΔP) across the pneumotachograph is given by the Poiseuille equation

$$\Delta P = \dot{V}\eta\ 8l/\pi r^4,$$

where $\dot{V}$ is gas flow, l and r are the respective length and radius of the resistive elements, and η is gas viscosity.

PULMONARY FUNCTION TESTING
GUIDELINES AND CONTROVERSIES

ISBN 0-12-788125-5

This equation applies to each of the capillary tubes, and an actual calculation of the pressure drop would require treating them as a group of resistances in parallel. This linear relationship between flow and pressure difference holds only for laminar flow. At the onset of turbulence, a second term proportional to $\dot{V}^2$ appears and the relationship becomes curvilinear. The resistance to turbulent flow depends upon the density as well as the viscosity of the gas.

The critical flow ($\dot{V}_c$) above which turbulence occurs can be predicted by calculating Reynolds number:

$$N_R = 2sr\rho/\eta,$$

where ρ is gas density, and s is the linear velocity of flow. For a cylindrical tube,

$$s = \dot{V}/\pi\, r^2$$

and, therefore,

$$N_R = 2\dot{V}\rho/\pi r\eta$$

If N_C is the critical value of Reynolds number, by rearranging the above equation we obtain

$$\dot{V}_c = N_C\pi rn/2\rho$$

For gas flow in a long cylindrical tube, the theoretical critical value of Reynolds number is roughly 2000. At the maximum recommended flows, the various models of pneumotachograph heads give Reynolds numbers of less than 1000, but even with this margin of safety there is some departure from a linear relationship between pressure drop and flow (1, 2).

Six different-sized heads are available for the Fleisch pneumotachograph. These can be used in a wide variety of applications from small animal studies to the measurement of maximum respiratory flows in humans. With gases of greater density or lower viscosity than air, Reynolds number will be greater, and therefore the maximum flows must be appropriately reduced, or changes must be made in the design of the head to permit higher flows (3). By contrast, little departure from linearity is seen when flow is measured in gas mixtures containing a high fraction of helium, even at flows well above the maximum recommended for the pneumotachograph head. This is because the low density and high viscosity of helium results in a low Reynolds number.

CALIBRATION AND TESTS OF LINEARITY OF RESPONSE

Usually the manufacturer will provide information on the linearity of the instrument and on the maximum flow at which reasonable linearity can be assumed. It is possible to improve the linearity of the output, thereby extending the useful working range of flows by electrical attenuation of the pressure transducer output at higher flows. Alternatively, in microprocessor-based systems, the flows can be corrected by a mathematical expression that reproduces the empirical relationship between flow and pressure transducer output. It is important for the user to realize that such "built-in linearization" is valid only for the gas composition and geometric arrangement for which the system was designed. If the pneumotachograph is used to measure flow in a "home-made circuit" that alters the upstream geometry, the linearizing function may not be effective at higher flows, and, especially with helium-containing gas mixtures, it may actually magnify the error.

Changes in the upstream geometry alter the linearity of the pneumotachograph if they produce turbulent flow, as might occur with sudden changes in the diameter of tubing and connectors close to the resistance element. Even if there is no turbulence, the velocity profile of the moving gas may be changed, so that a greater or lesser proportion of the faster moving molecules is directed through the outer channels of the pneumotachograph, where the pressure drop is sensed. Problems with upstream geometry are minimal if the resistance element can be placed downstream from a straight cylindrical tube of the same diameter whose length is at least five times the diameter. In some clinical applications, this arrangement would produce an unacceptably large dead space. The purpose of the screen and truncated conical tubing provided with most commercial pneumotachographs is to improve linearity by manipulating the velocity profile and reducing turbulence while keeping the dead space small.

The calibration curve of the pneumotachograph under steady-flow conditions is easily measured. It requires a Tissot spirometer, a vacuum cleaner to provide high airflows, and a stopwatch. The vacuum cleaner draws air (or any other gas to be tested) from the spirometer through the pneumotachograph, which is mounted in series with it, with care being taken to reproduce the upstream geometry under which the device will be used. A T-tap between the pneumotachograph and the vacuum cleaner can be used to vary the flow through the pneumotachograph.

Using such a setup, Finucane et al. (1) have shown that the linearity of the Fleisch pneumotachograph is influenced by the upstream geometry and that the pressure drop may deviate from linearity by 7–14% within the nominal range of flows of the pneumotachograph. Therefore, it is important to establish a calibration curve using the actual geometry of the system in which the pneumotachograph will be used.

Once the calibration curve is established, a one-point calibration can be done regularly (at least once a day). Separate calibration factors should be measured for flow in each direction if the pneumotachograph is to be used to measure inspiratory and expiratory flow. Calibration can be done with flowmeter tubes or, if an analog or digital integrating device is available, by injecting a known volume of air through the pneumotachograph at varying speeds to be sure the device is correctly linearized.

EFFECT OF GAS VISCOSITY

The pressure drop across the pneumotachograph at a given flow is proportional to the viscosity of the gas. The respiratory gases (N_2, O_2, CO_2, and H_2O) do differ significantly in their viscosities, oxygen being about 37% more viscous than carbon dioxide.

Because viscosity is affected by the interaction between gas molecules, the viscosity of a gas mixture cannot be exactly predicted by calculating the weighted average of the viscosities of the gases composing the mixture, but such calculations can be made with an acceptably small error for mixtures of N_2, O_2, CO_2, and H_2O (4, 5). Similar calculations with gas mixtures containing a high fraction of helium give completely unusable results.

EFFECT OF TEMPERATURE

If ambient air is drawn through the pneumotachograph, it is warmed as it passes through the heated resistance element. This warming of the gas increases the volume of flow and also increases the viscosity slightly. Therefore, the pressure drop across the pneumotachograph will be greater than it would if the device were calibrated with the heater off. Since the fractional changes in gas volume and gas viscosity per degree Celsius are known (being $\frac{1}{273}$ or 0.00366 and about 0.0025, respectively), it should be possible to calculate a factor to correct the pneumotachograph if it were calibrated unheated at room temperature and used heated to measure the flow in gas at 37° C. The difficulty with this approach is that the inspired air increases in temperature as it traverses the heated resistance element, and the total pressure drop across the resistance will be a function of the integral of the instantaneous values of flow along the length of the capillary tubing, which changes as the gas warms and expands. The profile of flows versus distance along the tubing will itself vary with the flow rate, since the warming will not be completed until a greater length of tubing has been traversed at a higher flow rate. Attempts have been made to estimate the correction, but these require assumptions about the pattern of heat transfer that may be difficult to verify (4, 5). Turney and Blumenfeld (4) have proposed an elegant computer-based method for accurate correction of instantaneous flows, with changes in temperature being detected by thermistors located in the pneumotachograph and changes in gas composition detected by a mass spectrometer continuously sampling the gas close to the flowmeter. While this method might be useful for specific research purposes, it obviously is impractical for most applications of the pneumotachograph, whose greatest advantages are its simplicity and convenience. A less complex approach might be to preheat the inspired gas before it reaches the resistance element. Smith (6) has used this method, but it has not been generally applied.

Apart from its effect on the absolute accuracy of flow and volume measurements, a difference in the physical properties of inspired and expired gas will cause an apparent difference in inspired and expired volume, which, in turn, will produce a continuous offset of the zero volume if flow is integrated during steady-state breathing. In order to determine the magnitude of this error, Barrès and Gauge (7) measured and integrated flow through a pneumotachograph mounted over an enclosed container of warm water. Air was moved in and out of the container through the pneumotachograph by means of a pump simulating inspiration of air under ambient conditions and expiration of saturated air at 37° C. They found that the expired volume was only about 2.5% higher than the inspired volume when the ambient temperature and humidity were 23° C and 65%, respectively. They suggested that the unexpectedly small effect of temperature is explained by very efficient heat exchange between the pneumotachograph walls and the inspired air, so that it reaches its final temperature before transversing more than a fraction of the resistance element. Therefore, they recommended against applying a correction for ATPS to BTPS to the inspired gas volume which would introduce a greater error than would occur without the correction. While it is unlikely that the explanation of Barrès and Gauge is correct, their caution against the arbitrary use of a correction factor for ATPS to BTPS should be remembered by all users of the pneumotachograph. Ideally, an empirical correction factor should be determined by measuring the apparent increase in flow under steady-state conditions when air at ambient temperature is drawn through the heated pneumotachograph over the full range of flow rates likely to be measured. The relationship between correction factor and flow rate will be curvilinear, but once it is established, the correction can be applied to each flow data point before flow is integrated to volume in any microprocessor-based recording system. If only an analog integrator is available, it is probably best to follow the recommendation of Barrès and Gauge and ignore the correction altogether.

One minor effect of temperature change, which was considered in the analysis of Turney and Blumenfeld (4), is the change in cross-sectional area of the pneumotachograph when it is heated. This would tend partially to offset the increase in pressure drop due to volume expansion as the gas warms in traversing the resistance element.

FREQUENCY RESPONSE

Finucane et al. (1) have studied the frequency characteristics of the pneumotachograph during periodic flow. Because of inertia of the gas in the capillary tubes, flow lags behind the change of pressure, but the delay is small, an estimated 8° phase lag and 1% loss of amplitude at 10 Hz in air, though it is considerably greater with denser gases. A further deterioration in frequency response is introduced by tubing and fittings between the flow transducer and the manometer. In fact, as recently shown by Jackson and Vinegar (8), the frequency response of pneumotachographs is largely dependent upon the response characteristics of the associated pressure transducer and interconnecting fittings. Additional problems with frequency response may occur when a pneumotachograph is used in a system in which there are large pressure transients, as when the device is used to monitor flow in a positive pressure ventilator (9, 10). These errors are especially important when the differential pressure manometer is asymmetrical in design, with significant volume differences between the two sides of the transducer (10).

RECOMMENDATIONS

From the previous discussion, it is clear that pneumotachography is a good deal more complex than is generally supposed, and that the technical problems in obtaining accurate flow measurements have received rather less attention than they deserve in the pulmonary physiology literature. Short of the elaborate approach used by Turney and Blumenfeld (4), it is doubtful that an error of the order of 1–2% can be eliminated entirely, and therefore it is important for those using this very convenient device to recognize its limitations. The following measures will keep the error to a minimum.

1. Flowmeters should be calibrated in the system in which they will be used over the entire range of flows that will be measured.
2. Changes in the system may necessitate recalibration and re-evaluation of the linearity of the flowmeter.
3. If flow is to be measured in two directions, the upstream and downstream geometries of the system should be similar.
4. If possible, the calibrating gas should reproduce the temperature, humidity, and composition of the gas whose flow will be measured.
5. If the pneumotachograph is used to monitor expired volume and is calibrated with room air at ambient temperature, the heater should be on and the pneumotachograph warm. A conversion factor for ATPS to BTPS should not be applied if the pneumotachograph is used to measure inspiratory flow or inspired volume.
6. If only inspiratory flow is to be measured in a non-rebreathing system, the device should be calibrated and used with the heater off, and a correction factor for ATPS to BTPS should be applied if appropriate.

This chapter has discussed a number of problems that must be considered when a pneumotachograph is used to measure flow and volume, but we do not wish to leave the reader with the impression that the pneumotachograph is inherently less accurate than the conventional spirometer. Tashkin and associates (11) have recently pointed out that, during a forced expiration, the cooling of the expired gas in its passage from the mouthpiece to a water spirometer varies with expiratory flow. As a result there can be significant errors in the calculation of certain spirometric indices, such as the $FEF_{25-75\%}$. These errors are avoided with a heated pneumotachograph that measures flow close to the mouth. This important difference between the performance of the conventional spirometer and the pneumotachograph would not be recognized if testing of the device were done with ambient air using hand-held or sinusoidal syringes. Obviously, there is a great need for better methods of evaluating the performance of devices that measure respiratory flow and volume under conditions reproducing those in which the instruments are actually used.

REFERENCES

1. Finucane KE, Egan BA, Dawson SV: Linearity and frequency response of pneumotachographs. *J Appl Physiol* 32:121-126, 1972.
2. Grenvik A, Hedstrand U, Sjögren, H: Problems in pneumotachography. *Acta Anaesthesiol Scand* 10:147-155, 1966.
3. Gelfand R, Lambertson CJ, Peterson RE, et al.: Pneumotachograph for flow and volume measurement in normal and dense atmospheres. *J Appl Physiol* 41:120-124, 1976.
4. Turney SZ, Blumenfeld W: Heated Fleisch pneumotachometer: A calibration procedure. *J Appl Physiol* 34:117-121, 1973.
5. von der Hardt H, Zywietz C: Reliability in pneumotachographic measurements. *Respiration* 33:416-424, 1976.
6. Smith WDA: The measurement of uptake of nitrous oxide by pneumotachography. 1. Apparatus, methods and accuracy. *Br J Anaesth* 36:363-378, 1964.
7. Barres G, Gauge P: Etude par le spirogramme électrique de l'influence de l'état physique du gaz sur le fonctionnement du pneumotachographe de Fleisch. *J Physiol (Paris)* 53:589-598, 1961.
8. Jackson AC, Vinegar A: A technique for measuring frequency response of pressure, volume and flow transducers. *J Appl Physiol* 47:462-467, 1979.
9. Kafer ER: Errors in pneumotachography as a result of transducer design and function. *Anesthesiology* 38:275-279, 1973.
10. Churches AE, Loughman J, Fisk GC, et al.: Measurement errors in pneumotachography due to pressure transducer design. *Anaesth Intensive Care* 5:19-29, 1977.
11. Tashkin DP, Patel A, Deutsch R, et al.: Is standard ATPS to BTPS correction of volumes and flow rates measured with a volumetric spirometer valid? *Am Rev Respir Dis,* suppl 121, 1980, p 412.

CHAPTER 10

Low-Density Gas Spirometry

ARTHUR DAWSON, M.D.

In the last few years, there has been increasing interest in comparing the flow-volume curves obtained from breathing air and from breathing a low-density gas containing 80% helium and 20% oxygen (''heliox''). This test may be a sensitive method of detecting mild airways obstruction and may also provide a means of determining whether the site of the obstruction is in the ''large airways'' or ''small airways.'' Although the clinical usefulness of heliox spirometry is controversial (1), it is regularly performed in some pulmonary laboratories, and therefore a discussion of the procedure seems appropriate.

The full theoretical explanation of how forced expiratory flow is affected when the density of the expired gas is reduced is quite complex, and it will not be reviewed here. The interested reader will find the subject discussed at length in several excellent articles (2–4). It will suffice to state that, during forced expiration, gas flow is turbulent in the trachea and its larger branches and laminar in the small peripheral airways. The resistance to turbulent flow decreases with a decrease in gas density, because less energy is lost in accelerating the low-density gas to form eddies. The resistance to laminar flow is independent of gas density. During a forced expiration, if the ''flow-limiting segment'' of the conducting airways is located in larger airways where flow is turbulent, maximum flow will increase with a low-density gas. In the course of a single forced expiration, as lung volume decreases, the flow-limiting segment moves upstream to smaller airways where flow is laminar. At the point of the expiration at which maximum flow is determined by the resistance of small airways with laminar flow, the air and heliox flow-volume curves can be superimposed. The lung volume at which maximum expiratory flow becomes independent of gas density is called the *volume of isoflow* (Viso$\dot{V}$) (5).

EQUIPMENT

In the earlier investigations of the effect of gas density on maximum expiratory flow, lung volume was measured with a volume-displacement body plethysmo-

PULMONARY FUNCTION TESTING
GUIDELINES AND CONTROVERSIES

ISBN 0-12-788125-5

graph. This may be preferable if such equipment is available, but ordinarily the heliox flow–volume curves will be measured on the same equipment that is used for routine spirometry, provided that its output can be presented in the flow–volume format. A pneumotachograph is not satisfactory, because its calibration is affected by the viscosity of the gas mixture. Even if the pneumotachograph is calibrated for a helium–oxygen mixture, the relative concentrations of nitrogen, oxygen, and helium will change in the course of the forced expiration, necessitating variable calibration factors. This problem can be avoided by having the patient perform the forced expiration into a bag-in-box system, so that the volume of gases exhaled into the bag displaces an equal volume of air from the box, which then can be accurately measured with a pneumotachograph. If flow is measured at the mouth with a spirometer, it must be recognized that—owing to compression of the intrathoracic gas—the change in lung volume as measured with a volume-displacement plethysmograph will not be identical to the integrated expiratory flow from the mouth and that the discrepancy may differ with air and low-density gas. However, the difference seems to be insignificant at the relatively low flows and lung volumes at which density dependence is analyzed (5).

PROCEDURE

In the original study of Despas et al. (3), the helium–oxygen mixture was breathed for 10 minutes before the flow–volume curve was measured. This detracted a good deal from the possible usefulness of the method as a quick screening test, and in several later investigations forced expiratory flow was measured after three or four vital-capacity breaths of the low-density gas (5–7). The replacement of the alveolar gas with the helium and oxygen is less complete after the three-breath method than after a longer period of equilibration, and the maximum flow at 50% of the vital capacity was 3.6% less in nonsmokers and 4.7% less in smokers than after 10 minutes of breathing low-density gas (6). The Viso$\dot{V}$ shows only a minimal difference when the 10-minute equilibration method is compared with the three-vital-capacity-breath method; as pointed out by Hutcheon et al. (5), the less complete equilibration of the helium mixture would tend to shift the Viso$\dot{V}$ to a higher lung volume in patients with airways obstruction, thus increasing the sensitivity of the test. Fairshter and Wilson (8) carried this argument a step further and demonstrated that when Viso$\dot{V}$ was measured after a single breath of heliox, it was more sensitive in separating nonsmokers from smokers with small airways obstruction than the Viso$\dot{V}$ after three breaths of heliox. At this time, there is insufficient agreement among investigators to establish a specific recommendation regarding the duration of helium–oxygen breathing before measuring the expiratory flows.

The forced expiratory maneuver should be performed at least three times during air breathing. It should then be repeated at least three times after the heliox is breathed. If the purpose of the test is to distinguish "responders" from "nonresponders" on the basis of the percent increase in flow with heliox, the heliox should be administered as three vital-capacity breaths before the forced expiration from which the measurements are made. Only if this procedure is followed can the normal predicted values that follow be used. For the comparison of air and heliox curves, the measured vital capacities must agree within 5% and preferably should agree within 2.5% (8). The published studies have recommended that when the vital capacities obtained with air and heliox are not identical, the curves should be superimposed and matched at residual volume (RV) rather than at total lung capacity (TLC). In fact, it can be shown that the reproducibility of Viso$\dot{V}$ measurements is improved if the lower portions of the two curves close to the residual volume are visually superimposed.

CALCULATIONS

The change in flow with low-density gas may be reported in terms of various spirometric indices, but parameters for which satisfactory normal data have been reported are the $\Delta FEF_{50\%}$ (percent increase in maximum flow at 50% of the vital capacity), the $\Delta FEF_{75\%}$ (at 25% of the vital capacity measured from RV), and the Viso$\dot{V}$.

NORMAL VALUES

Dosman and associates have reported data for 66 nonsmokers aged 17–60 years (6). They report 47.3 ± 13.7% (mean ± SD) to be normal for the $\Delta FEF_{50\%}$ and 29.12 ± 23.4% for the $\Delta FEF_{75\%}$. Neither showed any significant decline with age in nonsmokers, though both declined with increasing ages of subjects who were smokers. Viso$\dot{V}$ expressed as a percentage of the vital capacity did rise significantly with increasing age, as shown by the regression equation: $\text{Viso}\dot{V} = 0.291A + 4.917 \pm 6.88$ SD. Hutcheon et al. (5) measured Viso$\dot{V}$ in 18 younger nonsmokers and reported a slightly lower mean value and a small SD (9.7 ± 3.9).

EXPECTED REPRODUCIBILITY

No data have been published on the reproducibility of the heliox flow–volume curve when individual subjects are tested on different days, but Li and associates recently reported a study of between-technician variations in the interpretation of the same series of curves obtained from normal volunteers (9). They suggested that a change of at least 3–5% may be necessary to be considered significant. They also recommended that in prospective studies "meticulously detailed written instructions for the testers be established and maintained."

One determinant of the variability of the test is the number of maximal respirations of heliox administered before the forced expiratory flow is measured. The greater the number, the more constant the expired helium concentration and therefore the better the reproducibility will be. As noted previously, the reproducibility of the Viso$\dot{V}$ is improved if the air and heliox flow–volume curves are matched on the lower portions of their descending limbs rather than at either TLC or RV (R. Fallat, personal communication 1980).

CONTROVERSIAL ISSUES

Clinical Usefulness

As in the case with measurements of closing volumes, the clinical usefulness of spirometric tests with low-density gases is controversial. This is an issue that, although not reviewed in depth in this text, needs to be carefully considered by laboratories contemplating use of the test for clinical purposes.

One Breath, Three Breaths, or 10 Minutes of Breathing Heliox

As discussed previously, there is no agreement concerning the optimal number of breaths of heliox to take prior to repeating spirometry. The data would seem to indicate that using only a single breath would increase the sensitivity for detection of airways disease.

REFERENCES

1. Meadows JA III, Rodarte JR, Hyatt RE: Density dependence of maximal expiratory flow in chronic obstructive pulmonary disease. *Am Rev Respir Dis* 121:47–53, 1980.
2. Schilder DP, Roberts A, Fry DL: Effect of gas density and viscosity on the maximal expiratory flow-volume relationship. *J Clin Invest* 42:1705–1713, 1963.
3. Despas PJ, Leroux M, Macklem PT: Site of airway obstruction in asthma as determined by measuring maximal expiratory flow breathing air and a helium-oxygen mixture. *J Clin Invest* 51:3235–3243, 1972.
4. Drazen JM, Loring SH, Ingram RH Jr: Distribution of pulmonary resistance: Effects of gas density, viscosity and flow rate. *J Appl Physiol* 41:388–395, 1976.
5. Hutcheon M, Griffin P, Levison H, et al.: Volume of isoflow: A new test in detection of mild abnormalities of lung mechanics. *Am Rev Respir Dis* 110:458–465, 1974.

6. Dosman J, Bode F, Urbanetti J, et al.: The use of a helium-oxygen mixture during maximum expiratory flow to demonstrate obstruction in small airways in smokers. *J Clin Invest* 55:1090–1099, 1975.
7. Brooks SM, Zipp T, Barber M, et al.: Measurements of maximal expiratory flow rates in cigarette smokers and nonsmokers using gases of high and low densities. *Am Rev Respir Dis* 118:75–81, 1978.
8. Fairshter RD, Wilson AF: Volume of isoflow: Effect of distribution of ventilation. *J Appl Physiol* 43:807–811, 1977.
9. Li K-YR, Tan LT-K, Chong P, Dosman JA: Between-technician variation in the measurement of spirometry with air and helium. *Am Rev Respir Dis* 124:196–198, 1981.

Single Breath Nitrogen Test: Closing Volume and Distribution of Ventilation

PHILIP M. GOLD, M.D.

INTRODUCTION

A single breath nitrogen test (SBN_2) is administered to assess (1) the behavior of the dependent airways and (2) the uniformity of gas distribution in the lungs. At the outset, it should be noted that a Workshop on Screening Programs for Early Diagnosis of Airway Obstruction conducted by the National Heart and Lung Institute, Division of Lung Diseases, in October 1973 concluded that "although closing volume and closing capacity are sensitive tests, they are probably of low specificity and moderate precision, and their validity as an early diagnostic test is unknown" (1). Although research programs continue to acquire data regarding methodology, precision, and the physiological and clinical significance of the measurement of closing volume, little has changed since 1973 to alter the conclusion expressed by the workshop. At present, perhaps the most clinically useful aspect of the test is the measurement of the slope of phase III to determine the uniformity of gas distribution.

To perform the SBN_2 test, the subject inhales, from residual volume (RV), a maximum volume of 100% O_2, then exhales back to RV. Changes in lung volume and N_2 concentration at the mouth are plotted against each other on a recorder. Inspiratory and expiratory flow rates are carefully controlled. Partially because of a gravity-dependent gradient in transpulmonary pressure from apex to base, the dependent regions of the lung tend to empty more fully than the apical regions, and the bulk of the 100% O_2 inspired from RV goes to the dependent lung zones. When this single breath of oxygen is exhaled, a characteristic pattern (N_2%/volume) can be observed (see Fig. 1). The first gases to emerge are (I) dead space gas and (II) a mixture of dead space gas and alveolar gas. Then follows a fairly uniform mixture of alveolar gas (phase III). Finally, in most but not all subjects, a sharp rise in N_2 concentration occurs, usually in the final one-third of the vital capacity (VC); this rise marks the onset of the "closing volume" (phase IV). During this fourth phase, it is assumed that dependent airways have closed, while gas continues to emerge from the nitrogen-rich upper regions.

PULMONARY FUNCTION TESTING
GUIDELINES AND CONTROVERSIES

ISBN 0-12-788125-5

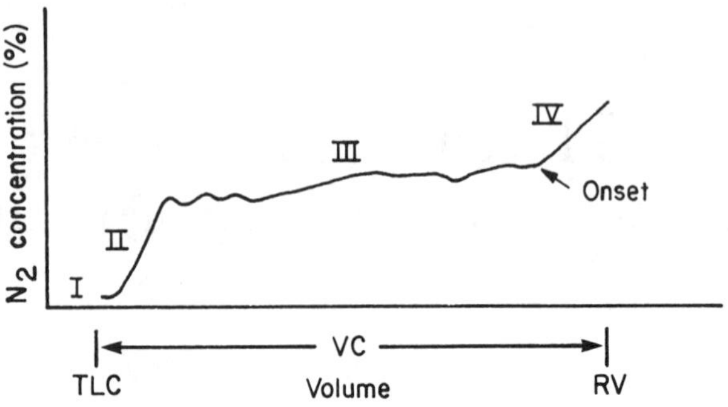

Fig. 1 *Sample curve.*

EQUIPMENT

1. Nitrogen analyzer or mass spectrophotometer. The recommended performance criteria are as follows: accuracy/linearity: 1.0% full scale; drift: 0.1% N_2/hr; resolution: 0.1% N_2; sampling rate: ≤20 ml/min; 90% response time (including signal delay): 0.05 second. Most recent models meet or exceed these criteria; however, a calibration curve should be constructed.
2. Volume-measuring device. Either a spirometer with electrical output (options include bellows, rolling seal, or water seal with potentiometer) or a pneumotachograph with an integrator is recommended. All devices should meet the American Thoracic Society (ATS) Snowbird Workshop criteria (2).
3. 20–30 liter bag-in-box system.*
4. 2 one-way valves or a two-way J-valve.*
5. Three-way mouthpiece valve. [If a five-way valve is available, it may be used in lieu of valves nos. 4 and 5; thus, the same system may be used for measuring single breath carbon monoxide diffusing capacity ($DL_{CO}SB$) and SBN_2.]
6. Feedback device for controlling flow (galvanometer, voltmeter, or oscilloscope).†
7. Rapid-responding X–Y–Y recorder. The second Y channel is used to record inspiratory and expiratory flow rates. (An X–Y recorder is less desirable, but will suffice.)
8. Oxygen source.
9. Compressed air source.*

Figure 2 exemplifies assembly of a SBN_2 system.

*These items are not essential, but facilitate repetition of the test without the necessity of rinsing the spirometer each time.

†Alinear (fixed-orifice type) resistors may be used in the circuit if subjects have difficulty keeping flows below 0.5 liter/sec. The recommended resistance is 12 cm H_2O *at* 1 liter/sec (3).

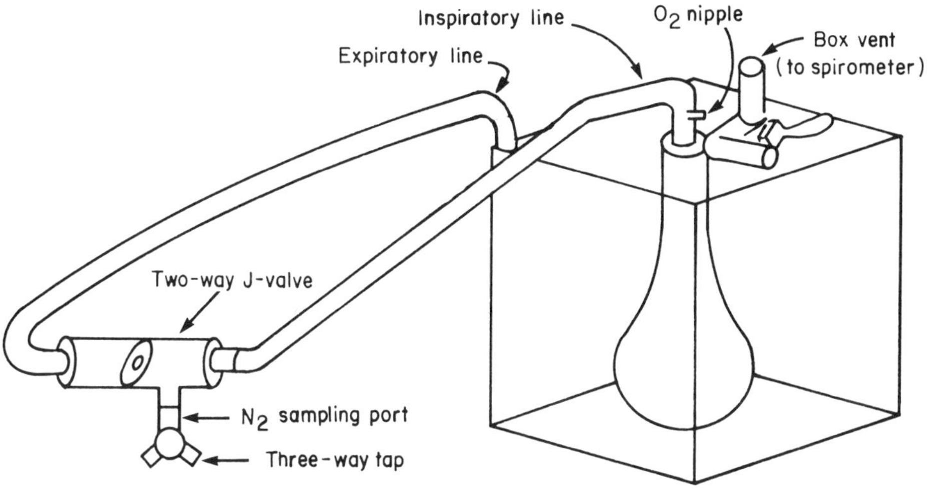

Fig. 2 *Example of a SBN_2 system.*

QUALITY CONTROL

Initially and at Regular Intervals

1. The volume system should be checked for accuracy, linearity, and freedom from leaks.

2. The nitrogen analyzer should also be checked for accuracy, linearity, and freedom from excessive drift. (See manufacturer's specifications.) For detection of closing volume alone, a 2-point calibration will suffice (0% N_2, room air). For the other applications [slope of phase III, single breath total lung capacity (TLC_{SB})] a 4–5-point calibration is recommended (0, 10, 20, 40, and 80% N_2). At the minimum, the meter should be checked at one other point between 0% and 80%, preferably in the 20–40% range. The Utah Biomedical Test Laboratory's evaluation of N_2 analyzers should be referred to for a more detailed discussion of problems with calibration (4).

Before Each Testing Period

1. The volume signal should be calibrated with a physical standard.
2. The flow signal should be calibrated with a rotameter at 0.5 liter/sec.
3. A 2-point calibration (at 0% and 80%) should be performed on the nitrogen analyzer.

PROCEDURE

Preparation

When only a spirometer is to be used for testing, rinse it several times with 100% O_2 until N_2 concentration at the mouthport is less than 0.1% during the expiratory flush.

When a bag-in-box system is to be used:

1. Disconnect the spirometer.
2. Turn the three-way mouthport valve so that the inspiratory line vents to the room.
3. Evacuate the balloon by introducing compressed air into the box via the vent. (The balloon contents will flow out through the three-way valve.)
4. Close the three-way valve, *vent the box,* and fill the balloon with oxygen.
5. Repeat steps 2 through 4 until the N_2 concentration at the mouthport is less than 0.1% during balloon evacuation.
6. Fill the balloon with enough O_2 for three SBN_2 maneuvers.
7. Connect the spirometer to the box, allowing enough volume for an inspiratory VC.

Test Procedure

1. With the three-way valve in the room air position, instruct the subject to breathe normally into the mouthpiece.
2. Tell the subject to take two deep breaths, then exhale to RV. Near RV, turn the three-way valve to the box position, activate the recorder, and observe the expired trace for cessation of flow. (If using a spirometer alone, turn the three-way valve *at* RV.)
3. Instruct the subject to inhale to total lung capacity (TLC), using a feedback device to keep the flow stable at $\leqslant$ 0.5 liter/sec (0.4 is ideal). When TLC is reached, tell the subject to exhale to RV, keeping the flow $\leqslant$ 0.5 liter/sec (no pause at TLC). When RV is reached, turn the valve back to the room air position.
4. Repeat the test twice; delay the repetition if the inspiratory–expiratory nitrogen concentration difference exceeds 5% when the subject is breathing room air.

CALCULATIONS

This entire section, except for the sample calculation of TLC, is from the National Heart and Lung Institute's suggested standardized procedures (3).

Criteria for Acceptability of Single Breath N_2 Closing Volume Curves

The following criteria must be met for acceptability; failure to satisfy any one of these leads to rejection of the curve:

1. Mean expiratory flow after the first 500 ml is expired must be $\leq$ 0.5 liter/sec (the subject is instructed to aim for 0.4 liter/sec).
2. Except for the first 500 ml of expiration during closing volume measurement, expiratory flow transients must not exceed 0.7 liter/sec. Unacceptable flow transients are defined as deviation from the required flow which persists during expiration of more than 300 ml.
3. Difference between inspired and expired VC must be less than 5%.
4. Differences in VC between blows must not exceed 10%.
5. There must not be a step change in the expired N_2 concentration with continued cardiogenic oscillations after the step. The causes of such step changes are obscure but are probably not related to airway closure. If such curves are accepted, the onset of phase IV will frequently be read as the volume at which the step occurs.

Measurements To Be Made from Acceptable Curves

Ideally, on all subjects, three acceptable tracings will be obtained. The mean of the three values is taken as the final value. When only two readable tracings are obtained, the mean of the two values is used. When only one readable tracing is obtained, the study should be rejected. Figure 1 depicts a sampling closing volume tracing.

Closing Volume (CV)

The onset of phase IV should be determined by the best-fit line drawn by eye through the latter half of phase III. The point of final departure from this line is the onset of phase IV. In some subjects, there is a sharp drop in N_2 concentration after the onset of phase IV. Occasionally, this can intersect the line drawn through phase III. Under these circumstances, the onset of Phase IV is taken as the first definite point of departure of the N_2 tracing from the best-fit line. The closing volume is the volume from the onset of phase IV to RV. CV is usually expressed as % of the expired VC.

Closing Capacity

Closing capacity (CC) is defined as closing volume (CV) plus RV and is usually expressed as a percentage of TLC.

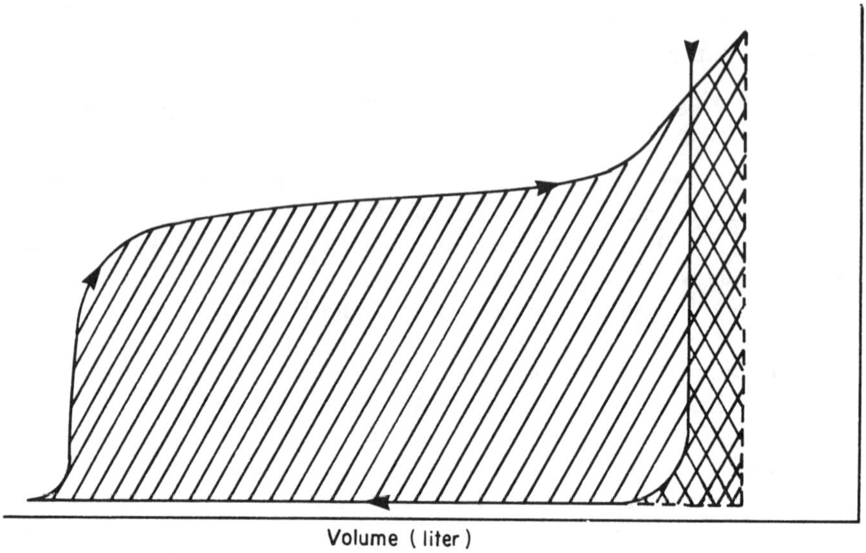

Fig. 3 *Area for sample calculation of TLC_{SB}.*

Total Lung Capacity

TLC can be calculated from the alveolar dilution equation, using the expired volume of nitrogen (V_EN_2) determined by planimetry or by electrical integration of the area under the single breath curve (3). For Eqs. 1–3, the following values are used: Area under expired N_2 curve (A) is 59.6 cm² (includes extrapolated cross-hatched area on the right of Fig. 3). N_2 calibration is 4.19%/cm. Volume calibration (BTPS) is 0.51 liter/cm. Volume expired (V_E) is 11.4 cm or 5.81 liter. Volume inspired (V_I) is 11.0 cm or 5.61 liter. Dead space (V_D) (subject's anatomical + instrument) is 0.26 liter. Alveolar N_2 concentration (F_AN_2) is assumed to be 0.80.

Calculation of mean expired N_2 (F_EN_2):

$$F_EN_2 = \frac{\frac{A}{\dot{V}_E}\left(N_2 \text{ calibration}\right)}{100} = \frac{\frac{59.6 \text{ cm}^2}{11.4 \text{ cm}}(4.19\%/\text{cm})}{100} = 0.2191 \quad \text{(Eq. 1)}$$

Correction of mean expired N_2 for dead space admixture ($F_A'N_2$):

$$F_A'N_2 = \frac{(F_EN_2)(V_E)}{\dot{V}_E - V_D} = \frac{(0.2191)\,(5.81)}{5.81 - 0.26} = 0.2294 \quad \text{(Eq. 2)}$$

Calculation of TLC:

$$TLC = \frac{(\dot{V}_I)(F_AN_2) - (\dot{V}_D)(F_A'N_2)}{F_AN_2 - F_A'N_2} = \frac{(5.61)(0.80) - (0.26)(0.2294)}{0.80 - 0.2294}$$

$$= 7.76 \text{ liter} \qquad \text{(Eq. 3)}$$

Residual Volume

RV can be derived by subtracting the recorded vital capacity from TLC.

Slope of Phase III

The slope of phase III is determined by the best-fit line, between 70% VC and the onset of phase IV.

The analysis of these curves cannot always be made in a totally objective manner. On some curves in particular, the onset of phase IV is difficult to determine, and when the same reader blindly reads such curves twice, there is not a very good agreement between the two measurements. This appears to be due to differences between individuals, because when a subject generates such a curve, it is likely that all curves that he generates will be difficult to analyze. On the other hand, if a subject generates a curve that is easy to analyze, in all likelihood, all curves obtained from him will be easy to analyze. Obviously, curve readers will have to use good judgment, and they may decide that some curves, although conforming to the criteria of acceptability, are unreadable and therefore must be rejected. It is impossible at present to establish a set of rigid rules governing such cases (4).

NORMAL VALUES

Buist and Ross have reported the results of closing volume measurements using the modified single breath nitrogen test in 284 healthy nonsmokers. No significant differences between the regression coefficients for men and women were observed (5). A subsequent collaborative study comparing the results of the single breath nitrogen test obtained in Winnipeg, Canada, Montreal, Canada, and Portland, Oregon, revealed similar age-related regression in nonsmokers and no significant differences related to geographic location, climate, air pollution, or occupation (6). Normal values reported by Knudson and colleagues (7) are similar. Using information obtained from 337 nonsmokers, Buist and Ross reported regression equations for the slope of phase III, (ΔN_2/liter, Delta nitrogen concentration per liter) versus age (8). Measurement values related to age and obtained with the single breath nitrogen test in asymptomatic, nonsmoking men and women are presented in Table 1.

Table 1 *Single Breath Nitrogen Test: Normal Values*

Reference	Population	Regression equation[a]
Buist and Ross (5)	284 Nonsmokers	$CV/\%VC = 0.318A + 1.919 \pm 4.61$ SEE
		$CC/\%TLC = 0.525A + 14.348 \pm 4.34$ SEE
Buist et al. (6)	95 Normal male	$CV/\%VC = 0.40A - 1.89 \pm 4.56$ SD
	nonsmokers	$CC/\%TLC = 0.53A + 13.25 \pm 4.00$ SD
		$\Delta\%N_2/\text{liter} = 0.001A + 0.81 \pm 0.59$ SD
	145 Normal female	$CV/\%VC = 0.40A - 2.90 \pm 4.56$ SD
	nonsmokers	$CC/\%TLC = 0.53A + 15.70 + 4.00$ SD
		$\Delta\%N_2/\text{liter} = 0.001A + 1.07 \pm 0.59$ SD
Knudson et al. (7)	All nonsmokers	
	Number / Age range	
	147 / 25–54	$CV/\%VC = 0.269A - 0.882$
	148 / 25–54	$CC/\%TLC = 0.471A + 11.942$
	189 / 8–19	$\Delta\%N_2/\text{liter} = 1.771 - 0.018H$
	239 / 20–54	$\Delta\%N_2/\text{liter} = 1.717 - 0.0002A - 0.018H$
	164 / 55+	$\Delta\%N_2/\text{liter} = 1.599 + 0.026A - 0.036H$
Buist and Ross (8)	All nonsmokers	
	137 Males	$\Delta\%N_2/\text{liter} = 0.710 + 0.01A \pm 0.43$ SEE
	203 Females (<60)	$\Delta\%N_2/\text{liter} = 1.036 + 0.009A \pm 0.57$ SEE
	(>60)	$\Delta\%N_2/\text{liter} = 0.058A - 1.777 \pm 1.30$ SEE

[a] H = height in inches; A = age in years.

REPRODUCIBILITY

The standard deviation of repeated measurements of CV and TLC (both in liters) is large, around 0.13 liter; thus, it is important that at least three measurements are obtained (9, 10). These variations are independent of the time or day that the test is performed (9, 10). In most cases, the range about the mean of three measurements of the slope of phase III should not be greater than $\pm 0.5\%$ N_2/liter (10).

TROUBLESHOOTING

The variability in absolute values for closing volume in the same individual from test to test can be attributed to the inherent variation in the expired volume at which the onset of airway closure occurs, reader difficulties in detecting the onset of phase IV, and variations in the expired vital capacity due to incomplete filling and/or emptying of the lungs (9). The volume at which phase IV occurs is critically influenced by the expiratory flow rate (11), and the slope of phase III varies with the inspiratory flow rate (12). Inability to control the expiratory flow within acceptable limits is probably the major source of imprecision in closing volume determinations. (In analyzing variability, it is helpful to have simultaneous measurements of flow and volume.) The sensitivity of the closing volume measurement in distinguishing between subjects is enhanced by taking the mean of three measurements. TLC measured by the single breath nitrogen test correlates well with that measured by helium dilution in a population of urban men and women free from abnormalities of gas distribution, for both smokers and nonsmokers, with and without symptoms (10). The single breath measurement will underestimate TLC in patients with airway obstruction (10).

CONTROVERSIAL ISSUES

In this chapter, the resident gas technique was described, because it was selected for standardization in epidemiological studies by the Division of Lung Diseases of the National Heart, Lung and Blood Institute. Factors influencing the division's choice included portability and general availability of equipment, relative procedural simplicity, field experience with the method, and the ability of the technique to measure total lung capacity from the single breath record. Simultaneous measurements using the bolus and resident gas techniques have shown either close similarities in results or a systematic tendency for the nitrogen closing volume measurements to be slightly lower than those determined by the bolus technique (7, 13, 14).

The method of performing the single breath nitrogen test presented in this chapter is a modification of the test described by Fowler (15). Using the Fowler test, the percent nitrogen difference between 750 ml and 1250 ml expired volume is reported as an index of the uniformity of distribution of ventilation (15, 16). Other methods have been used to assess the uniformity of the distribution of ventilation. These include the measurement of residual nitrogen following open circuit nitrogen washout (17, 18) and the determination of helium mixing time during closed circuit equilibration (19, 20). The scope of this review does not permit a detailed description of the methods for these tests, and the reader is encouraged to review the references cited.

REFERENCES

1. *Workshop on Screening Programs for Early Diagnosis of Airway Obstruction*. Division of Lung Diseases, National Heart and Lung Institute, October 1973.
2. Gardner RM, Baker CD, Broennle AM Jr, et al.: ATS statement—Snowbird workshop on standardization of spirometry. *Am Rev Respir Dis* 119:831–838, 1979.
3. Martin R, Macklem PT: *Suggested Standardized Procedures for Closing Volume Determinations (Nitrogen Method)*. Division of Lung Diseases, National Heart and Lung Institute, 1973.

4. Daniels AU, Couvillon LA, Lebrizzi JM: Evaluation of nitrogen analyzers. *Am Rev Respir Dis* 112:571-575, 1975.
5. Buist AS, Ross BB: Predicted values for closing volumes using a modified single breath nitrogen test. *Am Rev Respir Dis* 107:744-752, 1973.
6. Buist AS, Ghezzo, H, Anthonisen NR, et al.: Relationship between the single-breath N_2 test and age, sex, and smoking habit in three North American cities. *Am Rev Respir Dis* 120:305-318, 1979.
7. Knudson RJ, Lebowitz MD, Burton AP, et al.: The closing volume test: evaluation of nitrogen and bolus methods in a random population. *Am Rev Respir Dis* 115:423-434, 1977.
8. Buist AS, Ross BB: Quantitative analysis of the alveolar plateau in the diagnosis of early airway obstruction. *Am Rev Respir Dis* 108:1078-1087, 1973.
9. McFadden ER Jr, Holmes B, Kiker R: Variability of closing volume measurements in normal man. *Am Rev Respir Dis* 111:135-140, 1975.
10. Becklake MR, Leclerc M, Strobach H, et al.: The N_2 closing volume test in population studies: Sources of variation and reproducibility. *Am Rev Respir Dis* 111:141-147, 1975.
11. Hyatt RE, Rodarte JR: "Closing volume," one man's noise—other men's experiment. *Mayo Clin Proc* 50:17-27, 1975.
12. Make B, Lapp NL: Factors influencing the measurement of closing volume. *Am Rev Respir Dis* 111:749-754, 1975.
13. Travis DM, Green M, Don H: Simultaneous comparison of helium and nitrogen expiratory "closing volumes." *J Appl Physiol* 34:304-308, 1973.
14. Linn WS, Hackney JD: Nitrogen and helium "closing volumes": simultaneous measurement and reproducibility. *J Appl Physiol* 34:396-399, 1973.
15. Fowler WS: Lung function studies: III. Uneven pulmonary ventilation in normal subjects and in patients with pulmonary disease. *J Appl Physiol* 2:283-299, 1949.
16. Comroe JH Jr, Fowler WS: Lung function studies: VI. detection of uneven ventilation during a single breath of oxygen. *Am J Med* 10:408-413, 1951.
17. Cournand A, Baldwin ED, Darling RC, et al.: Studies on intra-pulmonary mixture of gases: IV. The significance of the pulmonary emptying rate and a simplified open circuit measurement of residual air. *J Clin Invest* 20:681-689, 1941.
18. Darling RC, Cournand A, Richards DW Jr: Studies of intrapulmonary mixture of gases: V. Forms of inadequate ventilation in normal and emphysematous lungs, analyzed by means of breathing pure oxygen. *J Clin Invest* 23:55-67, 1944.
19. Meneely GR, Kaltreider NL: The volume of the lung determined by helium dilution: Description of the method and comparison with other procedures. *J Clin Invest* 28:129-139, 1949.
20. Hathirat S, Renzetti AD Jr, Mitchell M: Intrapulmonary gas distribution; a comparison of the helium mixing time and nitrogen single breath test in normal and diseased subjects. *Am Rev Respir Dis* 102:750-759, 1970.

Measurement of Lung Volume: The Multiple Breath Nitrogen Method

ALFREDO A. JALOWAYSKI, PH.D.
ARTHUR DAWSON, M.D.

Gas dilution techniques may be used alone or in conjunction with plethysmography to measure functional residual capacity (FRC). When only dilution techniques are utilized, FRC may be underestimated in patients with obstructive lung disease, since the volume of some compartments of the lung may fail (partially or entirely) to equilibrate with the inspired gas mixture. If, however, thoracic gas volume (TGV) at FRC is measured simultaneously by plethysmography, the difference between the TGV and the dilution FRC gives an estimate of the volume of the "poorly ventilated space," a parameter of possible clinical importance. In addition, breath-by-breath analysis of the indicator gas concentration may be used to assess the efficiency of intrapulmonary gas mixing.

There are two commonly used gas dilution methods: the closed-circuit helium method and the open-circuit nitrogen method. Both methods require that the indicator gas used be physiologically inert and relatively insoluble in the blood and tissues. In the closed-circuit helium method, a foreign inert gas (helium) is rebreathed until an equilibrium concentration is reached in the lung. In the open-circuit nitrogen method, which is detailed in this chapter, the "resident gas," nitrogen, is eliminated during a period of breathing 100% oxygen. If the initial concentration of nitrogen in the lung is known or assumed and the total quantity of nitrogen washed out is measured, the initial volume of the lung can be calculated.

The open-circuit nitrogen method has two potential disadvantages relative to the closed-circuit helium method: the initial alveolar nitrogen concentration cannot be measured precisely and must therefore be estimated, and nitrogen is more soluble in tissues than helium. While little helium is "lost" to the blood and tissues during the closed-circuit equilibration, there is a significant contribution from tissue nitrogen to the total volume of nitrogen collected during the open-circuit washout. With the use of appropriate corrections, however, the magnitude of the error in estimating tissue nitrogen is probably small in relation to the overall accuracy of measurement of lung volume.

PULMONARY FUNCTION TESTING
GUIDELINES AND CONTROVERSIES

ISBN 0-12-788125-5

The classic 7-minute nitrogen washout test of Darling, Cournand, and Richards (1) gives a lower value for FRC than the closed-circuit helium method in patients with severe obstructive lung disease, but if the nitrogen washout time is prolonged, there is no significant difference between the results obtained with the two techniques (2). For assessment of the efficiency of intrapulmonary gas mixing, the washout curve generated from the open-circuit nitrogen method yields to mathematical treatment much more easily than the helium dilution curve.

EQUIPMENT

To measure lung volume, the volume of air expired during the washout period and the average nitrogen concentration in that volume must be determined. Therefore, the basic items of equipment are a nitrogen analyzer and a spirometer.

Nitrogen Analyzer

Nitrogen analysis was originally done with the Van Slyke–Neill apparatus (1), but mass spectrometers and gas chromatographs also have been used. Currently, most laboratories use the ionization chamber analyzers, which have the advantages of rapid response, stability, ease of use, and relatively low cost. These analyzers employ a vacuum pump, which continuously draws a sample of gas into a chamber where the gas is ionized by passing a high-voltage current through it. The ionized nitrogen emits a blue light that is detected by a filtered photocell; only light within the spectral region of nitrogen passes through the filter. The output of the photocell is amplified and displayed on a meter calibrated to indicate the nitrogen concentration.

A Manually Operated Open-Circuit System

The basic system for a manually operated open-circuit nitrogen washout is illustrated in Fig. 1. Oxygen is supplied from a compressed gas cylinder. Humidification is desirable, especially if a prolonged washout is to be done. A large bag (Douglas bag or neoprene meteorological balloon) provides a reservoir for the oxygen. The patient breathes through a flanged mouthpiece connected to a non-rebreathing valve while a vacuum pump continuously samples the gas from the exhalation side of the mouthpiece. Two taps are arranged so that the patient can breathe either room air from a spirometer or 100% oxygen from the bag. The spirometer tracing is observed, with the patient inspiring room air until he has established a stable respiratory pattern on the mouthpiece; when the patient is at his end tidal volume (FRC), the two taps are switched, so that the patient inspires

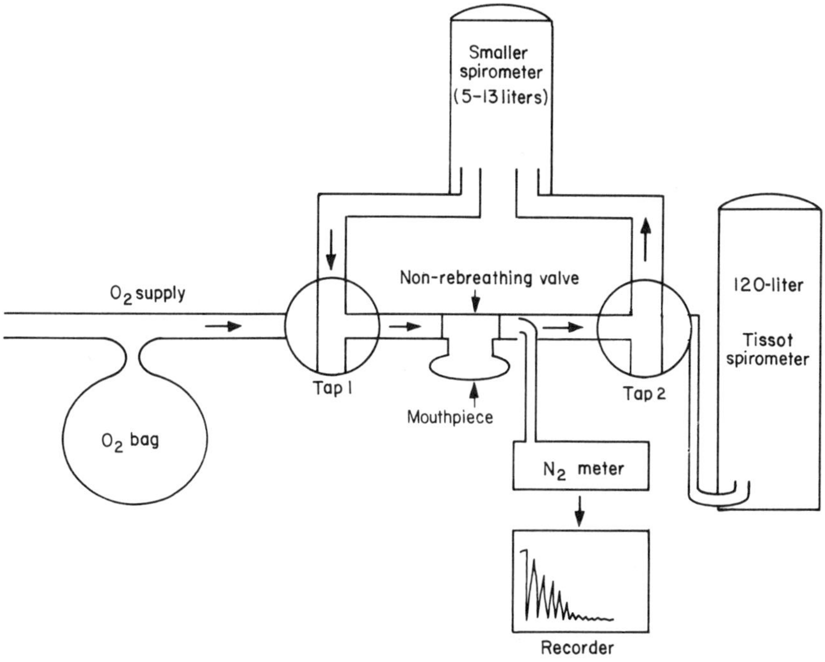

Fig. 1 *Manually operated open-circuit nitrogen washout system.*

100% oxygen, and the expired gas is collected in a 120-liter Tissot spirometer. The nitrogen concentration is displayed on a strip chart or X–Y recorder, so that the breath-by-breath washout curve can be analyzed.

An Automated Open-Circuit System

The fully automated open-circuit system (illustrated in Fig. 2) utilizes a solenoid valve, which allows the patient to breathe either room air or 100% oxygen through a demand valve. Flow at the mouth is recorded with a pneumotachograph. Flow and nitrogen concentration are sampled by an analog-to-digital converter (sample rate $\geq$ 25 Hz), the flow signal being suitably delayed to correct for the transit time from the mouth to the sampling point and for the lag time of the nitrogen analyzer. The microprocessor calculates the volume of nitrogen eliminated with each breath by summing the instantaneous values of the product of integrated expiratory flow and fractional nitrogen concentration. The end-tidal nitrogen concentration versus time (or versus total alveolar ventilation) is displayed on a cathode-ray tube or plotter. If desired, the solenoid valve can be controlled by the microprocessor in order to switch the patient from room air to oxygen automatically during an expiration.

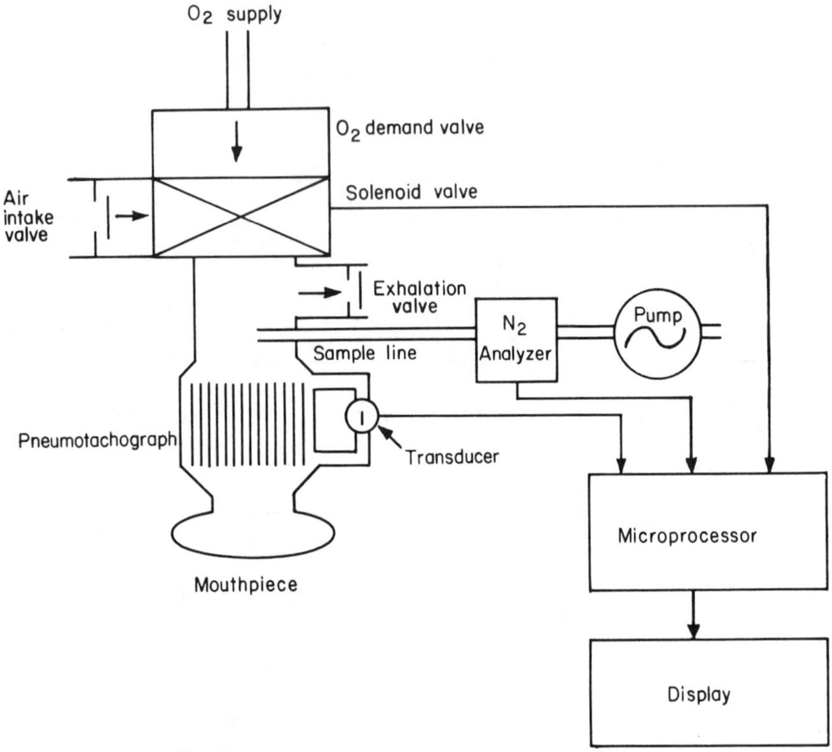

Fig. 2 *Automated open-circuit nitrogen washout system.*

QUALITY CONTROL

Minute leaks of nitrogen into the system are the primary cause of erroneous results with this test. Leaks in the tubing or the bell of the Tissot spirometer may be detected by closing all openings, adding a weight to the bell, and observing for any change in volume. If the temperature is constant, the volume should remain the same. The valves and fittings of the spirometer generally require little attention, but they should be cleaned and lubricated every 6 months, or when difficult turning or leakage is observed.

The mouthpiece valve should be removed after each use, placed in antiseptic solution for at least 5 minutes, rinsed in warm water, disassembled, and allowed to dry. The tubing connecting the spirometers to the system should be removed for weekly cleaning.

Tissot Spirometer Dead Space Calculation

Regular calculation (at least monthly) of the Tissot spirometer dead space is recommended. This is an excellent way to check for leaks.

1. The Tissot spirometer is washed 10 times with air, the gas analyzed for its nitrogen content, and the bell lowered fully.

2. A 15-liter anesthesia bag is filled with 100% O_2 and attached to the tubing at tap 2 (see Fig. 1). The bag is emptied completely into the Tissot spirometer to determine the volume of oxygen added (V_{BAG}).

3. The gases in the bag–spirometer system are mixed by alternately filling and emptying the bag from the spirometer at least 15 times. The bag is again emptied into the spirometer and the volume checked for leakage.

4. The nitrogen analyzer is connected to the outlet port of the spirometer, and the final nitrogen concentration is measured.

5. The dead space (V_{DS}) is calculated from the formula

$$V_{DS} = V_{BAG}\,[(F_2 - F_{BAG})/(F_1 - F_2)],$$

where F_1 and F_2 are the initial and final nitrogen concentrations in the Tissot spirometer and F_{BAG} is the initial nitrogen concentration in the oxygen-filled bag.

6. The dead space thus determined will only be valid if the position of the fully lowered Tissot bell and the level of water in the Tissot remain unchanged. Any changes necessitate repeat measurement of the dead space.

7. The dead space of the tubing and non-rebreathing valve between tap 1 and tap 2 (Fig. 1) can be determined by water displacement or estimated from the dimensions.

Performance of the Nitrogen Analyzer

Precise calibration and accurate performance of the nitrogen analyzer are essential for satisfactory results. If the mixed expired nitrogen concentration (F_{EN_2}) is 3%, an error of 0.1% in the nitrogen reading will cause a 3% error in the lung volume determination. If the mixed F_{EN_2} is 1.5%, the same error in the reading (0.1%) causes a 6% error in the FRC. Slight inaccuracies of the nitrogen analyzer are less critical with automated systems, since the final value of the lung volume is most affected by the initial breaths of the washout when the nitrogen concentration is relatively high.

Apart from inaccurate calibration, errors in the nitrogen analysis can result from insufficient warm-up time, plugging of the needle valve, excessive moisture in the analyzer, and malfunction of the vacuum pump.

The linearity of the nitrogen analyzer should be checked initially, whenever erroneous measurements are suspected, and periodically thereafter (arbitrarily recommended frequency is every 6 months). A satisfactory two-point calibration can be done by adjusting the meter to the factory specified value on room air, then closing the needle valve completely to obtain a zero N_2 reading (the pump evacuates the ionization chamber). Calibration with low-concentration ($\approx$5% and 10% N_2) gases will validate the linearity in the critical (0–10%) range of the analyzer.

ASSESSMENT OF ACCURACY

The best way to test the accuracy of the whole system is to perform periodic measurements of the spirometer dead space or the "FRC" of a 3- or 4-liter syringe. Another simple test is to measure the FRC of one of the laboratory staff whose lung volume is known.

PROCEDURE

For an ionizing-type nitrogen analyzer, the following procedure is suggested.

1. The output is connected to a time base recorder. A 2-point (room air, 0% N_2) calibration is performed on the analyzer, according to the manufacturer's instructions. When room air is drawn through the needle valve, the output signal is amplified to give a wide deflection (approximately 20 cm is ideal) on the Y axis. Zero N_2 is usually obtained by completely closing the needle valve to evacuate the ionizing chamber.
2. The 120-liter Tissot spirometer, 9-liter spirometer, and tubing are flushed with *air*.
3. Shortly before the test is begun, the oxygen reservoir bag is filled with 100% oxygen.
4. The procedure is thoroughly explained to the patient. The more relaxed the patient is, the more his end-expiratory volume will represent the true resting end-tidal volume (FRC).
5. The patient is connected to the mouthpiece, and his respiratory pattern is observed while he breathes room air on the smaller spirometer. The washout is not begun until he shows a stable tidal volume and respiratory frequency.
6. At the end of a normal expiration, the taps are turned so that the patient inspires 100% oxygen from the reservoir bag and expires into the Tissot spirometer.
7. The expired gas collection is ended when

   a. the expired nitrogen falls below 1.2%
   b. leaks are detected by a sudden rise in the expired nitrogen concentration
   c. the patient cannot continue
   d. the Tissot spirometer or collecting bag is full

A 7-minute collection is sufficient for normal adults or children. In patients whose ventilation is markedly uneven, the 7-minute washout often underestimates the FRC (2).

8. To end the test, the tap leading to the Tissot spirometer is closed. The patient is instructed to take a deep breath of O_2 and to blow out slowly for as long

as he can into the smaller spirometer. The end-expiratory nitrogen concentration is recorded as the "alveolar nitrogen," though it probably underestimates the true mean alveolar nitrogen when there are slowly ventilated spaces.

9. To achieve a uniform gas mixture in the Tissot, an evacuated 3-liter syringe should be carefully attached to tap 2 and alternately filled and emptied several times. [The fan may not effectively mix the gas in the Tissot metal side tube (approximately 500 ml) with the contents of the bell proper.]

10. The volume collected in the Tissot spirometer and its nitrogen concentration are then measured.

Note that the procedure and calculations described for the manual system differ from many previous descriptions in that the amount of nitrogen present in the dead space of the Tissot plus tubing at the beginning of the test (V_{D2}; see Calculations) needs to be estimated and subtracted in the calculations. This eliminates the necessity for washing out the Tissot with 100% O_2 before each determination (but washing out the Tissot with room air after each determination is still required).

CALCULATIONS

FUNCTIONAL RESIDUAL CAPACITY

The basic equation for calculation of the FRC using the manual method follows:

$$\mathrm{FRC(corr)} = \left[\frac{(V_E + V_{D1})(F_E - F_I) - (V_{D2})(F_N) - V_{TIS}}{F_{A1} - F_{A2}}\right]\left(K_{BTPS}\right)$$

where
V_E = volume expired into Tissot during washout, in liters
V_{D1} = volume of dead space in Tissot spirometer system distal to tap 2, in liters (see Fig. 1)
V_{D2} = volume of dead space in Tissot spirometer distal to tap 2 plus volume of tubing between tap 1 and tap 2, (equals $V_{D1} + \approx 0.2$ liter, depending on volume of tubing between mouthpiece and tap 2)
F_E = nitrogen concentration in Tissot system at end of washout
F_I = nitrogen concentration (present as impurity) in the oxygen source
F_N = nitrogen concentration in Tissot system at the beginning of washout
V_{TIS} = volume correction for tissue nitrogen, in liters
F_{A1} = initial alveolar nitrogen concentration (assumed to be 0.81)

F_{A2} = final "alveolar nitrogen concentration"
K_{BTPS} = correction factor for converting ATPS to BTPS
corr = corrected for BTPS

To help demonstrate the calculation of this equation, a sample calculation follows, using the values listed.

$V_E = 14.77 \quad V_{D2} = 4.33 \quad F_E = 0.316 \quad F_{A1} = 0.81 \quad K_{BTPS} = 1.075$
$V_{D1} = 4.13 \quad F_N = 0.796 \quad F_I = 0.004 \quad F_{A2} = 0.012 \quad V_{TIS} = 0.22$

$$\text{FRC (ATPS)} = \left[\frac{(14.77 + 4.13)(0.316 - 0.004) - (4.33)(0.796) - 0.22}{(0.81 - 0.012)} \right]$$

$$= 2.795 \text{ liters}$$

$$\text{FRC (BTPS)} = (2.795)\ (1.075) = 3.005 \text{ liters}$$

Volume Correction for Tissue Nitrogen

The volume correction for nitrogen elimination V_{TIS} sources other than the lungs (blood and tissues) is estimated to be about 30 ml per minute of washout time (3). Since tissue elimination does not continue at a constant rate during a prolonged washout time, a nonlinear function is required if a variable washout period is used. For such purposes, the following equation was derived from data of Emmanuel and associates (4).

$$V_{BN_2} = 0.1209\ t^{1/2} - 0.0665$$

where V_{BN_2} is the nitrogen (in liters) eliminated by a 70-kg man and t is the washout time in minutes. If it is assumed that the nitrogen elimination is proportional to body weight W in kilograms, the final equation becomes

$$V_{TIS}\ (0.1209\ t^{1/2} - 0.0665) \cdot (W/70)$$

"Switch-In" Volume Correction

The volume of nitrogen collected during the washout period is used to calculate the volume of air contained in the lung at the end of the expiration prior to switching the patient to oxygen breathing. The operator should observe the respiratory tracing on the spirometer, and turn the taps only after the patient has established a stable tidal volume and end-expiratory level. If the volume at the point of switching differs from the average end-expiratory volume observed, the calculated FRC should be corrected by an appropriate amount.

Correction of the Pneumotachograph for Viscosity

If a pneumotachograph is calibrated on room air and used either in a manual system or as described in the automated system, it will give incorrect readings during oxygen breathing, because the viscosity of oxygen is about 12% greater than the viscosity of air. Therefore, if inspired volumes are used in the calculations, the calibrating factor for the pneumotachograph should be multiplied by 1.12.

Correction of expired volume is more difficult, because the expired gas consists of a mixture of oxygen, nitrogen, carbon dioxide, and water vapor. The increased viscosity of oxygen is offset by the low viscosities of carbon dioxide and water vapor. The viscosity of a gas mixture can be estimated approximately from the equation

$$\eta^{-1/2} = F_1\eta_1^{-1/2} + F_2\eta_2^{-1/2} + \ldots F_n\eta_n^{-1/2}$$

where F_1 and F_2 are the fractional concentrations and η_1 and η_2 the viscosities of the component gases. At 37° C the viscosities of O_2, N_2 and CO_2 are 211, 182, and 154 micropoises, respectively, whereas the "effective viscosity" of H_2O is 104. The viscosity of room air is 188.6. In theory, the maximum error of the pneumotachograph would occur during phase I of the single breath nitrogen washout curve (see Chapter 8) when the expired gas contains only oxygen saturated with water vapor. Using the equation for viscosity of a gas mixture with $F_{O_2} = 0.94$ and $F_{H_2O} = 0.06$, the viscosity would be 200.8, or 6.5% above the viscosity of room air. However, since during phase I the expired gas contains no significant amount of nitrogen, it can be ignored when measuring lung volume.

The most important correction will apply to phase III of the expired nitrogen curve (the alveolar plateau), at which point the composition will be roughly 5% CO_2, 6% H_2O, and the remainder a mixture of oxygen and nitrogen in a ratio that can vary from as much as 0.88 to 0.01 to as little as 0.12 to 0.77. When the oxygen fraction is 0.88, the viscosity of the mixture would be about 197, or 4.7% above room air. During the initial breaths of the washout, the viscosity of the expired gas is lower than that of room air (when the F_{N_2} is 0.77, $\eta = 177$ or 93.8% of room air, and when the F_{N_2} is 0.50, $\eta = 183.7$ or 97.4% of room air). These initial breaths have the greatest effect on the final value of the FRC, because they contain most of the total expired nitrogen. Therefore, during the initial breaths the volume of nitrogen washed out will be underestimated, and during the later breaths it will be overestimated. The error in the final calculated FRC will depend on how rapidly the nitrogen is washed out. If the elimination is rapid, the FRC will be underestimated, and if delayed, it will be overestimated. In either case, the error probably will not exceed ±3%.

If a microprocessor is available that can apply a correction factor to each instantaneous value of flow, the following equations can be used. Even though the equation for viscosity of a gas mixture is alinear in form, if the F_{CO_2} is assumed at 0.05 and the F_{H_2O} at 0.06, this regression equation fits the calculated data well.

$$\eta = 197.1 - 26.5F_{N_2}$$

If these coefficients are divided by 188.6, (the viscosity of room air), the following equation is the correction factor K by which each instantaneous value of flow should be multiplied.

$$K = 1.045 - 0.1405F_{N_2}$$

Calculation of the Anatomical Dead Space

In systems using a pneumotachograph, since a rapid recording of the volume expired and the instantaneous nitrogen concentration is available, the anatomical dead space can be estimated by the method of Fowler (5). The details of this calculation will not be described here. The first several breaths of the washout can be used for multiple calculations, so long as the end expiratory nitrogen concentration remains above 30%. This permits rejection of those expirations with a small tidal volume whose phase III is too small for an accurate calculation of its slope. Calculation of the anatomical dead space is necessary to calculate the alveolar ventilation, a value used in some methods of analysis of the efficiency of pulmonary gas mixing.

Efficiency of Gas Mixing

If the lung were uniformly ventilated, and if tidal volume and frequency were constant during the washout, a plot of the logarithm of nitrogen concentration versus time would be a straight line. The less uniform the distribution of ventilation, the more time will be required for the nitrogen concentration to fall to a specific value.

Many methods have been devised to estimate the efficiency of intrapulmonary gas mixing based on the multiple breath washout curve. The simplest is to record the alveolar nitrogen concentration after 7 minutes of washout. It should be 1.5% or less in a healthy adult. The lung clearance index of Bouhuys (6) is defined as the total ventilation required to wash out the alveolar nitrogen concentration to 2% divided by the FRC. This calculation allows for variations in tidal volume and respiratory frequency.

Although other calculations have been devised to analyze the multiple breath nitrogen clearance curve, none has been generally accepted for clinical use. Some recent references are supplied for the interested reader (7–9).

NORMAL VALUES

There has been no study of lung volumes by the nitrogen washout method in a large number of normal subjects. Nearly identical values are obtained with the nitrogen method and the closed-circuit helium method in normal individuals (3), and, therefore, the same normal predicted values can be used for both methods.

At the end of 7 minutes of nitrogen washout, the end-tidal nitrogen concentration should be less than 1.5% in a normal adult, and the 2-minute nitrogen concentration should be less than 2% in normal children (10).

EXPECTED REPRODUCIBILITY

Duplicate tests of the FRC in normal subjects should agree within 200–400 ml in adults and 100–200 ml in children, whether the tests are done within hours or days.

TROUBLESHOOTING

The two most common sources of error are leaks in the system and malfunction of the nitrogen analyzer (see Quality Control). Isolated erroneous results usually are due to a leak at the mouthpiece. This can sometimes be detected by observing sudden jumps in the end-tidal nitrogen concentration, but a small leak from an inadequate seal of the lips around the mouthpiece may escape notice unless the patient is carefully observed. It may be necessary to help some patients to keep their lips tightly closed. If the test has to be restarted, it is important to wait until the nitrogen stores in the alveoli and the tissues are repleted. Fifteen minutes should be sufficient time for a patient whose washout is not excessively slow, but 30 minutes may be necessary after a prolonged nitrogen washout test.

In computerized systems, inaccurate calibration of the pneumotachograph or incorrect adjustment of the time lag between pneumotachograph and nitrogen analyzer can cause errors. Also, obstructions in the nitrogen sampling line or needle valve, pump malfunction, or a change in the dead space (e.g., a change in the type of mouthpiece) can cause errors because of a change in the time lag between the pneumotachograph flow signal and the instantaneous nitrogen concentration. Such errors may be difficult to detect and correct, so frequent quality control testing is essential.

CONTROVERSIAL ISSUES

Assumed Value of the Initial Alveolar Nitrogen

There is no way of measuring the average alveolar nitrogen concentration at the beginning of the washout, so it must be estimated. The value of 0.81 represents a reasonable estimate for a fasting normal person. Since this concentration varies with the respiratory quotient, 0.80 or 0.79 might represent better estimates if the test is done with nonfasting patients. In patients with obstructive lung disease, there may be poorly ventilated regions in the lung where the nitrogen concentration is much higher. However, the underestimate of the initial alveolar nitrogen is probably offset by an underestimate of the final alveolar nitrogen, since the end-expiratory nitrogen will not be representative of the higher nitrogen concentration in poorly ventilated units. Therefore, the error in the value of $F_{A1} - F_{A2}$ will be relatively small (1). There is no entirely satisfactory solution to this problem, but a possible compromise is to use 0.81 for fasting normal subjects and patients with a prolonged washout time, 0.80 for nonfasting subjects without much delay in the washout, and 0.79 for subjects who hyperventilate during the test ($\dot{V}_E$ greater than 10 liters/min).

Can the Nitrogen Washout Test Be Hazardous?

In some patients with markedly impaired ventilatory drive, it is theoretically possible that significant depression of respiratory drive could occur during the 15 minutes of oxygen breathing required for the prolonged nitrogen washout test. This is unlikely to be a significant concern in the diagnostic pulmonary laboratory, where most of the patients tested are ambulatory or at least sufficiently well to be transported by wheelchair.

Does Breathing High Concentration of O_2 Alter the FRC?

Although most studies have concluded that FRCs determined by the nitrogen washout method give comparable results to other methods, a recent study noted decreases in FRC (an average of 12%) in all 44 subjects after they breathed high concentrations of O_2 for 3–5 minutes (11). Acceptance of these conclusions must await confirmation by additional studies.

REFERENCES

1. Darling RC, Cournand A, Richards DW Jr: Studies on the intrapulmonary mixture of gases: III. An open circuit method for measuring residual air. *J Clin Invest* 19:609–618, 1940.
2. Ross JC, Copher DE, Teays JD, et al.: Functional residual capacity in patients with pulmonary emphysema. *Ann Intern Med* 57:18–28, 1962.
3. Hickman JB, Frayser R: A comparative study of intrapulmonary gas mixing and functional residual capacity in pulmonary emphysema, using helium and nitrogen as the test gases. *J Clin Invest* 37:567–573, 1958.
4. Emmanuel G, Briscoe WA, Cournand A: A method for determination of the volume of air in the lungs: Measurements in chronic pulmonary emphysema. *J Clin Invest* 40:329–337, 1961.
5. Fowler WS: Lung function studies: II. The respiratory dead space. *Am J Physiol* 154:405–416, 1948.
6. Bouhuys A: Pulmonary nitrogen clearance in relation to age in healthy males. *J Appl Physiol* 18:297–300, 1963.
7. Fleming GM, Chester EH, Saniie J, et al.: Ventilation inhomogeneity using multibreath nitrogen washout: Comparison of moment ratios and other indexes. *Am Rev Respir Dis* 121:789–794, 1980.
8. Light RW, George RB, Meneely GR, et al.: A new method for analyzing multiple-breath nitrogen washout curves. *J Appl Physiol* 48:265–272, 1980.
9. Lewis SM, Evans JW, Jalowayski AA: Continuous distributions of specific ventilation recovered from inert gas washout. *J Appl Physiol* 44:416–423, 1978.
10. Zelkowitz PS, Giammona ST: Cystic fibrosis. Pulmonary studies in children, adolescents, and young adults. *Am J Dis Child* 117:543–547, 1969.
11. Garfinkel F, Fitzgerald R: The effect of hyperoxia, hypoxia, and hypercapnia on F.R.C. and occlusion pressure in human subjects. *Respir Physiol* 33:241–250, 1978.

CHAPTER 13

Closed Circuit Helium Dilution Method of Lung Volume Measurement

L. POWELL ZARINS, RCPT

INTRODUCTION

Closed circuit helium dilution is one of the most commonly used methods for the measurement of static lung volumes. The procedure is simple to perform, does not require expensive recording devices, adapts to modular systems, and can be used for bedside measurements. It also allows the functional residual capacity (FRC) to be related directly to other static lung volumes, e.g., residual volume (RV) and total lung capacity (TLC). However, the method is time-consuming, especially when duplicate measurements are required, and it may significantly underestimate thoracic gas volumes in subjects with severe obstructive airway disease.

To perform the dilution procedure, the subject breathes tidally into a spirometer containing a known concentration of helium. Oxygen is added to replace what is consumed metabolically, and CO_2 is absorbed chemically. The gases in the subject's lungs equilibrate with the gases in the spirometer, causing a drop in the system helium concentration; the magnitude of the drop is related to the size of the subject's lung volume at FRC. Recordings of the rate of change of helium concentration (%He/time) may be used to evaluate the efficiency of gas mixing during quiet breathing.

EQUIPMENT

SPIROMETER

The spirometer should be equipped with a blower and a soda lime canister. The dead space of the spirometer should be as small as possible, but the bell should still be capable of recording an inspiratory capacity (IC) of at least 5 liters. Some authors suggest filling the inside of the spirometer with paraffin to reduce the dead space; however, this may change its response characteristics. Alterna-

PULMONARY FUNCTION TESTING
GUIDELINES AND CONTROVERSIES

ISBN 0-12-788125-5

tively, some manufacturers provide a small bell for use during the dilution procedure.

Helium Meter

While mass spectrometers and acoustic helium analyzers can provide quite accurate helium analysis for single breath procedures, they would be impractical for multiple breath dilutions. The gas lost through the sampling port could not be recovered, and this would cause a continual slight drop in system helium concentration. In contrast, thermal conductivity meters return all sampled gas to the system, allowing easy determination of helium equilibration. The thermal conductivity meter should be linear (±0.2% He) over the range of 0–15% helium. Microprocessor systems that automatically calculate the FRC are also available.

Gases

Either 100% helium or 80% helium–20% oxygen (heliox) may be used. In either case, an additional tank of 100% oxygen is also required.

QUALITY CONTROL

The system should be checked before each test for freshness of the dessicant and CO_2 absorber. The spirometer water level should be kept constant to ensure uniform apparatus dead space. All thermal conductivity meters are influenced by changes in concentrations of the background gases (N_2, O_2, CO_2) and are susceptible to damage by excessive moisture. Thus, the dessicant and CO_2 absorber should be renewed before the indicators have completely changed color. If the helium analyzer requires both a CO_2 absorber and a dessicant, the CO_2 absorber should precede the dessicant, since water is a chemical end product of most CO_2 absorbers. If the meter is bypassed when not in use, the dessicant requires less frequent changing.

Leaks

With the blower on, add to the spirometer a mixture of helium and air sufficient to produce a ¾ scale deflection of the helium meter. Next, close the valve at the mouthpiece and place a test weight (110–150 gm, usually supplied by the manufacturer) on the top of the spirometer. Start the kymograph at the slowest paper speed. Except for the initial pen movement caused by compression of the spirometer contents, the volume tracing should remain steady. The spirometer helium concentration should also remain stable (±0.05%) over a 10-minute interval.

Blower Balancing

The blower speed affects the time required for equilibration of helium concentration. The circulation setting will vary among spirometers; values of 500–750 ml/sec are representative. Some spirometers may need to be counter-weighted, so that the bell is stable with respect to atmospheric pressure when the system is open to the room. However, excessive system pressure can cause an artifact in the helium meter, which is often powered by its own pump within the analytical cell.

Linearity of the Meter

Perform the recommended electrical or physical calibration procedure in the manufacturer's maintenance manual.

Linearity of the System

With the blower on, add to the spirometer at 4:1 mixture of helium and oxygen sufficient to cause at least ¾ scale deflection of the meter. Next, bottom the bell, close the mouthpiece valve, and record the helium concentration. Carefully add about 1 liter of air, either by opening the valve and raising the bell or by injecting the air with a calibration syringe. Close the valve quickly and record the helium concentration after equilibration. Continue to add air in 1-liter increments, recording the meter readings after each addition. The exact amount of air added each time can be measured from the spirometer paper. Determine the apparatus dead space (See Calculations) after each addition. No trend in either direction (steady increase or decrease in calculated volume) greater than 5% should be seen (see Table 1).

Table 1 *Sample Linearity Calculations*

Volume added (liter)	He observed (%)	Calculated dead space (liter)
0.0	13.28	—
1.2	10.71	5.00
1.9	9.62	4.99
3.1	8.23	5.05
4.2	7.20	4.97
4.8	6.82	5.07

PROCEDURE

Selection of Oxygen Supply Method

Two methods for adding oxygen are described in the literature: the "simplified" bolus method of Meneely et al. (1) and the volume-stabilized method of McMichael (2). With the former method, a bolus of oxygen (a 7- to 10-minute supply) is added to the spirometer after the initial helium concentration reading is recorded. The subject then rebreathes the spirometer gas until the bolus of oxygen initially added is consumed, as indicated by the return of the subject's end-tidal point to the baseline level, and a final helium concentration reading is taken. With the volume-stabilized method, oxygen is supplied continuously; the flow is adjusted during the procedure to match the subject's oxygen uptake.

While both methods for supplying oxygen are considered accurate, the simplicity of the bolus method is offset by several disadvantages. The oxygen supply may be consumed before equilibration takes place, in which case it may be necessary to add more. Also, the constantly changing inspired oxygen concentration (F_IO_2) may affect breathing patterns (3). Finally, there is less assurance that equilibration has actually occurred, because the volume of the system is changing continually. In contrast, the volume-stabilized method requires adjustment of the oxygen supply during the procedure, but the study may be carried out as long as necessary and the F_IO_2 remains stable.

Equipment Preparation

Warm up equipment, check blower balance and water level, change dessicant and CO_2 absorber if necessary, and add test gases to the spirometer. The exact amounts of test gases added will vary according to the apparatus dead space, the range of the helium meter, and the method of oxygen supply. Ideally, the initial helium concentration should produce at least a ¾ scale deflection of the meter, and the spirometer capacity should be adequate to allow the measurement of an inspiratory capacity or expiratory reserve volume at the end of the procedure. Oxygen should be added to bring the F_IO_2 to 21%.

Subject Preparation

To achieve a steady rate of O_2 consumption, the subject should sit quietly prior to testing. Instruct the subject to breathe in a manner that ensures a stable breathing level, representative of the subject's usual FRC. Explain the importance of a tight seal around the mouthpiece and demonstrate the inspiratory capacity maneuver, if it is to be used during the test.

Helium Dilution Procedure

1. Attach noseclips and instruct the subject to breathe quietly on the two-way valve. Record the initial helium concentration.
2. At the subject's end-tidal point, as determined by observation of the thoracic cage movements or by detection of cessation of flow at the valve, turn the valve from the room air position to the spirometer position.
3. The procedure varies at this point, depending on which method of oxygen supply is used.
   a. If the O_2 bolus technique is used, observe the spirometer tracing, which will rise steadily to the baseline level as oxygen is consumed. When the baseline level is reached, instruct the subject to perform an expiratory reserve volume (ERV) maneuver, and switch the two-way valve back to the room air position. Allow time for gas equilibration within the system, and record the final meter reading.
   b. If the volume-stabilized method is used, adjust the oxygen flow to maintain a constant spirometer volume at the end-tidal point. To speed equilibration, ask the subject to perform an inspiratory capacity (IC) maneuver every 30 seconds; observe the meter reading after each maneuver. When no change greater than $\pm 0.05\%$ is seen in helium concentration after two maneuvers 30 seconds apart (allowing time for meter lag), record one final IC maneuver and switch the valve back to the room air postion. Again allow time for system gas equilibration before recording the final meter reading.

The output from the helium meter can be graphed by a recorder, and only the initial and final readings need to be hand-recorded. If a recorder is not available, it is advisable to record the readings by hand every 15 seconds during the procedure. It may also be possible to record a vital capacity at the end of the dilution procedure, thus relating the FRC to both the TLC *and* the RV. However, care must be taken not to exceed the volume limits of the spirometer.

CALCULATIONS

Determination of the Apparatus Dead Space

The original Meneely method (1) required exact helium volumes and concentrations for calculation of the dead space volume of the apparatus (V_{ds}). Since some of the meters presently in use display expanded scale units instead of percent concentration readings, it is now common practice to use the ratio of the final concentration to the drop in concentration for these calculations.

Check the water level; calibrate and zero the meter. Bottom the spirometer bell. Add enough helium (along with one part O_2 for every four parts He) to cause at least a ¾ scale deflection of the meter. Bottom the spirometer bell and record the meter reading (C_1). Carefully add a volume of air by raising the bell smoothly, then quickly close the valve (V added). Record the second meter reading (C_2). Repeat this procedure three times and calculate the mean of three estimates as follows:

$$V_{ds} = \frac{C_2 \text{ (V added)}}{C_1 - C_2}$$

The apparatus dead space should be recalculated whenever the large CO_2 absorber is changed. Laboratories that use electronic spirometers or the O_2 bolus method may wish to incorporate the dead space measurement into the dilution procedure, as described by Ruegg and Reynolds (4). This practice would allow rapid and frequent checks of system dead space. However, measurement discrimination may be adversely affected by the low (less than 10%) helium concentration at the beginning of the helium dilution procedure, unless additional helium is carefully added to the spirometer prior to beginning the dilution.

Determination of FRC

FRC is calculated from the following equation:

$$\text{FRC (uncorr)} = \frac{(C_1 - C_2)\,(V_{ds} + V_{added})}{C_2} - V_{mp}$$

where C_1 is the initial helium meter reading; C_2 the final helium meter reading; V_{ds} the apparatus dead space; V_{added} the volume of air and helium added to the spirometer at the beginning of the procedure; and V_{mp} the volume of the mouthpiece deadspace.

Errors may occur in switching subjects into the closed system; subjects may also exhibit erratic breathing patterns, which may complicate the procedure. Three cases are presented, with suggestions for handling them.

Case 1

The subject is switched into the spirometer system at a point above his end-tidal level; his end-tidal point remains stable throughout the procedure (see Fig. 1). If using the bolus method, terminate the study at the switch-in level of the tidal breath. If using the volume-stabilized method, maintain the switch-in level throughout the study. With both methods, when reporting the FRC, subtract the amount of air in excess of the true FRC (BTPS). In both cases illustrated (Fig. 1a

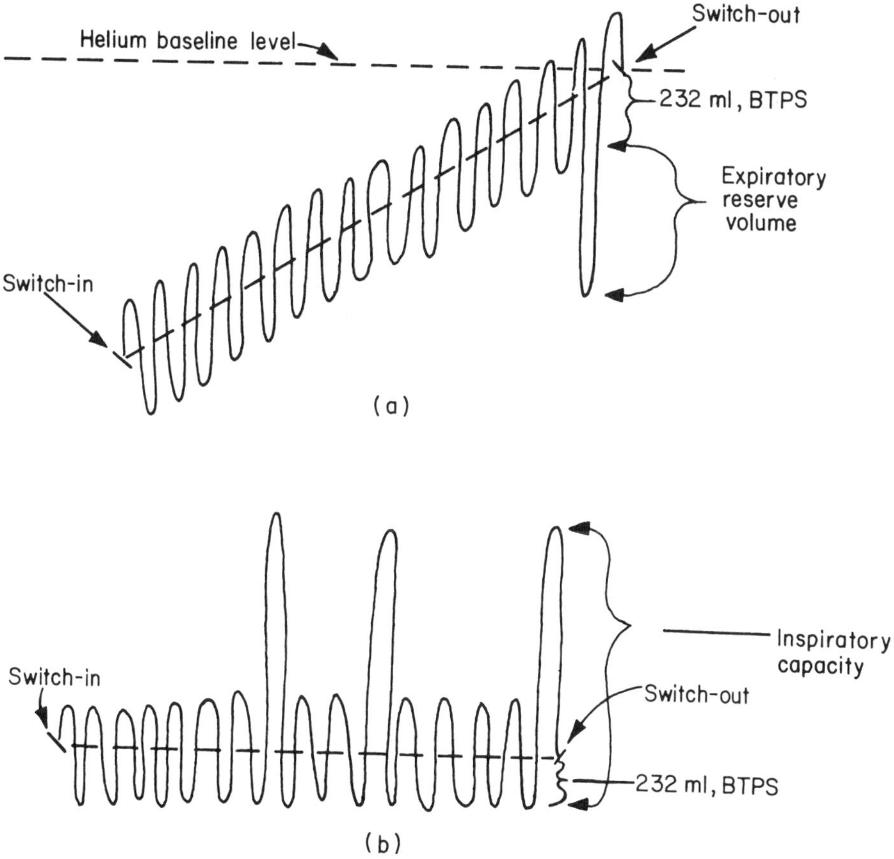

Fig. 1 *(a) Switching error using oxygen bolus method. (b) Switching error using volume-stabilized method.*

and 1b), 232 ml should be subtracted from the calculated FRC; the inspiratory capacity and expiratory reserve volumes, respectively, should be calculated from the actual end-tidal point.

Case 2

The subject is switched into the spirometer system at the end-tidal point; however, his end-tidal level fluctuates erratically during the procedure. With both O_2 supply methods, one should coach the patient to relax his chest muscles during expiration, so that his breathing level stabilizes by the end of the procedure. With the bolus method, the study must be terminated when the subject's end-tidal point crosses the baseline level, regardless of how much it has deviated from the beginning level. Record an expiratory reserve volume before switching out. With the volume-stabilized method, it is possible to correct for fluctuations in end-tidal point by adding or withholding oxygen; try to keep the level very stable during the last minute of the procedure and record an inspiratory capacity before switching out.

Case 3

The subject was switched into the system at the end-tidal point, the end-tidal point was stable during the procedure, but the valve was switched out above the end-tidal point. No correction is required with either method. Once true equilibration has occurred, helium concentration is independent of bell position.

Corrections to the FRC

There are numerous "corrections" that can be applied to the calculated FRC (see Controversies). Regardless of which of these corrections is valid, the laboratory should either follow the calculation protocol of the authors of the study used to predict normal lung volumes or, conversely, correct those normal predictive values so that they correspond to the laboratory's protocol. Otherwise, errors in prediction may occur.

NORMAL VALUES

The following are the most widely used studies offering normal static lung volumes. None of the studies excluded smokers, and although it was not consistently specified by all authors, it is assumed that all of the subjects were whites of European descent.

1. Boren, Kory, and Syner (5). Test site: several VA hospitals. Altitude: 0–1524 m (0–5000 ft). Subjects: 422 males. Method: Meneely et al. (1). Posture: Semirecumbent. Corrections: −75 ml nitrogen increment; −125 ml helium absorption; + standard BTPS correction.
2. Goldman and Becklake (6). Test site: Johannesburg, South Africa. Altitude: 1737 m (5700 ft). Subjects: 44 males, 50 females. Method: McMichael (2); Briscoe et al. (7). Posture: Seated. Corrections: −30 ml respiratory quotient; −70 ml helium absorption; + BTPS correction. (Reported FRC's include mouthpiece dead space.)
3. Grimby and Soderholm (8). Test site: Goteborg, Sweden. Altitude: sea level. Subjects: 152 males, 58 females. Method: Soderholm (9). Posture: seated. Corrections: −100 ml helium absorption; + BTPS correction.
4. Needham, Rogan, and McDonald (10). Test site: Aberdeen, Scotland.

Altitude: sea level. Subjects: 183 men, 141 women. Method: Bates and Christie (11). Posture: seated. Corrections: None (*no* BTPS correction).

EXPECTED REPRODUCIBILITY

The published standard deviations of repeated helium dilution FRC measurements range from 90 to 160 ml (1, 12, 13). The system variability alone, as calculated from repeated apparatus dead space measurements, accounts for 80 ml of this value (12). Schaaning et al. (12) estimated the "95% tolerance limits" for detecting a real change in FRC at 340 ml, based on two sets of duplicate measurements. In a study in progress at the University of California, San Diego, the inspiratory capacity was measured in 57 healthy males immediately before the end of the dilution procedure; TLC was calculated as the sum of the FRC and IC, as recommended by Hathirat et al. (14). The 95% confidence limits (mean difference between duplicate measurements, ±2 SD) for detecting a change in TLC were ±340 ml; for FRC these limits were ±520 ml. These results indicate that the TLC may be more reproducible than the FRC and should be measured directly whenever possible. A 5-minute interval is recommended between studies; severely obstructed subjects may require an even longer interval.

TROUBLESHOOTING

The most common problem encountered is leakage of gas between the mouth and valve, around the noseclip, or occasionally through a perforated eardrum. This leakage will cause a steady rate of fall in helium concentration, with no trend toward equilibration. The CO_2 absorber, when chemically exhausted, will permit buildup of CO_2 in the system, causing changes in the subject's respiratory pattern, and also introducing some error in helium meter readings. Moisture in the helium meter or excessive blower pressure in the system will also cause fluctuating or erroneous meter readings.

CONTROVERSIAL ISSUES

Corrections to the Measured FRC

BTPS Factor

Although the practice is not universal (10), the majority of investigators correct the calculated lung volume from ATPS to BTPS. Studies to resolve this issue definitively have not been published. (This correction adds about 8% to the FRC.)

Helium Absorption

Some helium is absorbed into the bloodstream during the rebreathing procedure; estimates of the quantity absorbed vary. The average correction is −60 ml.

Respiratory Quotient (RQ), Nitrogen Increment

Because oxygen uptake usually exceeds CO_2 output in the lung, the helium concentrations in the lung are higher than those in the spirometer. In addition, the concentrations of background gases (N_2, O_2) are altered during the rebreathing procedure, and thus there is more nitrogen in the spirometer at the end of the test than in the beginning. The average *combined* correction for these two factors is −100 ml (1).

These corrections were evaluated as part of a study in progress at the University of California, San Diego. In 125 healthy subjects, ages 20–80, the mean plethysmographic FRC was 3065 ml, and the mean helium FRC (uncorr) was 2920 ml. The helium FRC (uncorr) values were then corrected to BTPS, and 100 ml was subtracted for He absorption and RQ. These are approximately the same corrections reported by Goldman and Becklake (6). The mean corrected helium FRC was 3050 ml. If the plethysmographic results are used as primary standards, the good agreement between the two FRC methods (plethysmograph-corrected He) seems to validate the simultaneous application of the BTPS, He absorption, and RQ corrections. However, the absolute correction to the mean FRC, + 130 ml, would not be considered clinically significant.

Criteria for Cessation of Test

The NIH Epidemiology Standardization Project (15) recommended that, with the volume-stabilized method, studies be terminated after 7 minutes or at that point when helium concentration does not change by more than 0.02% in a 30-second interval. As some meters may not be able to discriminate such a small concentration drop, it is recommended that tests be terminated when there is no change greater than 0.05% over a 60-second interval. This should be the equivalent of the NIH standard. (Allow time for meter lag.)

Usefulness of Inspiratory Capacity Maneuvers

During the dilution procedure, the ventilatory pattern can influence the equilibration time and, in some cases, the accuracy of the results, especially when the subject has poorly communicating airspaces. Two papers in the literature (12, 16) indicate that when vital capacity maneuvers are performed during the study, the helium FRCs compare well with the plethysmographic FRCs in obstructed subjects. However, this has not been documented in patients with severe chronic obstructive lung disease or bullous emphysema. Studies to date have not defined which, if any, indices of airways obstruction correlate well enough with the degree of unreliability of helium dilution values to serve as good "contraindicators" for the procedure.

Full vital capacity maneuvers may be difficult to obtain and may cause airway closure in some subjects. Therefore, we recommend incorporation of *inspiratory* capacity maneuvers. They will shorten the period required for equilibration and may increase the accuracy of the measurement. Since they may also alter the oxygen consumption rate and the shape of the dilution curve, however, they should be omitted in studies in which the rate of oxygen consumption or gas mixing is being calculated.

Effect of the CO_2 Absorber on Measured ERV

One equipment manufacturer recommends correcting the expiratory reserve volume by +5% for the expired CO_2 that is removed by the chemical absorber (17). When a calibration syringe containing 5% CO_2 is injected into a blower-driven spirometer circuit equipped with a CO_2 absorber, a 5% drop in measured volumes can indeed be demonstrated. In practice, however, the drop in measured volume is probably related to the mean expired CO_2, the surface area of the absorber, and the speed with which the expired air is introduced into the circuit. Therefore, accurate corrections for CO_2 absorption may require evaluation with the specific equipment and rates of expiration used in clinical testing. We suggest that each laboratory evaluate its own system until more specific data become available.

REFERENCES

1. Meneely GR, Ball CO, Kory RC, et al.: A simplified closed circuit helium dilution method for the determination of the residual volume of the lungs. *Am J Med* 28:824–831, 1960.
2. McMichael J: A rapid method of determining lung capacity. *Clin Sci* 4:167–173, 1939.
3. Garfinkel F, Fitzgerald RS: The effect of hyperoxia, hypoxia, and hypercapnia on F.R.C. and occlusion pressure in human subjects. *Respir Physiol* 33:241–250, 1978.
4. Ruegg WR, Reynolds GP: A procedure for the measurement of lung volumes by helium dilution. *Analyzer* 10:18–22, 1980.
5. Boren HG, Kory C, Syner JC: The Veteran's Administration-Army cooperative study of pulmonary function: II. The lung volume and its subdivisions in normal man. *Am J Med* 41:96–114, 1966.
6. Goldman HI, Becklake MR: Respiratory function tests; normal values at median altitudes and the prediction of normal results. *Am Rev Tuberc* 79:457–467, 1959.

7. Briscoe WA, Becklake MR, Rose TF: Intrapulmonary mixing of helium in normal and emphysematous subjects. *Clin Sci* 10:37-51, 1951.
8. Grimby G, Soderholm B: Spirometric studies in normal subjects: III. Static lung volumes and maximum voluntary ventilation in adults with a note on physical fitness. *Acta Med Scand* 173:199-206, 1963.
9. Soderholm B: The hemodynamics of the lesser circulation in pulmonary tuberculosis. *Scand J Clin Lab Invest*, suppl. 26, 31-32, 1957.
10. Needham CD, Rogan MC, McDonald I: Normal standards for lung volumes, intrapulmonary gas-mixing, and maximum breathing capacity. *Thorax* 9:313-325, 1954.
11. Bates DV, Christie RV: Intrapulmonary mixing of helium in health and in emphysema. *Clin Sci* 9:17-27, 1950.
12. Schaanning CG, Gulsvik A: Accuracy and precision of helium dilution technique and body plethysmography in measuring lung volumes. *Scand J Clin Lab Invest* 32:271-277, 1973.
13. Holmgren A: Determination of the functional residual volume by means of the helium dilution method. *Scand J Clin Lab Invest* 6:131-136, 1954.
14. Hathirat S, Renzetti AD, Mitchell M: Measurement of the total lung capacity by helium dilution in a constant volume system. *Am Rev Respir Dis* 102:760-770, 1970.
15. Ferris BG (principle investigator): Epidemiology standardization project. *Am Rev Respir Dis* 118 (pt 2):1978.
16. Reichel G: Differences between intrathoracic gas measured by the body plethysmograph and functional residual capacity determined by gas dilution methods. *Prog Respir Res* 4:188-193. 1969.
17. *Instructions for Use of the Godart Pulmonet Type 114*. Godart Manufacturing Co., Bilthoven, Holland.

CHAPTER 14

Body Plethysmography

L. POWELL ZARINS, RCPT
JACK L. CLAUSEN, M.D.

Plethysmography is the most rapid and accurate method of measuring absolute lung volumes. The plethysmograph ("body box") measures the total compressible gas volume in the thorax, and its accuracy is not affected by the presence of poorly ventilated airspaces, which often causes the gas dilution techniques to underestimate lung volume.

A body box also provides a method of measuring *airway* resistance (R_{aw}), which, along with pulmonary tissue resistance (R_{ti}) and chest wall resistance (R_{cw}), make up the total *respiratory* resistance (R_L). *Respiratory* resistance ($R_{aw} + R_{cw} + R_{ti}$) can be measured without a plethysmograph by the forced oscillation technique, but suitable instrumentation has not been readily available. *Pulmonary* resistance ($R_{aw} + R_{ti}$) can also be measured without a plethysmograph, but the necessity of introducing an esophageal balloon limits the clinical application of the method. *Airway* resistance, however, may be measured rapidly and noninvasively with standard plethysmographic equipment.

In clinical laboratories, the constant-volume variable-pressure type of plethysmograph ("pressure box") is most commonly used. It consists of a large chamber, a pneumotachograph, and three transducers, which measure changes in box pressure (ΔP_{box}), mouth pressure (ΔP_{mo}), and flow at the mouth ($\dot{V}$). The subject, seated in the closed chamber, breathes through a special mouthpiece–shutter assembly. At end-expiration, the shutter is closed to occlude the mouthpiece, and the subject is asked to rhythmically compress and decompress his thorax by panting lightly against the closed shutter. While the shutter is closed, no airflow occurs within the airways, so mouth pressure changes (ΔP_{mo}) are equal to alveolar pressure changes (ΔP_{alv}). Also, during this maneuver, the changes in box pressure reflect the changes in thoracic volume, and are proportional to the changes in alveolar gas pressure. The linearity of the inverse relationship of mouth pressure and box pressure is preserved (for small changes in pressure), because conditions in the respiratory system are isothermal. Thus, Boyle's law ($P_1 V_1 = P_2 V_2$), can be applied to these pressure–volume changes to

PULMONARY FUNCTION TESTING
GUIDELINES AND CONTROVERSIES

ISBN 0-12-788125-5

calculate the volume being compressed, the subject's thoracic gas volume (TGV).

For measurements of airway resistance, the same shallow panting technique is employed, in order to keep the subject's glottis open and prevent respiratory temperature artifacts in the box. While the subject pants through the open mouthpiece, flow at the mouth and the corresponding cyclical changes in box pressure are recorded. The shutter is then closed briefly for TGV measurement. The ratio of alveolar pressure to thoracic compression ($\Delta P_{mo}/\Delta P_{box}$, shutter closed) is divided by the ratio of airflow at the mouth to thoracic compression ($\dot{V}/\Delta P_{box}$, shutter open). The quotient represents the airway resistance.

"Pressure" boxes measure compressive volume changes of the thorax from the changes in plethysmographic pressure during panting; "volume" or "flow" plethysmographs measure changes in thoracic volume directly with a spirometer or an integrated pneumotachograph connected to an outlet in the box wall. The volume signal thus obtained must be modified by a special circuit to correct for transient box pressure increases caused by the impedance of the spirometer or pneumotachograph. Both large and small thoracic volume changes at high and low frequencies can be measured with volume boxes. For example, inspiratory capacity or forced expiratory flow rates can be recorded immediately after measurement of the TGV. However, the advantages of volume boxes are offset by the cost and complexity of the required equipment, so they have not been widely used for routine clinical applications. Therefore, the remainder of this chapter will apply to variable-pressure plethysmographs only.

EQUIPMENT

Plethysmographic equipment may be purchased either as a package or as separate components. Generally, it is not advisable to attempt to select and assemble components for a plethysmographic system unless the compatibility of all equipment has been demonstrated.

The box itself is usually constructed of Plexiglas or special plywood, and carefully engineered to meet the acoustic criteria required for accurate measurements. The pneumotachograph selected for airway resistance measurements should be linear over the range of 0.2 to 1.5 liter/sec. Both solenoid and air-actuated shutter assemblies are available; the latter is quieter. The distal end of the shutter assembly must interface smoothly with the pneumotachograph to avoid turbulence or jet-streaming of the air entering the pneumotachograph. Three differential-pressure transducers are needed, to measure ΔP_{box} (range = ± 2 cm H_2O for a 530-liter box), ΔP_{mo} (range = ± 25–50 cm H_2O), and $\dot{V}$ (appropriate pressure range for the pneumotachograph selected). A rapid-response instrument for displaying or recording X–Y data plots is also needed.

From the image on a storage oscilloscope, direct measurements of angles can be made, using a special transparent rotating protractor. For recordings of the actual angles, either Polaroid photographs of oscilloscope images or recorders utilizing light-sensitive paper and a cathode-ray tube may be used. Although mechanical (servo-type) recorders can also be used, they may introduce distortion at high frequencies. Several calibrating devices are required: a 30-cc variable-speed oscillating piston pump for the box-pressure transducer, a slant-gauge manometer or U-tube for the mouth-pressure transducer, and a rotameter for the pneumotachograph (0–1.5 liter/sec).

Microprocessor systems are available for semiautomatic control of the shutter and recording system. These systems may be designed for automated calculation of data.

QUALITY CONTROL

Component Evaluation and Calibration

Body Box

The solenoid or hand-operated vent should be opened whenever the box door is opened or closed. Otherwise, the transducer may be damaged by the excessive pressure change. Also, to lessen the effect of atmospheric pressure fluctuations, the atmospheric side of the box transducer may be damped by connecting it to a container, such as a 20-liter (5-gallon) water bottle, that has a high-resistance vent open to the room [e.g., an 18-gauge needle or cotton-stuffed tubing (1)]. Most non-air-conditioned boxes also require the installation of a high-resistance thermal leak to compensate for the observed steady increase in box pressure caused by the subject's body heat. The leak usually consists of a piece of small-bore tubing (e.g., 6.3 mm internal diameter) that vents to the atmosphere. The length of the tubing must be determined experimentally, so that after a subject has been closed in the box for 30 to 60 seconds, the thermal drift is minimal, whereas the pressure signals from the 30-cc calibration pump are equivalent at 1, 2, and 3 Hz. The stability of the signals between 1 and 3 Hz should be checked periodically, as door seals may develop leaks with aging.

Calibration of Transducers

Transducers should be checked initially and at regular intervals (every 6 months) for linearity and freedom from drift and excessive noise. Daily, each transducer should be calibrated physically (e.g., using a 30-cc piston pump for box pressure, a rotameter for flows, and a manometer for mouth pressure), using ranges encountered in clinical measurements. If an X–Y display is used for calculations, and the relationship P_{mo}/P_{box} is defined as an angle, the gains of the channels should be set so that most TGV angles encountered in clinical use will be near 45°. To measure lung volumes in the 1–4 liter range, the following are representative calibration settings for a 550-liter pressure box: P_{mo}: 2.5 cm deflection for 5 cm of water; $\dot{V}$: 2.5 cm deflection for 1 liter/sec flow; P_{box}: 5 cm deflection during calibration with a 30-cc oscillating pump.

Pneumotachograph-Shutter Assembly

One may determine the resistance of the entire assembly from the mouthpiece to the distal end of the pneumotachograph by measuring the pressure drop across it at flows of 0.2, 0.5, and 1.0 liter/sec. This resistance (R_{sys}) is subtracted from the subject's calculated airway resistance (see Calculations section). R_{sys} must be checked periodically, since the fine screens of some pneumotachographs may become partially occluded.

Evaluation of the Entire System

Accuracy of Volume Measurements

To evaluate the accuracy of volume measurements, the recommended approach is to use an isothermal lung model as a reference standard. A description of a suitable lung model follows:

Assemble a rigid 3- to 4-liter container with two outlets (e.g., 4-liter glass Erlenmeyer flask with two-holed rubber stopper; see Fig. 1). If both outlets of the container are on the top, attach small-diameter tubing from one outlet to the bottom of the container (see Fig. 1). Measure the volume of the container (± 2%) by water displacement and fill it evenly with a known volume (mass/density) of metal wool (copper, steel, or aluminum), which will absorb the heat of compression. If the total weight of the wool is insufficient or the mesh of the wool is too coarse (not enough surface area), temperature increases will not be prevented, and plethysmographic estimates of the flask volume will be erroneously low. Attach a 60- to 100-cc rubber bulb to the flask outlet that has tubing extending into the bottle, and connect the other flask outlet as closely as possible to the mouthpiece-shutter assembly. The volume within the bulb and tubing should be included in the calculation of total flask volume. A seated subject holds the lung model inside the closed box. P_{mo}/P_{box} is displayed on the X–Y loop screen. When the shutter is closed, the subject holds his breath and compresses the lung model by squeezing the bulb at approximately 2 Hz. Several volume measurements are recorded, and the measured volume is calculated as if it were TGV, except that ambient pressure is not corrected for water-vapor pressure (i.e., 1030 cm H_2O is used instead of 970 cm H_2O at sea level). Compare the known gas volume of the system (subtract the volume of the metal wool) with the

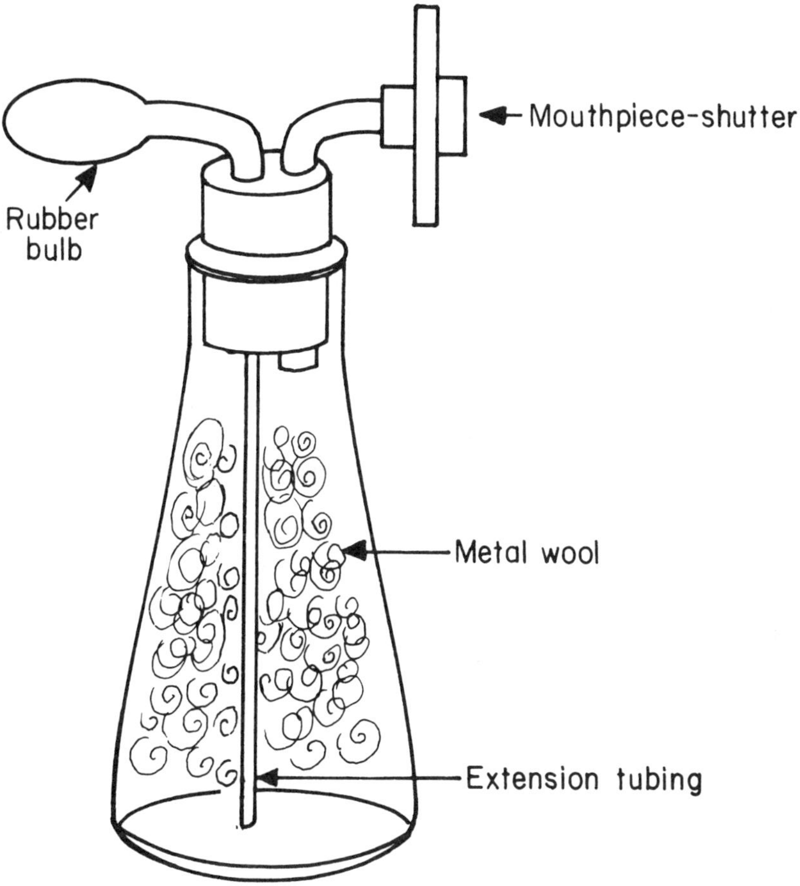

Fig. 1 *Lung model.*

plethysmographically measured volume. If the volume of the lung model is underestimated, pressure changes secondary to increases in temperature may be occurring. To correct this, add more metal wool to the flask and repeat the measurements. (It is instructive to construct a graph of wool added/volume measured). Known volumes and measured volumes should agree within 5%.

An oscillating pump may be substituted for the bulb if the crankshaft end of the piston is open to the box. Most standard body box calibrating pumps do not meet this requirement (see reference 2 for more details).

Accuracy of Airway Resistance Measurements

The following procedure demonstrates the ability of the body box system to accurately measure known increases in airway resistance, as suggested by

DuBois et al. (3). However, because of the possible effects of external resistive loads on lung volumes and airway resistance, this method may not be valid for resistances greater than 5 cm H_2O/liter/sec.

Materials Obtain several 9–10 cm length cardboard tubes of the same diameter as the pneumotachograph (disposable mouthpieces work well), a large number of nonheparinized glass micro-hematocrit tubes, a similar number of wooden sticks (e.g., handles of cotton swabs), and a small amount of ordinary glue.

Methods To construct a flow resistor, fill one of the cardboard tubes with a 50:50 mixture of wooden sticks and hematocrit tubes evenly dispersed. Apply glue as needed but avoid occluding the glass tubes. With a differential-pressure transducer, measure the pressure drop across the resistor at flows of 0.2, 0.5, and 1.0/liter/sec. Construct additional resistors, varying the proportion of tubes and sticks in order to cover a resistance range of 0.5–5.0 cm H_2O/liter/sec. The resistances should be constant (± 10%) at flow rates between 0.2 and 0.5 liter/sec. To measure the resistances with the plethysmograph, measure the resistance of a normal subject panting through an empty cardboard tube inserted between the subject and the mouthpiece connector of the pneumotachograph–shutter assembly. Then substitute each of the resistors in turn, measuring the resultant increases in total resistances. The predicted increases should agree within 20% of those measured by the plethysmograph for resistances less than 5 cm H_2O/liter/sec.

PROCEDURE

At least once a day, physically calibrate the transducers. Seat the subject in the box and demonstrate the shutter mechanism and proper panting technique. Encourage him to relax his chest during tidal breathing so that his end-tidal point will represent his usual FRC. Adjust the noseclips and mouthpiece, vent the box, and close the door.

Display $\dot{V}/P_{box}$ (“open loops”) on the oscilloscope screen. When the subject is breathing tidally, the $\dot{V}/P_{box}$ tracing usually moves in a counterclockwise loop, going off the screen to the right with the increase in box pressure during inspiration, and returning onto the screen with expiration. Both the TGV and R_{aw} panting maneuvers should begin at the point when the tracing returns to zero flow at the end of expiration. Expiration of heated air during tidal breathing may cause some artifact in the box pressure signal. Wait for the box pressure to stabilize; a slight inflection point may be noted when the subject pauses at FRC. Observation of the synchronization of the subject's thoracic movements with the tracing on the screen helps to identify the end-expiratory point. At end-expiration, ask the subject to pant lightly. If the loops are of appropriate size and frequency (± 0.5–1.0 liter/sec, 1–2 Hz), record two of them, then close the shutter, change the Y-axis input from $\dot{V}$ to P_{mo} and record one or more TGV ("closed" loops). Repeat three times.

For FRC measurement, display P_{mo}/P_{box} on the screen. At the subject's end-tidal point, close the shutter and ask him to pant. Record one or two loops; repeat three times. TLC may be measured directly by measuring the inspiratory capacity with a spirometer or integrating the flow signal from the pneumotachograph immediately after the TGV panting maneuver (4). If an external spirometer is used, vent the box during the inspiratory capacity maneuver. Otherwise, the pressure changes may be uncomfortable to the patient and may damage the transducer.

CALCULATIONS

Measurement of Angles

The "shutter-closed" loops (TGV) are usually linear, although a small amount of hysteresis is occasionally observed. These angles should be drawn from endpoint to endpoint (Fig. 2a).

In normal subjects, the "shutter-*open*" (R_{aw}) loops are usually linear (inspiratory and expiratory resistances are the same) with only a small amount of hysteresis. In some patients, loops have a sigmoid shape secondary to turbulence at higher flow rates, and a variety of different angles may be drawn. In the case illustrated (Fig. 2b), the resistances calculated at the two different flow rates shown would be 2.0 and 4.0 cm H_2O/liter/sec. Therefore, it is necessary to standardize (or specify) the flow rates at which resistance is measured; it is recommended that resistances be calculated at 0.5 liter/sec.

Figure 2c illustrates the R_{aw} loops of a patient whose resistance during expiration is significantly larger than during inspiration. If a single value of resistance is reported, choose the inspiratory value; otherwise, both inspiratory and expiratory values should be identified.

Figure 2d illustrates the two different angles that could be constructed for measuring the expiratory resistance at 0.5 liter/sec in a loop with hysteresis during expiration. Although hysteresis can result from technical problems, it is a typical finding in patients with obstructive airway disease. Expiratory hysteresis as shown in Fig. 2d is frequently seen in patients with emphysema. To increase the sensitivity and improve consistency in resistance measurements, the angle should be constructed through the later part of expiration if expiratory resistance is measured from such a tracing (see Controversies).

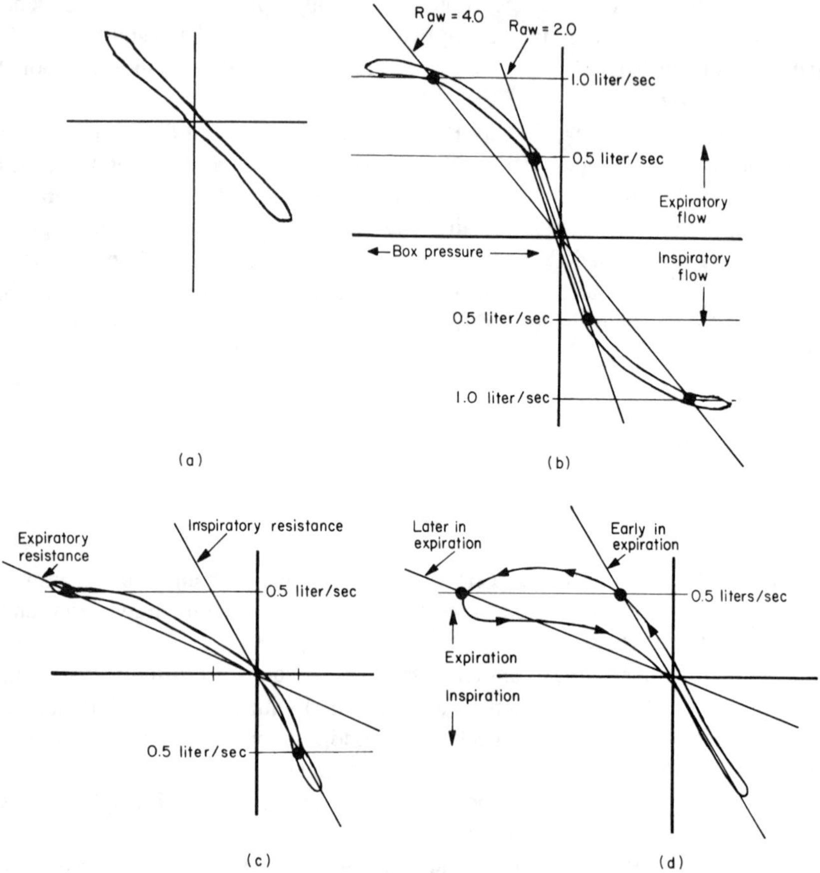

Fig. 2 *Plethysimographic loops for (a) TGV and (b,c,d) R_{aw}.*

Equations

$$R_{aw} = \left[\left(\frac{P_{mo\ (c)}}{P_{mo\ (d)}} \right) \left(\frac{\dot{V}_{(d)}}{\dot{V}_{(c)}} \right) \left(\frac{\tan P_{mo}/P_{box} <}{\tan \dot{V}/P_{box} <} \right) \right] - R_{sys}$$

$$TGV = \frac{\left(\frac{P_{box\ (c)}}{P_{box\ (d)}} \right) \left(\frac{P_{mo\ (d)}}{P_{mo\ (c)}} \right) (P_{atmos} - P_{H_2O})\ (SVC)}{\tan\ (P_{mo}/P_{box} <)}$$

where

$P_{mo\ (c)}$ = calibration pressure (cm H_2O)

$P_{mo\ (d)}$ = calibration signal deflection (mm)
$P_{box\ (c)}$ = calibration volume (cc)
$P_{box\ (d)}$ = calibration signal deflection (mm)
$\dot{V}_{(c)}$ = calibration flow (liter/sec)
$\dot{V}_{(d)}$ = calibration signal deflection (mm)
$<$ = observed angle
R_{sys} = resistance of the system
P_{atmos} = atmospheric pressure, cm H_2O
P_{H_2O} = water vapor pressure at 37° C cm H_2O
SVC = subject volume correction (see the following equation)

Unless the box calibration is done with the subject sitting inside, the following correction factor should be used:

$$SVC = \frac{\text{Box volume (liters)} - \dfrac{\text{Subject's weight (kg)}}{1.07}}{\text{Box volume (liters)}}$$

where 1.07 is the assumed density of human body.

Sample Calculations

$P_{mo(c)} = 5.0$ cm H_2O $\quad P_{box(c)} = 30$ cc $\quad \dot{V}_{(c)} = 1.0$ liter/sec
$P_{mo(d)} = 27$ mm $\quad P_{box(d)} = 49$ mm $\quad \dot{V}_{(d)} = 24$ mm
Box volume = 530 liters $\quad$ Subject's weight = 80 kg $\quad P_{atmos} = 1010$ cm H_2O
Tan $P_{mo}/P_{box} <(32°) = 0.625$ $\quad$ Tan $\dot{V}/P_{box} <(63°) = 1.96$
$R_{sys} = 0.4$ cm H_2O/liter/sec $\quad P_{H_2O} = 63$ cm H_2O

$$R_{aw} = \left[\left(\frac{5.0}{27}\right)\left(\frac{24}{1.0}\right)\left(\frac{0.625}{1.96}\right)\right] - 0.4 = 1.02 \text{ cm } H_2O\text{/liter/sec}$$

$$TGV = \frac{\left(\frac{30}{49}\right)\left(\frac{27}{5.0}\right)(1010 - 63)\left[\frac{530 - (80/1.07)}{530}\right]}{0.625} = 4300 \text{ ml}$$

The mean of three TGV angles is used in calculations. However, the airway resistances should not be determined from mean angles, but calculated separately and the mean of three values determined. Alternatively, the airway resistance measured at the TGV that is closest to the subject's FRC may be selected for report.

Airway resistance, in a normal individual, is known to decrease with increasing lung volume. To provide a volume-standardized airway resistance measurement, the conductance (G_{aw}, the reciprocal of resistance) is divided by the TGV at which the R_{aw} was measured, to yield the specific conductance, SG_{aw}.

NORMAL VALUES

Static Lung Volumes

There are no published studies available that used the plethysmograph for measurements of lung volumes in adequately defined groups of normal adult subjects. Since FRCs determined by plethysmographic and helium dilution techniques agree well in normal subjects, the regression equations derived from gas dilution techniques can be used. (See Chapter 13.)

Airway Resistance

Currently, there are not enough studies of airway resistance in nonsmoking healthy adults for derivation of satisfactory normal limits. In a study of 60 healthy females aged 20–26, Brunes and Holgren (5) reported a mean R_{aw} of 1.51 ± 0.40 (± 1 SD), and a mean SG_{AW} of 0.25 ± 0.07. R_{aw} was not significantly related to the height, weight, body surface area (BSA), or static lung volumes.

Skoogh reported a significant correlation between G_{aw} (measured at TLC minus 55% VC) and TGV in 56 nonsmoking adults (6). However, the observed scatter limits the usefulness of predicting normal values for G_{aw} based on TGV; R_{aw} at FRC was not reported.

From reviews of published and unpublished data (5–7) the following normal ranges are suggested:

$$R_{aw} = 0.2\text{–}2.5$$
$$G_{aw} = 0.4\text{–}5.0$$
$$SG_{aw} = 0.112\text{–}0.400$$

REPRODUCIBILITY

FRC

DuBois et al. (8) reported that the range of coefficients of variation for repeated measurements of FRC in three subjects was 1.8–2.8%. Pelzer and Thompson (9) studied the variability of TGV measurements ("spontaneous panting volume") on the same day. Using the mean of 4 angles, the coefficients of variation were 3.8% in trained and 6.1% in untrained subjects.

R_{aw}

Pelzer and Thompson (9) also studied the variability of airway resistance in a mixed group of both trained and untrained subjects on the same day. Again using the mean of 4 angles, they reported a mean coefficient of variation of 11.1% for G_{aw} and 10.2% for SG_{aw}.

CONTROVERSIAL ISSUES

Measurement of Resistance from Loops with Hysteresis

Criteria for measuring the angle of a resistance loop when there is significant hysteresis are not established (10, 11). This can be a particular problem when hysteresis appears during expiration, as illustrated in Figure 2d. In such patients, selecting the deceleration phase for resistance measurements offers the potential advantage that by selecting the higher resistance, the test will be more sensitive for identifying abnormal function. A contrasting viewpoint is that since hysteresis may be secondary to differences in pressure and flow time constants, taking measurements from these "distorted" loops with hysteresis may not give valid values of resistance, and therefore should not be attempted. Currently the most common practice seems to be to measure the angles from a "best-fit" straight line drawn through the curve in the more linear portion near zero flow. This may result in improved reproducibility (especially when panting maneuvers vary in magnitude) but may also reduce the diagnostic sensitivity or specificity of the measurements.

Significance of Intra-abdominal Gas

Although early studies indicated that intra-abdominal gas was not measured during plethysmographic measurements of TGV (8), more recent studies have shown that in some subjects "accessory muscle-panting" may result in increases in TGV due to inclusion of compressible intra-abdominal gas (12, 13). With standard panting techniques, this error is usually not significant.

Accuracy of Plethysmographic Measurements of TGV in Patients with Severe Airways Obstruction

The accuracy of plethysmographic measurements of TGV is dependent upon the validity of the assumption that mouth pressure changes are equal to alveolar pressure changes during panting against a closed mouthpiece. Brown et al. noted that in subjects with asthma, measurements of TLC derived from TGV panting maneuvers done near RV were significantly larger than TLC measurements derived from TGV panting maneuvers done near TLC, and this difference increased after induced bronchospasm (14). This data suggested that alveolar pressure changes may be underestimated during bronchospasm, leading to erroneously high measurements of TGV. From simultaneous measurements of esophageal and mouth pressures, Rodenstein et al. also concluded that plethysmographic measurements of lung volume may be erroneously high in patients with obstructive airway disease; they hypothesized the error to be resultant from volume changes in compliant airways during panting, resulting in flow and consequent pressure losses across obstructed airways (15). In our laboratory, we have occasionally noted spuriously high measurements of thoracic gas volumes by plethysmography in patients with severe obstruction; subsequent measurements of thoracic volumes by radiographic techniques confirmed these errors. In these instances, it was possible that at least some of the error was attributable to relatively small leaks in the shutter assembly, which might cause significant errors in patients with very high airway resistances.

The frequency with which clinically significant overestimates of lung volumes occurs has not been defined. Clinical experience and studies that have compared plethysmographic and radiographic measurements of thoracic volumes would suggest that significant errors may occur only in patients with induced bronchospasm or severe obstruction.

Accuracy of Resistance Measurements during Tidal Breathing

DuBois et al. (3) suggested rapid shallow panting during resistance measurements; the purpose was to minimize glottal closure and differences between inspiratory and expiratory gas temperatures. Also, the accuracy of most non-air-conditioned constant-volume plethysmographs is frequency dependent, because of the built-in "thermal leak" described earlier. Attempts have been made to facilitate resistance measurements during tidal breathing; these have involved either attaching a rebreathing bag to the pneumotachograph or making gas temperature corrections electronically (16). However, resistance during tidal breathing may be higher than that during panting, possibly because TGV is lower during tidal breathing (16). In addition, the range of normal values for resistance during quiet breathing has not been established. Therefore, we recommend careful consideration before tidal breathing measurements of resistance are used clinically, in order to ascertain whether the results are the same as those measured during panting, and, if they are not, to demonstrate that the differences seen are real, and not caused by equipment artifact.

REFERENCES

1. Leith DE, Mead J: *Principles of Body Plethysmography*. National Heart and Lung Institute Publication, November 1974.

2. Kanner RE, Morris AH (eds): *Clinical Pulmonary Function Testing*, ed. 3. Salt Lake City, Utah, Intermountain Thoracic Society, 1975, III: 13–15.
3. DuBois AB, Botelho SY, Comroe JH: A new method for measuring airway resistance in man using a body plethysmograph. *J Clin Invest* 35:327–335, 1956.
4. Hulse CM, Durie RH, Murphy EM: X-Y-T recorder with body plethysmograph for determining functional residual capacity from thoracic gas volume, letter. *Chest* 76:117–118, 1979.
5. Brunes L, Holmgren A: Total airway resistance and its relationship to body size and lung volumes in healthy young women. *Scand J Clin Lab Invest* 18:316–324, 1966.
6. Skoogh BE: Normal airways conductance at different lung volumes. *Scand J Clin Lab Invest* 31:429–441, 1973.
7. Briscoe WA, DuBois AB: The relationship between airway resistance, airway conductance and lung volume in subjects of different age and body size. *J Clin Invest* 37:1279–1285, 1958.
8. DuBois AB, Botelho SY, Bedell GN, et al.: A rapid plethysmographic method for measuring thoracic gas volume. *J Clin Invest* 35:322–326, 1956.
9. Pelzer AM, Thompson ML: Effect of age, sex, stature and smoking habits on human airway conductance. *J Appl Physiol* 21:469–476, 1966.
10. Alpers JH, Guyatt AR: Significance of a looped appearance of the flow; alveolar pressure relationship of the lung as examined by the whole body plethysmograph. *Clin Sci* 33:1–10, 1967.
11. Lord PW, Edwards JM: Variation in airway resistance when defined over different ranges of airflows. *Thorax* 33:401–405, 1978.
12. Habib MP, Engel LA: Influence of the panting technique on the plethysmographic measurement of thoracic gas volume. *Am Rev Respir Dis* 117:265–271, 1978.
13. Brown R, Hoppin FG Jr, Ingram RH Jr, et al.: Influence of abdominal gas on the Boyle's Law determination of thoracic gas volume. *J Appl Physiol* 44:469–473, 1978.
14. Brown R, Ingram RH Jr, McFadden ER Jr: Problems in the plethysmographic assessment of changes in total lung capacity in asthma. *Am Rev Respir Dis* 118:685–692, 1978.
15. Rodenstein D, Stanescu DC, Cauberghs M, et al.: Failure of body plethysmography to accurately measure lung volume in bronchial obstruction (Abstract). *Am Rev Respir Dis* 123 (pt 2):88, 1981.
16. Barter CE, Campbell AH: Comparison of airways resistance measurements during panting and quiet breathing. *Respiration* 30:1–11, 1973.

GENERAL REFERENCES

1. Comroe JH: Retrospectroscope: Man-Cans. *Amer Rev Resp Dis* 116: 945–950, 1091–1099, 1977.
2. Hemingway A: *Measurement of airway resistance with the body plethysmograph*. Springfield, Ill., Charles C Thomas, 1973.

CHAPTER 15

Estimation of Lung Volumes from Chest Radiographs

JACK L. CLAUSEN, M.D.
L. POWELL ZARINS, RCPT

Total lung capacity (TLC) and functional residual capacity (FRC) may be estimated from chest radiographs. Several studies have compared radiographic TLCs with plethysmographic TLCs and have shown that the *mean* difference between paired measurements in large groups of subjects is small, usually less than 200 ml (1-3), but occasionally larger (4). Thus, the radiographic methods offer a convenient alternative to the more cumbersome and technical physiological techniques in epidemiological settings. However, examination of the scattergrams from some of the previously mentioned studies has also shown that occasional large (greater than 1.5 liter) misestimations of lung volume occur with the radiographic techniques. The possibility of such inaccuracies limits the clinical or individual diagnostic usefulness of these methods, although they may be appropriate for retrospective or serial studies of trends in lung volume, where absolute accuracy is not essential. (See Controversies.)

Of the radiographic techniques available for estimation of lung volumes, the two most commonly used are the "ellipsoid" method of Barnhard et al. (5) and the planimetry method of Harris et al. (1). The former method assumes that, because of the elliptical shape of the lungs, they may be divided into sections that may be geometrically treated as cylindroids. The volume of each section is determined from measurements of the major and minor diameters [from posterior-anterior (PA) and lateral chest X rays] and the height of each section. The volumes of all sections are summed and corrected for radiographic magnification. The cardiac, infradiaphragmatic, pulmonary tissue, and blood volumes are then estimated and subtracted; the remainder represents the radiographic lung volume. (See Figs. 1a and 1b.)

Harris et al.'s planimetry technique is based upon equations empirically derived by regressing the surface areas of the radiographic lung fields against

PULMONARY FUNCTION TESTING
GUIDELINES AND CONTROVERSIES

ISBN 0-12-788125-5

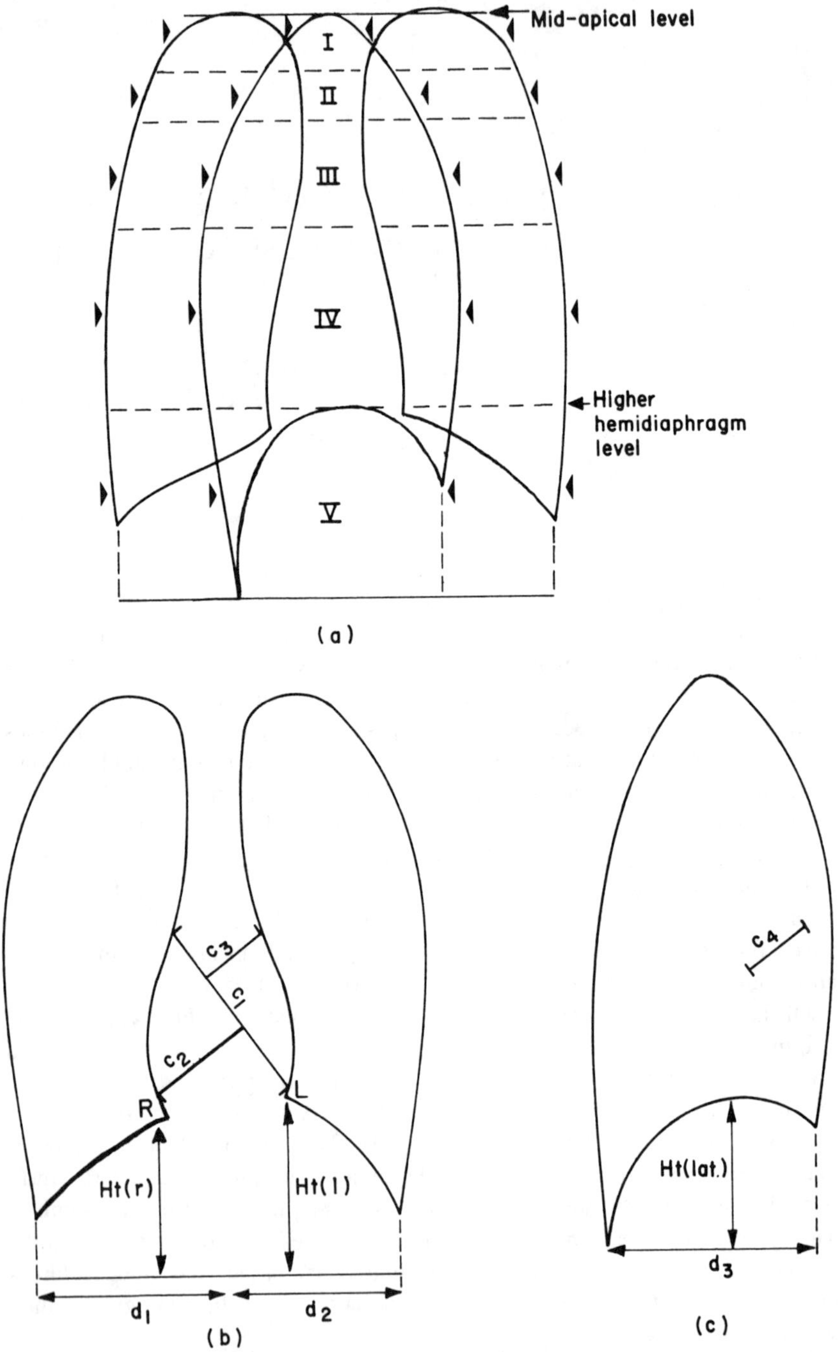

Fig. 1 *(a) PA and lateral outlines superimposed for delineation of zones I–V in the ellipsoid method. (b) Diaphragm and heart measurements using the ellipsoid method. (c) Lateral diaphragm and heart measurements using the ellipsoid method.*

plethysmographic measurements of TLC in the same subjects. These surface areas are usually measured with a planimeter. Computerized systems of varying complexity (2, 6, 7) which directly calculate surface areas have been described and may be worthwhile for studies of large numbers of subjects. Recently, regression equations for planimetry have been developed for measuring either FRC or TLC in supine subjects, using portable chest radiographs (8).

The comparability of the various methods of TLC measurement may vary according to the type and severity of the pulmonary disorder being studied, since there are inherent differences between the quantities being measured (*thoracic lung volume* by radiography, *compressible gas volume* by plethysmography, and *communicating gas volume* by inert gas methods). In patients with obstructive disease, TLC measurements by radiographic and plethysmographic techniques usually produce comparable results, whereas lung volumes measured by inert gas methods may be underestimated because of "noncommunicating" airspaces (5). In contrast, in patients with significant space-occupying disease of the intrathoracic space (e.g., pleural effusion, severe interstitial fibrosis, or pneumonia), the radiographic TLC may be much larger than the TLC measured by plethysmography or gas dilution, although this is not a consistent finding (9, 10). While the X-ray techniques may be less sensitive in detecting reductions of the TLC in these restricted subjects, it could be argued that it may be more appropriate to relate parameters such as airway resistance or lung elasticity to the *actual* thoracic lung volume rather than to the compressible gas volume, especially in research investigations of lung mechanics.

EQUIPMENT AND SPECIFICATIONS

Both the Barnhard and Harris methods specify 72-inch (183-cm) target-to-film distances for PA and lateral chest X rays; the equations from the portable supine technique of Ries et al. (8) require distances of 38 inches (97 cm) for AP and 72 inches (183 cm) for lateral films. In theory, the target-to-film distance for the ellipsoid measurements may be varied if the magnification factor is adjusted accordingly. However, literature validating the accuracy of such modification is scanty (11).

For planimetry, it is convenient if the instrument measuring arm is long enough to include the entire lung surface on the lateral film in one measurement (e.g., K & E model #620005).

QUALITY CONTROL

The planimeter should be calibrated according to the manufacturer's instructions before use. A clear understanding of the boundaries of the radiographic lung fields (especially mediastinal outlines) is essential for accurate and reproducible results. Persons learning this technique should compare thoracic outlines and computed volumes with those done by experienced personnel. The patient and the X-ray technician should be aware of the necessity for a maximal inspiration during the radiographic exposures.

PROCEDURE

The patient should be instructed in the technique of inhalation to maximal lung volume. Breathholding at TLC is instinctively accomplished by most patients by relaxing against a closed glottis. Although not specified in the original descriptions of the techniques, this is probably the most acceptable method.

CALCULATIONS

Ellipsoid Method

Using a view box, place a transparency over the PA film. A grease pencil or felt-tip pen may be used for tracing.

1. The right and left lung fields are outlined similarly (see Fig. 1a). Start at the apex and trace the mediastinal and cardiac borders, continue along the margins of the hemidiaphragms, and return along the internal margins of the ribs to the apex. Draw two horizontal lines, one at the level midway between the two apices and the other at the level of the higher hemidiaphragm.
2. From the PA view of the heart, draw the long diameter of the heart, C_1, defined as the longest possible line from the junction of the superior venous pedicle with the right heart margin to the left heart margin (Fig. 1b). From this line extend perpendiculars (C_2, C_3) to the farthest point of the right and left heart borders.
3. Replace the PA film with the lateral film. Align the highest hemidiaphragm of the lateral film with the diaphragmatic horizontal line previously drawn (from the PA film). Trace the lateral lung fields, starting at the posterior costophrenic angle, following the interior margins of the posterior ribs, tapering smoothly to a conical cap at the line of the mid-apical level (previously drawn from the PA film). Taper smoothly down the interior rib margins to the anterior end of the higher hemidiaphragm, then follow this hemidiaphragm back to the posterior costophrenic angle.
4. On the lateral view of the heart, draw C_4, the longest possible diameter roughly perpendicular to the long axis (Fig. 1c). With a marking pen, make small dashes to indicate the bases of the first two lung zones, one 2.75 cm down from

the mid-apical horizontal, and the other 2.75 cm beneath it. Measure the distance from the bottom of the second zone to the horizontal line at the top of the highest hemidiaphragm, and divide this distance into two parts (zones III and IV). Draw a final horizontal line at the level of the posterior costophrenic angle on the lateral film, which represents the base of zone V. Drop perpendiculars to this horizontal line where needed, as indicated by dotted lines in Fig. 1a. With a bold-colored pen, indicate the midpoints of each of the zones just delineated (e.g., for the first zone, the midpoint would be 1.38 cm down from the mid-apical horizontal line; see the arrowheads on Fig. 1a).

5. On a worksheet [see sample worksheet (Fig. 2)] enter the height, PA midpoint width, and lateral midpoint width of each of the five lung zones, and record the length of the cardiac axes (C_1-C_4).

6. To measure the infradiaphragmatic space, first divide the length of the base of zone V on the PA film by 2 (Fig. 1b: D_1, D_2). Measure the distance from the base of zone V to the highest point on each hemidiaphragm [Ht(R), Ht(L)]; then measure the length of the base of zone V on the lateral film (D_3).

7. Follow the calculations as indicated on the worksheet (Fig. 2). For clarity, the outlines traced are separated into three figures (Figs. 1a, b, and c); however, all tracings can be made on one tranparency. It is not necessary to draw dotted lines for each lung zone; only the two horizontals (mid-apical and higher hemidiaphragmatic) indicated are essential, and the other zone limits can be shown by a simple slash mark. The actual measurements are made at the midpoints (arrowheads on Fig. 1a), and with this simplified procedure, both PA and lateral measurements can be made at the same time. Note that the orientation of the lateral film can influence the measurements; no guidelines have been published to standardize this orientation. We arbitrarily have chosen to align the lateral margins of the PA and lateral films in the vertical plane independent of the orientation of the thorax.

Planimetry Method

1. Trace the right and left PA lung fields using the same boundaries as for the ellipsoid method.

2. To outline the lateral film, at the level *halfway* between hemidiaphragms, draw a line from the anterior rib margins to the posterior margins of the vertebral bodies (Fig. 3). Follow the posterior margins of the vertebral bodies to the apex and back down the ribs to the anterior level of the diaphragms. (Note that the diaphragmatic and posterior lung boundaries differ from those used in the ellipsoid method.) The lateral apex cannot usually be visualized and thus must be drawn intuitively in a smooth conical shape.

3. With a planimeter, measure the surface area of the right PA, left PA, and lateral lung fields. Sum these areas.

Name Doe, John

I.D. # 00987653

Date of study 12-1-79

Age 36 Ht 188 cm Wt 85 kg

Body Surface area 2.11 m^2

Measurement (CM)	Zone I	Zone II	Zone III	Zone IV	Zone V
(1) PA width	18.1	23.1	26.0	27.1	26.9
(2) LAT width	7.4	14.5	21.3	22.2	19.8
(3) Height	2.75	2.75	9.0	9.0	8.5
Zone volumes [=(1)(2)(3)]	368	921	4984	5415	4527

C_1 17.7 C_2 6.2 C_3 4.0 C_4 11.0

D_1 12.25 D_2 12.25 D_3 18.2 Ht(R) 8.5 Ht(L) 4.9

Total lung zone volumes = (16215)(0.572)* = 9275
* = zone volume correction factor (0.572)

Cardiac area = $(C_1)(C_2 + C_3)(C_4)$ = 1986

Diaphragm area (L) = $(D_2)(D_3)$ [Ht(L)] = 1092

Diaphragm area (R) = $(D_1)(D_3)$ [Ht(R)] = 1895

Subtotal = (4973)(0.381)** = 1895
** = cardiac and diaphragm volume correction factor (0.381)

Tissue volume (5.94 ml/kg body weight) = 505

Blood volume (230 ml/m^2 body surface area) = 485

Total subtractions = 2885

TLC = total lung zone volumes minus total subtractions = 6390

Fig. 2 *Ellipsoid worksheet.*

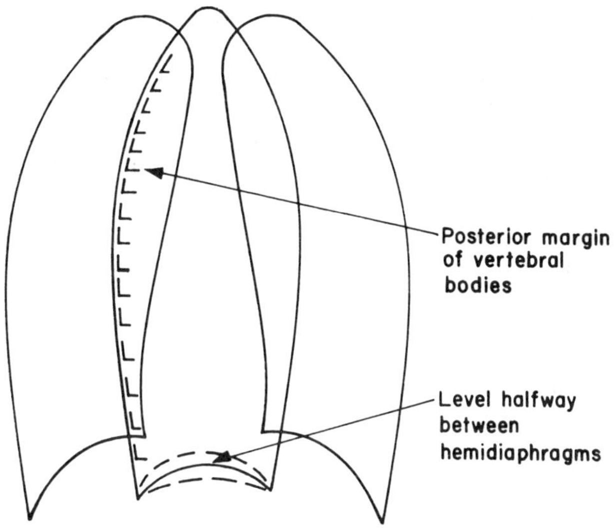

Fig. 3 *Planimetry outline.*

4. By Harris's equation,

$$TLC = 8.5S - 1200$$

where S is the surface area in square centimeters (1).

NORMAL VALUES

Normal predictive values using radiographic techniques have not been established in adequate numbers of subjects. Predictive equations derived from gas dilution techniques are currently the best available alternatives (see Chapter 13).

EXPECTED REPRODUCIBILITY

Studies of the reproducibility of measurements from repeat radiographs in the same subject are not available. The between-observer reproducibility in measuring lung volumes from the same radiograph will depend upon the experience and training of the observers. When 10 radiographs were measured by the ellipsoid method, then remeasured 10 days later by the *same* observer (all markings erased each time), the greatest difference was found to be −277cc (3). Repeated planimetry measurements of the same outline should agree within ±1.0%.

TROUBLESHOOTING

The most common source of error is failure of the subject to have inspired fully to TLC at the time of the radiographic exposure. In addition, systematic errors will result if guidelines defining the boundaries of the lung fields are not followed. A small amount of imprecision is unavoidable, since these boundaries are often not clearly defined because of underexposed radiographs or radiographically dense parenchymal or pleural abnormalities. Also, relatively small alterations in the distance between the subject and the X-ray film can cause very appreciable errors due to image magnification.

CONTROVERSIAL ISSUES

Comparison of Ellipsoid and Planimetric Methods

It has not been established which of the two radiographic techniques (ellipsoid or planimetric) is the method of choice. While much time can be saved by modifying the ellipsoid method, as described in the section on calculations, this method still demands more effort per measurement than the planimetry technique if done manually, and would involve more programing steps if done by computer. To evaluate the comparative accuracy of the two methods, TLCs were measured in 48 normal subjects by plethysmographic, ellipsoid, and planimetric techniques (9). The mean values for TLCs by all three methods were essentially identical (6.17, 6.09, and 6.06 liters, respectively). The correlation coefficients between plethysmographic and X-ray techniques were 0.932 for the ellipsoid and 0.965 for the planimetry methods. Thus, when data from large groups are averaged, either method would be acceptable, with the planimetry method being preferred for TLC measurements because it is simpler, and the ellipsoid method being preferred for studies of regional changes of lung volume, an application for which it would be clearly superior.

Clinical Use of Radiographic Techniques

Whether or not either radiographic technique is sufficiently accurate for a clinically useful measurement of TLC in individual patients has not been established. Differences between plethysmographic and ellipsoidal radiographic measurements of greater than 25% in normal subjects have been reported (3–5). In the previously mentioned study of 48 normal subjects (9), 11 of the ellipsoid radiographic TLCs differed from the plethysmographic TLC by more than 10%; this was the case with only 3 of the planimetric measurements. In three instances, the ellipsoid measurement was in error by more than 15%, whereas no planimetric result was this inaccurate. These findings indicate that although the ellipsoid technique was previously considered to be the more accurate of the two methods, planimetry may be at least equally accurate, and it is certainly much simpler. Either radiographic method has been reported to give more accurate results than the inert gas methods of lung volume measurements in groups of patients with severe chronic obstructive pulmonary disease (COPD) (4, 10); however, the need for measurement accuracy must be weighed carefully against the hazards of additional radiation exposure. Since routine radiographs are usually within 500 ml of the true TLC (12), they may give a reasonable clinical estimate of the degree of hyperinflation without the need to take special TLC radiographs.

We conclude that the radiographic techniques would be most clinically useful (1) in retrospective studies of changes in total or regional lung volume, when previous pulmonary function tests are unavailable; (2) in prospective studies of changes in lung volume, when radiographs would be required anyway for medical management; and (3) in special cases (i.e., tracheotomy patients) where an estimate of total lung capacity is needed and a more accurate method is not available or applicable.

REFERENCES

1. Harris TR, Pratt PC, Kilburn KH: Total lung capacity measured by roentgenograms. *Am J Med* 50:756–763, 1971.
2. Barrett WA, Clayton PD, Lambson CR, et al.: Computerized roentgenographic determinations of total lung capacity. *Am Rev Respir Dis* 113:239–244, 1976.
3. Lloyd HM, String TS, Dubois AB: Radiographic and plethysmographic determination of total lung capacity. *Radiology* 86:7–14, 1966.
4. Ferris BG: Principal investigator. Epidemiology standardization project. *Am Rev Respir Dis* 118 (pt 2): Appendix 6, p. 104, 1978.
5. Barnhard HJ, Pierce JA, Joyce JW, et al.: Roentgenographic determination of total lung capacity. *Am J Med* 28:51–60, 1960.
6. Bencowitz HZ, Shigeoka JW: Radiographic total lung capacity determination aided by a programmable calculator. *Am Rev Respir Dis* 122:791–794, 1980.
7. Pierce RJ, Brown DJ, Holmes M, et al.: Estimation of lung volumes from chest radiographs using shape information. *Thorax* 34:726–734, 1979.
8. Ries AL, Clausen JL, Friedman PJ: Measurements of lung volumes from supine portable chest radiographs. *J Appl Physiol* 47:1332–1335, 1979.
9. Clausen JL, Zarins L, Ries AL: Measurements of abnormal increases in pulmonary tissue in restrictive lung disease. *Am Rev Respir Dis* 117 (suppl):322, 1978.
10. Miller RD, Offord KP: Roentgenologic determination of total lung capacity. *Mayo Clin Proc* 55:694–699, 1980.
11. Gamsu G, Shamas DM, McMahon J, et al.: Radiographically determined lung volumes at full inspiration and during dynamic forced expiration in normal subjects. *Invest Radiol* 10:100–108, 1975.
12. Crapo RO, Montague T, Armstrong J: Inspiratory lung volume achieved on routine chest films. *Invest Radiol* 14:137–140, 1979.

CHAPTER 16

Pulmonary Diffusing Capacity for Carbon Monoxide

ANTONIUS L. VAN KESSEL, B.S., RCPT

The gas transfer factor for carbon monoxide, also referred to as the pulmonary diffusing capacity (DL_{CO}), is a parameter used to evaluate the transfer of gas from the distal air spaces into the pulmonary capillaries. To measure DL_{CO}, very low concentrations of carbon monoxide (CO) are inspired; from the ratio of the CO concentrations of the inspired and expired gas, the disappearance rate of CO is calculated and expressed as a function of the driving pressure:

$$DL_{CO} = \dot{V}_{CO}/(P_1 - P_2), \text{ ml/min/torr*} \qquad \text{(Eq. 1)}$$

where $\dot{V}_{CO}$ is the uptake of CO per minute, P_1 the partial pressure of CO in alveoli, and P_2 the partial pressure of CO in plasma in pulmonary capillaries.

Because hemoglobin has such a high affinity for CO, the partial pressure of CO in the plasma (P_2 in Eq. 1) can be considered 0, and the pressure gradient ($P_1 - P_2$) can be simplified to P_A, the partial pressure of the inspired (alveolar) CO. As a second consequence of the CO–Hb affinity, DL_{CO} is independent of the velocity of pulmonary capillary blood flow. However, it is influenced by those abnormalities of ventilation and perfusion that decrease the ''effective'' surface area for gas exchange, and also by deficiencies or disorders of the hemoglobin system.

The physical determinants of the rate of CO transfer are the CO driving pressure (PACO), the surface area and thickness of the capillary walls, and the diffusion coefficient for CO. The chemical determinants are the red cell volume (V_c) and the reaction rate of CO with Hb (θ). θ varies with the partial pressure of inspired oxygen. Thus, when DL_{CO} is measured at two different inspired oxygen levels, the two chemical components of resistance to CO transfer, V_c and θ, may

*In S.I. units, moles/sec/kPa.

PULMONARY FUNCTION TESTING
GUIDELINES AND CONTROVERSIES

ISBN 0-12-788125-5

be separated; the contribution of the physical components, expressed cumulatively as the *membrane diffusion factor* (D_m) may also be estimated (1,2) (see Fig. 1). Although this refinement of the D_{LCO} technique (estimation of V_c, θ, and D_m) is not widely applied, it is not beyond the technical capabilities of most pulmonary laboraties, and may be of interest in certain cases (3).

The remainder of this chapter deals with the more commonly utilized methods of D_{LCO} measurement: (1) single-breath, (2) steady-state, and (3) rebreathing techniques. Each method has specific advantages and limitations.

SINGLE-BREATH TECHNIQUE

This technique was initially introdued by Krogh (4) and Bohr in the early part of this century and later refined by Forster et al. (5), Ogilvie et al. (6), and McGrath and Thomson (7). The patient is connected to a spirometer with a ''balloon-in-box'' system, inhales a maximum breath from residual volume (vital capacity) of a gas containing 0.3% CO and a tracer gas, and is instructed to hold his breath for 10 seconds. During exhalation, an alveolar sample is collected in a small bag and analyzed for CO concentration (F_ACO). The CO uptake during the time of breath holding can then be calculated from the inspired and expired CO concentrations.

The decrease in F_ACO during breath holding is exponential in time because the disappearance rate of CO is proportional to the CO concentration gradient, which is continuously changing.

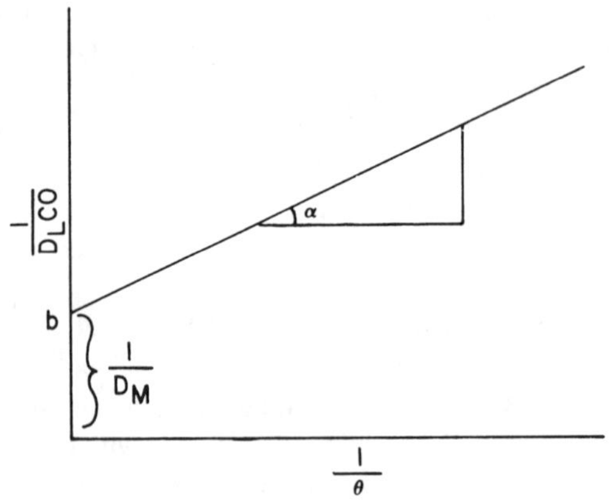

Fig. 1 *Graphical representation of the relationship $1/(D_{LCO}) = 1/D_m + 1/\theta V_c$, where D_{LCO} is the total pulmonary diffusing capacity, D_m the pulmonary membrane diffusing capacity, θ the reaction rate of CO with Hb, V_c the pulmonary capillary blood volume, and α the slope ($1/V_c$).*

$$F_ACO_t = F_ACO_0 \cdot e^{-Kt} \qquad \text{(Eq. 2)}$$

where F_ACO_t is alveolar CO concentration at time t, F_ACO_0 the initial alveolar CO concentration, t the breath-holding time in seconds, and where

$$K = \frac{DL_{CO} \times (BP - 47)}{V_A \times 60} \qquad \text{(Eq. 3)}$$

where BP is barometric pressure in millimeters Hg, and V_A the alveolar volume. By taking the logarithm of Eq. 2 and rearranging Eq. 3, with appropriate substitutions one can develop the following relationship:

$$DL_{CO} = \frac{V_A \times 60}{(BP - 47) \times t} \ln \frac{F_ACO_0}{F_ACO_t} \qquad \text{(Eq. 4)}$$

In practice, the V_A is obtained from the ratio of the inspired and expired inert gas concentrations, and the F_ACO_0 is corrected to represent the "effective" inspired alveolar CO concentration.

The single-breath DL_{CO} test has several advantages: It takes little time to perform, requires minimal cooperation from the patient, and blood samples are not needed. The disadvantages of the method are that breath holding at maximum lung volume is not a normal breathing state, and some patients with small vital capacities may not be able to produce an alveolar gas sample that is representative of the F_ACO at the time of collection. Maldistribution of ventilation may distort F_ACO but less so than with the steady-state method. Also, the method does not lend itself well to exercising patients and patients with severe dyspnea. Nevertheless, the single breath DL_{CO} technique is probably the most widely used.

STEADY-STATE TECHNIQUE

With the steady-state or Filley method, the patient breathes a mixture of 0.1% CO in air for several minutes through a one-way valve system. During the last 2 minutes, the exhaled air is collected in a neoprene bag (either a weather balloon or a more expensive version of the Douglas bag) and analyzed for O_2, CO_2, and CO concentrations (Rapidly responding analyzers are required.) During the collection, an arterial blood sample is drawn and analyzed for PCO_2 (8).

The amount of CO transferred from the alveoli to the capillary blood per unit time ($\dot{V}_{CO}$) can be calculated from the inspired and expired gas concentrations and the volume of gas exhaled [$\dot{V}_E$ at standard conditions (STPD)]. The mean alveolar CO concentration (F_ACO) can be estimated by rearranging the Bohr gas equation for dead space volume divided by tidal volume (V_D/V_T), knowing mixed expired CO_2 (F_ECO_2), mixed expired CO (F_ECO), arterial PCO_2 (F_aCO_2) and inspired CO (F_ICO). If one assumes that V_D/V_T for CO_2 is the same as that for CO, then we can write

$$\frac{V_D}{V_T} = \frac{F_ACO_2 - F_ECO_2}{F_ACO_2} = \frac{F_ACO - F_ECO}{F_ACO - F_ICO} \quad \text{(Eq. 5)}$$

This can now be solved for alveolar CO concentration

$$F_ACO = F_ICO - \frac{F_ACO_2}{F_ECO_2}(F_ICO - F_ECO) \quad \text{(Eq. 6)}$$

and

$$P_ACO = F_ACO \times (BP - 47) \quad \text{(Eq. 7)}$$

This value can now be used to calculate DL_{CO}.

Since the steady-state DL_{CO} test is performed under normal (tidal) breathing conditions, it is compatible with anesthesia, sleep, and exercise protocols. Despite this advantage, the steady-state method is not widely used because the results are more subject to error than those of the single-breath method, particularly in patients with either uneven distribution of ventilation and/or patients with ventilation-perfusion ($\dot{V}/Q$) abnormalities; it is then difficult to ascertain whether a decrease in DL_{CO} by the steady-state method is a function of impairment of the $\dot{V}/Q$ ratio or an alteration of the gas transfer characteristics of the lungs. The main source of difficulty is the estimation of alveolar CO concentrations. Other disadvantages of this method are the necessity for an arterial blood sample, and the technique's sensitivity to changes in breathing pattern, e.g., hyperventilation. (Although the so-called "end-tidal" steady-state method does not require arterial blood samples, it suffers from many more sources of error.)

REBREATHING TECHNIQUE

The rebreathing method requires the patient to rebreathe the test gas from a balloon, the volume of which approximately equals the patient's forced expiratory volume at one second (FEV_1). The patient expires to residual volume (RV) before the tap is switched, then rebreathes from the balloon, which should be emptied with each inspiration. The period of rebreathing is 30–45 seconds at a controlled rate of 30 breaths/min. The rebreathing method for measuring DL_{CO} is less reproducible and requires considerable patient cooperation, but is less influenced by uneven distribution of ventilation than the steady-state or single-breath techniques (9). The rebreathing technique is the least useful method in most circumstances. For a more complete review of the history and development of DL_{CO} testing, see Comroe's article (10).

CLINICAL APPLICATIONS

The clinical usefulness and specific indications for DL_{CO} measurements are not well defined. In part, this is because of the variety of different testing procedures in use, and in part because of the complexity of the physiologic determinants of the rate of uptake of CO. Also, as with many other pulmonary function tests, controversies about the usefulness of the DL_{CO} remain unresolved because of the paucity of investigations that have adequately studied this issue. The most common applications include the evaluation of patients with diffuse interstitial processes (e.g., sarcoid and diffuse interstitial fibrosis) and the assessment of patients with suspected emphysema. Theoretically, the DL_{CO} may also be reduced in patients with regional reductions of pulmonary vascular blood volume as may occur with pulmonary emboli or pulmonary vasculitis. The relationship between hemoglobin concentration and predicted (or observed) DL_{CO} is important to understand so that a low DL_{CO} which is solely attributable to severe anemia is not misinterpreted as secondary to nonexistant lung disease. Although there are more direct methods for assessing anemia than with the DL_{CO}, this test may have potential applications in the evaluation of patients with suspected intrapulmonary hemorrhage. For a more complete review of the clinical applications, the reader is referred to the work of Bates et al. (11) and Morton and Ostensoe (12).

EQUIPMENT

Even though few conceptual changes have been made in the approach to measure the gas transfer factor for CO, there is now a much greater selection of equipment available than several years ago when DL_{CO} methods were developed. While it is not feasible to include in this chapter the methodology for all apparatus and instrument combinations, an attempt will be made to describe the broad range of equipment that is readily available and commonly used in pulmonary laboratories throughout the country, and several references are included (13–17).

Equipment Requirements for the Steady-State Method

1. CO analyzer. There are three different types of instruments available which can measure low CO concentrations accurately: the infrared analyzer, the gas chromatograph, and the electrochemical cell. Table 1 summarizes the various features of each instrument. For the purpose of the steady-state method, the CO analyzer needs to be calibrated in absolute units in order to calculate the CO uptake in milliliters per minute.
2. Blood gas analyzer to measure arterial CO_2 tensions.
3. Oxygen analyzer for the purpose of measuring inspired and exhaled oxygen concentrations. The analyzer should have a resolution high enough to enable it to read a change of 0.02% of O_2 accurately. Blood-gas electrodes are therefore not suitable for this purpose. Acceptable methods are gas chromatography, mass-

Table 1 *Operating Characteristics of CO Analyzers*

	Ease of operation and maintenance	Response time	Sample size (ml)	Price range	Linearity	Versatility	Specificity	Output modes	Portability	Misc.
Infrared analyzer	Very easy	1 sec	500 or less	$8000 and up	No	For CO	CO_2 and H_2O vapor interfere and need to be absorbed	Analog or digital; easy to interface with computer.	ac, not portable	
Gas chromatograph	Requires more maintenance and operation skills	1–6 min	1–3	$2000 and up	Variable	Can be used for CO_2, N_2, Neon, O_2, CO,	H_2O causes column deterioration and must be absorbed	Graphical, peak-height represents CO concentration. Difficult to automate or interface with computer.	ac or dc, but not portable	
Electrochemical	Very easy	30 sec	500 or less	under $2000	Variable	For CO only	Not affected by H_2O vapor or CO_2	Analog output only. Can be interfaced with computer using A–D converter.	ac or dc, portable (4.1 kg)	Very susceptible to alcohol vapors. Needs replacement cell periodically.

spectrometry, para-magnetic, polarographic, or fuel-cell analysis and the micro-Scholander technique. (See Chapter 5 for a discussion of the advantages and limitations of the various O_2 analyzers.)

4. CO_2 analyzer to measure exhaled CO_2 concentration. An infrared CO_2 analyzer is the best instrument for measuring CO_2 gas concentrations.

5. Instrument to measure the exhaled gas volume. A simple dry-test or wet-test gas meter will suffice.

6. A two-way breathing valve (small dead space).

7. Assorted items such as stopcocks, tubing, neoprene balloons or Douglas bags for exhaled gas collection, and a stopwatch.

8. Test gas. At sea level use 0.1% CO in air. Above sea level use 0.1% CO in O_2 enriched air so that the PO_2 equals 150 torr at that altitude.

Equipment for the Single-Breath Method

A single-breath DL_{CO} system can be assembled with separate components. It is convenient, however, to buy a complete assembly. Some systems available may include all the necessary gas analyzers; others consist of the breathing circuit only.

The technique and methodology described here requires all of the following equipment components:

1. spirometer
2. kymograph with appropriate speed to discriminate 10 seconds accurately
3. box-balloon system (Donald-Christie type box)
4. five-way breathing valve
5. assorted stopcocks, tubing, valves, and neoprene balloons
6. Test gas. At sea level use 0.3% CO, 10% He (or 0.3% Ne), 21% O_2, and the remainder N_2. Above sea level use 0.3% CO, 10% He (or 0.3% Ne), O_2 concentration equivalent to a PO_2 of 150 torr at that altitude, and the remainder N_2
7. CO gas analyzer (see previous section)
8. He analyzer
9. CO_2 analyzer (see previous section)
10. CO, He, and CO_2 analyzers may be replaced by a gas chromatograph

QUALITY CONTROL

Quality control can be divided into two major categories: instrumentation performance and methodology or procedural errors. The latter will be discussed in the methods section of this chapter.

The accuracy of spirometers can easily be checked with the use of a 3-liter syringe; kymograph paper speeds should be verified with the aid of an accurate stopwatch. Leak testing and helium meter linearity checks should be performed as described in Chapter 10. Gases stored in Douglas bags or neoprene balloons should be analyzed promptly to minimize concentration changes resulting from diffusion through the wall.

Accurate calibration of the CO analyzer is of utmost importance. Most CO analyzers are alinear in response and require multiple-point calibration. Since the degree of alinearity changes with time, complete, full-scale recalibration should be repeated on at least a weekly basis.

The simplest calibration procedure involves sequential dilution with room air of the CO test gas using a calibrated (at 100 ml intervals) 1-liter syringe as described by Kanner and Morris (18). The accuracy of this method depends on the absolute precision of the CO concentration in the test gas as well as on the ability of the technologist to prepare accurate CO mixtures. Figure 2 suggests a simple set-up for the dilution procedure. For each dilution step, it is preferable to first fill the syringe with pure test gas (stopcock in position as shown in Fig. 2), then turn the stopcock 180° clockwise, and slowly push out gas from syringe to the desired mark. Next, disconnect syringe carefully from stopcock and fill with air to the 1-liter mark. Plug syringe with rubber stopper until ready to analyze its content for CO concentration. (Alternatively, dilutions may be prepared by adding boluses of test gas and room air to an evacuated anesthesia balloon, using an oiled 100-ml glass syringe and small stopcock.) Start the calibration procedure with pure (100%) test gas and set the CO analyzer to the highest meter reading. Subsequent dilutions should be 90%, 80%, etc., until pure (CO free) room air is used to verify the zero reading. Finally, plot the meter readings versus the percentage of CO concentrations as calculated from the dilution factors. As mentioned before, complete full-scale calibration should be performed at least weekly or more frequently if significant changes in the calibration curve are

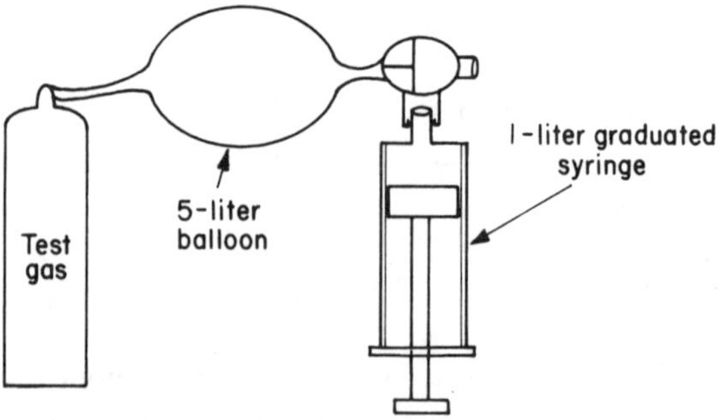

Fig. 2 *Simple calibration set-up for CO and He analyzers.*

evident. Zero point and test gas values should be checked before each DL_{CO} test. This method of calibration can be used for both single-breath and steady-state test gas mixtures.

Gaensler and co-workers (19) have described a CO calibration technique for infrared and electrochemical analyzers, which either permits relative calibration without a standardized gas mixture suitable for single-breath DL_{CO} methods, or absolute calibration with a standardized gas mixture, a requirement for the steady-state DL_{CO} test. The method is based on the dilution of pure test gas by the addition of 100% N_2. Accurate readings of reduced O_2 concentration in the mixture provide the basis for calculating and plotting decreased CO concentrations of the test gas. The method is reported to be highly accurate but requires a more complicated set-up and additional equipment (e.g., an O_2 analyzer with absolutely linear characteristics) as compared to the previously described simple dilution technique. Okuba and Lenfant (20) have reported a similar method specifically designed for calibrating a gas chromatograph for CO analysis.

When all individual analyzers and other instruments are properly prepared and calibrated, a simulated volume-dilution test should be performed to ascertain accurate results of the overall procedure. This can best be done using either a 3-liter syringe (19) or, better, a second spirometer with known dead space as lung models. Using the test procedures described in the next section with a simulated lung, one should be able to check the overall performance of the DL_{CO} set-up by comparing the calculated volume of the test lung with the actual values.

PROCEDURE

This section describes the methodology of manually operated systems for both the single-breath and the steady-state (Filley) techniques. Automated systems are useful for large volume laboratories because they may save the operator's time. It is a misconception, however, to equate "automation" with "accuracy" unless the technologist has a working knowledge of the fundamental principles of operation of the individual instruments used and a thorough understanding of the methodology of the testing procedure.

METHODOLOGY

All equipment should be ready before the patient is brought into the laboratory. This policy lowers the anxiety level of both the patient and technologist and reduces the margin of technological and methodological error. Patients should be given a 5-minute rest period prior to a DL_{CO} measurement to minimize the effects of increased or redistributed pulmonary capillary blood volume.

Steady-State Testing Procedure*

1. Fill balloon A with test gas (see Equipment) and connect to breathing assembly.
2. Calibrate CO, O_2, and CO_2 analyzers and carefully analyze the inspired gas mixture (F_ICO, F_IO_2, and F_ICO_2) directly from balloon A.
3. Prepare equipment for arterial puncture.
4. Have patient, seated comfortably, breathe through the mouthpiece connected to breathing valve and place nose clip on patient.
5. Turn T-shaped stopcock on balloon A so that patient breathes the CO gas mixture.
6. Turn T-shaped stopcock on balloon B so that exhaled air is directed into the room for 1 minute.
7. During the second minute, collect exhaled air in balloon B, then flush out the bag and reconnect to T-shaped stopcock. This step is necessary to fill the dead space of collection assembly with the patient's expirate. During the third and fourth minute, the patient exhales into the room.
8. At the beginning of the fifth minute, turn the stopcock and collect exhaled gas into balloon B for the final 2 minutes. Time with stopwatch and observe and record breathing frequency.
9. During gas collection, draw an arterial blood sample; seal, label, and ice the blood sample.
10. At the end of collection, turn T-shaped stopcock to seal balloon B and disconnect patient from mouthpiece.
11. Analyze exhaled gas mixture for CO, CO_2 and O_2 concentration (F_ECO, F_ECO_2, F_EO_2).
12. Measure total volume of collected air with gas meter.
13. Analyze arterial blood sample for blood-gas parameters.

Single-Breath Testing Procedure**

1. Open tap A (box vent) and evacuate the balloon through tap B using wall vacuum or a vacuum pump.
2. Fill balloon through tap B to near capacity with test gas. Close both taps.
3. Turn valve C to position 1 and fill spirometer with approximately 7 liters of air by pulling up the spirometer bell.
4. Turn valve C to position 2 and apply pressure by hand to the top of the spirometer bell. This action will flush out the dead space of the inspiratory breathing circuit. (Steps 3 and 4 should be repeated several times whenever the inspiratory circuit is contaminated with room air.)

*See Fig. 3.
**See Fig. 4.

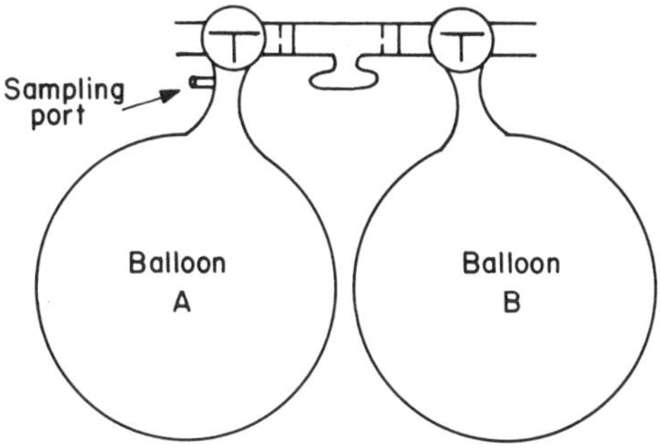

Fig. 3 *Breathing assembly for steady-state $D_{L_{CO}}$ measurements. Balloon A contains test gas; balloon B is used to collect exhaled air.*

5. Repeat step 3; then attach a small anesthesia balloon (2 liters) to the mouth opening of valve C. Clamp off the neck of the balloon and evacuate it.

6. Turn valve C to position 2, release clamp on balloon, and push test gas into the small balloon by pressing on the spirometer bell.

7. Analyze content of small balloon for CO and He concentration (see step 17 if gas chromatograph is used). Attach sample balloon to position 4 outlet of valve C. Evacuate it.

8. Turn valve C to position 1 and pull up spirometer bell to refill spirometer to approximately 7 liters. Turn valve C to position 3.

9. Place nose-clip on patient's nose. Connect mouthpiece to valve C. Have patient breathe room air in a relaxed, sitting position.

10. Start kymograph; a speed of 160 mm/min is preferred.

11. Instruct patient to exhale maximally (RV). Turn valve C to position 2 and have patient inhale a maximal breath (vital capacity, VC) from the balloon-in-box. Instruct patient to hold breath for about 10 seconds. The breath-holding time is estimated by the operator from the vertical lines on the kymograph (e.g., at a speed of 160 mm/min, the time interval between two vertical lines on Collins paper is 12 seconds) or from a stopwatch.

12. At the end of the 10-second breath-holding period, turn valve C to position 1 and instruct patient to exhale rapidly and completely. The initial portion of the exhaled air will return to the spirometer (see Fig. 4) indicating on paper the end of the breath-holding period as well as the size of the wash-out volume, which should be standardized. (See Calculations.)

13. Now quickly rotate valve C to position 4 so that the exhaled alveolar air can be collected in the small anesthetic balloon.

14. When a standardized volume has been collected, turn valve C to position 1 to allow patient to breathe into spirometer, thus indicating on paper the time period for sample collection.

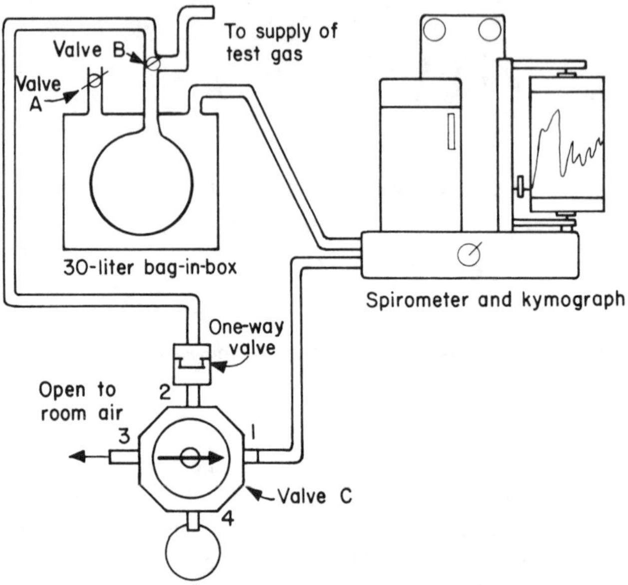

Fig. 4 *Suggested instrument set-up for single-breath $D_{L_{CO}}$ measurements. See test for step-by-step instruction of the procedure.*

15. Clamp off upper part of balloon; stop kymograph motor; remove noseclip, and disconnect patient from mouthpiece.

16. Analyze contents of balloon for He and CO concentrations (F_ECO_2 may also be measured if feasible).

17. If a gas chromatograph is used for CO and Ne concentrations, the initial (inspired) sample should be saved and analyzed sequentially with the expired sample in order to minimize problems with drift of the gas chromatograph.

18. Rinse out spirometer circuit between tests (valve in position 1.)

Procedural Quality Control

Heavy smokers have as much as 10–12% carboxy-hemoglobin in their blood. The assumption that back pressure for CO in mixed venous blood entering the pulmonary capillary bed is zero may not be valid for heavy smokers. The steady-state method is more subject to error than the single-breath technique in patients who smoke heavily. In any case, patients should be instructed not to smoke for at least 4 hours prior to the $D_{L_{CO}}$ procedure. Resting $D_{L_{CO}}$ measurements should be performed with the patient in a sitting position. A simple method to measure CO back pressure is to use the lungs as a tonometer. Just before the $D_{L_{CO}}$ test, have the patient hold his breath at FRC, then collect an alveolar sample after washing out the dead space. Determine the CO concentration with a CO analyzer. Single-breath $D_{L_{CO}}$ measurements should be repeated, allowing a 5-minute interval between the two tests. Results should agree within 10%, and the average value of the two tests reported. $D_{L_{CO}}$ measurements should not be performed on patients who have been breathing oxygen-enriched mixtures immediately prior to the test. A 20-minute interval is recommended between shunt studies (or nitrogen washouts) and $D_{L_{CO}}$ tests.

For the single-breath technique, the method of gas analysis must be taken into consideration before the results can be calculated. When helium katharometers are used, it is necessary to pass the gas samples through chemical absorbants to remove CO_2 and water vapor before analysis. The removal of CO_2 from expired gas samples has the effect of concentrating the other gases, including helium, in the sample. Thus, when alveolar volume (V_A) is calculated from the helium dilution ratio before and after breath holding, the *expired* helium reading (F_EHe) should be corrected to represent the "true" alveolar concentration. (See Calculations for the correction formula.)

Water vapor must also be removed from gas samples prior to infrared CO analysis, and, even though some analyzers are fitted with special optical filters that allow accurate CO analysis is the presence of CO_2, it is recommended that the CO_2 be removed anyway. This step ensures that the He and CO in the expired sample are concentrated to the same extent, and, since these two concentrations (F_EHe and F_ACO_t) appear as terms in the numerator and denominator, respectively, of the log expression of the $D_{L_{CO}}$ formula (Eq. 8), any additional corrections for CO_2 removal would be self-canceling, and therefore unnecessary (19).

$$\ln \frac{F_ACO_0}{F_ACO_t} = \ln \frac{(F_ICO)\ (F_EHe)}{(F_ACO_t)\ (F_IHe)} \qquad \text{(Eq. 8)}$$

(See the next section for complete definition of terms.)

Often the helium katharometer and infrared CO analyzer are set up in series, and the gas samples are passed through CO_2 absorber and dessicant, in that order, prior to analysis (18).

When gases are analyzed by the gas chromatography method, CO_2 is separated, but not removed, and therefore *no* special correction should be applied to the F_EHe.

CALCULATIONS

Sample Calculation for Steady-State Method

Measured data

Gas concentrations are as follows: $F_IO_2 = 0.2108$, $F_ICO_2 = 0.0003$, $F_ICO = 0.00123$, $F_EO_2 = 0.1753$, $F_ECO_2 = 0.0317$, and $F_ECO = 0.00087$. Arterial blood gases have the following partial pressures and pH; $PaO_2 = 84.5$ torr,

$PaCO_2$ = 42.0 torr, and pH = 7.40. Breathing frequency is 28 breath/min; measured volume (uncorrected for volume loss due to gas analysis), 11200 ml; collection time, 2 minutes; room temperature, 24° C; and barometric pressure, 760 torr.

Calculated data

Volume correction for gas used to analyze exhaled gas concentration (F_ECO, F_EO_2, F_ECO_2) is 1600 ml. $\dot{V}_E$ at ATPS is the total of the measured volume plus the volume correction divided by collection time.

$$\dot{V}_E \text{ (ATPS)} = (11200 + 1600)/2 = 6400 \text{ ml/min}$$

$\dot{V}_E$ at STPD is V_E at ATPS multiplied by STPD factor.

$$\dot{V}_E \text{ (STPD)} = 6400 \times 0.9 = 5760 \text{ ml/min}$$

$$F_EN_2 = 1 - (F_EO_2 + F_ECO_2) = 1 - (0.1753 + 0.0317) = 0.7930$$

$$F_IN_2 = 1 - (F_IO_2 + F_ICO_2) = 1 - (0.2108 + 0.0003) = 0.7889$$

$$\dot{V}_{CO} = \dot{V}_E(\text{STPD}) \times \left[\left(F_ICO \times \frac{F_EN_2}{F_IN_2} \right) - F_ECO \right]$$

$$= 5760 \times \left[\left(0.00123 \times \frac{0.7930}{0.7889} \right) - 0.00087 \right] = 2.1104 \text{ ml/min}$$

$$PACO = (BP - 47) \times \left[F_ICO - \frac{F_ACO_2}{F_ECO_2} \times (F_ICO - F_ECO) \right]$$

where

$$F_ACO_2 = PaCO_2/(BP - 47) = 42/713 = 0.0589$$

$$PACO = 713 \left[0.00123 - \frac{0.0589}{0.0317} (0.00123 - 0.00087) \right] = 0.40 \text{ torr}$$

$$DL_{CO} = \frac{\dot{V}_{CO}}{PACO} = \frac{2.1104}{0.40} = 5.3 \text{ ml/min/torr}$$

Sample Calculation for Single-Breath Method

Measured data

Barometric pressure is 760 torr; room temperature, 24° C; breath-holding time (from Fig. 5), 10.5 seconds; and vital capacity (ATPS, from Fig. 5), 4000 ml. Gas concentrations are as follows: F_ECO_2 = 0.042, F_IHe = 0.106, F_EHe = 0.073, F_ICO = 0.003, F_ECO = 0.00095,

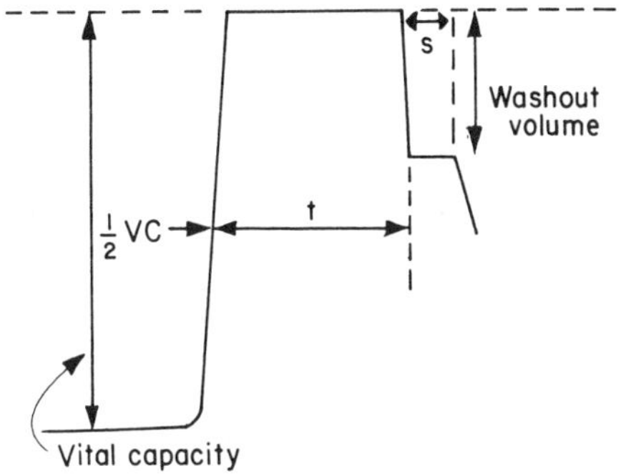

Fig. 5 *Determination of breath-holding time (t) as recommended by Gaensler (19). The kymograph speed in this example is 160 mm/min or 32 mm/12 seconds. The breath-holding time is measured from the point of mid-inspiration (half of vital capacity) to the onset of alveolar gas collection. Washout and sample collection time is designated by s.*

Calculated data

VC (STPD) = VC (ATPS) × STPD factor = 4000 × 0.9 = 3600 ml.

For calculation of V_A, the $F_E He$ should be corrected for the amount of CO_2 absorbed using the catharometer reading multiplied by $(1 - F_E CO_2)$, or

$$F_E He \text{ (corrected)} = 0.073 \times (1 - 0.042) = 0.0699$$

(If CO_2 analysis is not feasible, assume an $F_E CO_2$ of 0.05 (19). Do not correct $F_E He$ when analysis is done by chromatography.)

$$V_A \text{ (STPD)} = \frac{VC \text{ (STPD)}}{F_E He/F_I He} = \frac{3600}{0.0699/0.106} = 5459 \text{ ml.}$$

For the purpose of making a valid comparison of V_A and VC obtained from the single-breath DL_{CO} procedure with the actual total lung capacity (TLC) and VC of the patient, one should convert both DL_{CO} volumes (V_A and VC) to BTPS conditions. If we assume that the inhaled CO concentration dilutes to the same extent as the inert He, we can calculate $F_A CO_0$, i.e., the initial alveolar CO concentration at time 0 of the breath-holding period.

$$F_A CO_0 = F_I CO \times \frac{F_E He}{F_I He} = 0.003 \times \frac{0.073}{0.106} = 0.00206$$

Now

$$DL_{CO} = \frac{V_A \text{ (STPD)} \times 60}{(BP - 47) \times t(\text{sec})} \ln \frac{F_A CO_0}{F_A CO_t} = \frac{5459 \times 60}{713 \times 10.5} \ln \frac{0.00206}{0.00095}$$

$$= 43.75 \times 0.774 = 33.9 \text{ ml/min/torr}$$

NORMAL PREDICTED VALUES

There are many studies of normal predicted values in the literature from which regression formulae or tables for DL_{CO} can be compiled. There appears to be a wide range of values even when similar methods are used. This variation may, in part, be attributed to differences in technique or to different criteria of population selection.

Table 2 summarizes regression formulas from several references for DL_{CO} obtained by the single-breath technique (SB). To aid in the decision of which normals values to adopt, one should test a limited number of normal persons in the laboratory (e.g., 10–100) and compare these results with different published predicted normal values. Based upon this experience, we at Stanford University Medical Center have selected the data published by Bates, Macklem, and Christie (11), originally developed by McGrath and Thomson (7), for single-breath DL_{CO}. We derived the following regression formulas from these data (Eqs. 9 and 10; see also formulas derived from Bates et al. (11) and McGrath et al. (7) in Table 2). For males

$$DL_{CO}\ (SB) = (0.456\ H - 0.33A - 37.98) \times 0.07\ Hb \qquad (Eq.\ 9)$$

and for females

$$DL_{CO}\ (SB) = (0.42\ H - 0.262 - 36.16) \times 0.07\ Hb \qquad (Eq.\ 10)$$

where A is age in years; H, height in centimeters; and Hb, hemoglobin in grams per 100 ml.

Dinakara et al. (25) found that CO uptake changes approximately 7% per gram Hb. The regression formulas used at Stanford (Eqs. 9 and 10) reflect this hemoglobin correction factor (0.07 Hb), which can also be used for the other DL_{CO} prediction formulas. By applying the Hb correction factor to the predicted value instead of the observed value for DL_{CO}, one can identify a decreased DL_{CO} as a gas exchange abnormality not based on alteration in Hb but on other gas transfer abnormalities of the lungs.

Normal predicted values for steady-state DL_{CO} measurements in adults are approximately 33% lower than single-breath normal predicted values, when Filley's data are compared with McGrath's (7,8).

Normal DL_{CO} values for children have been reported by a number of investigators. Polgar and Promadhat (26) have reviewed five such publications and compiled the data.

It appears that the work of Bucci et al. (27) provides the best pediatric data for single-breath values and that of Weng and Levison (28) for steady-state values. Regression formulas for these normal predicted values are as follows:

Bucci: $DL_{CO}\ (SB) = \text{antilog}\ (0.656\ H + 0.308)$

Weng: $DL_{CO}\ (SS) = -17.556 + 0.228\ H$

Table 2 *Predicted Normal Values for D_LCO (SB) in Adults*

Reference	No. of Subjects	Age range	Regression equations[a]	Comments
Ogilvie et al. (6)	16 males 12 females	8–72 18–68	18.85 BSA − 6.8 0.874 H (in.) − 31.6 0.149 W (lb.) + 5.2	$D_{L_{CO}}$ found not to be age or sex dependent. Smoking habits not reported.
Burrows et al. (21)	84 males 51 females	18–89	males: 15.5 BSA − 0.238A + 6.8 females: 15.5 BSA − 0.117A + 0.5 both: 3.46 TLC (STPD) + 7.0	Sample consisted of 41 "normals," 25 patients "free of pulmonary disease," and 69 patients with "localized pulmonary lesions." Smoking habits of subjects not reported.
Marks et al. (22)	10 males 3 females	20–35	16.5 BSA	
Bates et al. (11) from McGrath et al. (7)	39 males	15–75	males: 0.456H (cm) − 0.3A − 37.98 females: 0.42H (cm) − 0.262A − 36.16	Sample included smokers, but reported "no obvious effect of smoking." See text for explanation of the development of the regression formulas. (Female regression equations were apparently derived from male data.)
Gelb et al. (23)	50 males 30 females	20–90	13.67 + 4.36 TLC (BTPS) − 0.2A	All subjects were nonsmokers.
Crapo and Morris (24)	123 males 122 females	15–91 17–84	males: 0.416H (cm) − 0.219A − 26.34 females: 0.256H (cm) − 0.144A − 8.36	Study done at an altitude of 1400 m. (F_IO_2 was 25%, equivalent of P_IO_2 of sea level studies.) All subjects were nonsmokers.

[a] H is height; W, weight; A, age; BSA, body surface area.

In contrast to adult predicted normal values, children's normals are independent of sex or age and are based on height only.

REPRODUCIBILITY

The expected reproducibility for $D_{L_{CO}}$ measurement, like many other pulmonary function tests, depends in part on the competence and persuasive skills of the technologist.

Gaensler (19) reviewed $D_{L_{CO}}$ data from 1840 persons and reported "that inadequate inspiration, poorly flushed circuits, misreading of analytical meters, and inadequate CO calibration curves were the most important sources of variation."

These variations were almost certainly due to the technologist, not the equipment or the patient. Automation per se will not eliminate these types of problems and is therefore not a satisfactory substitute for a well-trained and motivated technologist.

Factors that reportedly influence variations in $D_{L_{CO}}$ measurements include alveolar volume, breath-holding time, wash-out volume, size of alveolar sample (19,29), diurnal factors (30), Valsalva and Müller maneuvers (31), and blood transfusions (32).

Cadigan et al. (29) published data which indicate that, in a group of patients with capillary-block syndrome, the coefficient of variation (c.v.) for $D_{L_{CO}}$ (SB) is 2.6% if the alveolar volume at which $D_{L_{CO}}$ is measured is larger than 95% of TLC as obtained by adding the RV (N_2 wash-out) to the largest VC of each patient. In contrast, the c.v. of serial $D_{L_{CO}}$ measurements in a similar group of patients studied two years earlier was 10.7%. In the latter group, however, V_A was uncontrolled and reportedly fluctuated as much as 40%. The author reports a c.v. of 3.2% in normal subjects if V_A was held *constant* but not necessarily higher than 95% of TLC values.

Daly and Roe (33), in a retrospective study on normal males employed in industry report a c.v. of 4.2% for $D_{L_{CO}}$ (SB) measurements. These subjects had been instructed to inhale maximally but no effort was made to correlate V_A with TLC. His conclusion was that $D_{L_{CO}}$ is not greatly influenced by a constant V_A nor by breath-holding time. My experience is that when patients are properly coached to inhale maximally from RV, the coefficient of variation of paired observations is less than 5%.

Even though the disappearance rate of CO from the pulmonary alveoli to the capillary blood is exponential in nature, good reproducibility will be obtained if the breath-holding time is kept between 9 and 11 seconds (6, 29, 34). The method of calculating breath-holding time is important (19) and should be standardized as illustrated in Fig. 5. However, it should be noted that this calculation is not strictly consistent with the protocols of any of the normal studies recommended in the previous section, and may cause small discrepancies if inspiration or expiration are unduly prolonged. (All the cited normal studies measured breath-holding time from the beginning of inspiration to the beginning of sample collection.)

Valsalva and Müller maneuvers may cause a change in pulmonary capillary blood volume and therefore can influence the DL_{CO} (S.B.) measurement (31). To minimize the effects of these respiratory gymnastics, the patients should be instructed to simply relax against the closed four-way valve without making deliberate efforts to hold their breath at maximum lung capacity.

According to Cinkotai (30), DL_{CO} falls during the day at a rate of 1.2% per hour between 9:00 a.m. and 5:00 p.m. and at 2.2% per hour between 5:00 p.m. and 9:00 p.m. This phenomenon may affect reproducibility if one compares data obtained at different times of the day.

To improve reproducibility, standard techniques should be employed. Inspiration and expiration should be as rapid as possible. The total time allotted for wash-out and sample collection (s in Fig. 5) should be less than 4 seconds (6). If a longer time is observed, it should be noted on the report, especially when serial DL_{CO} measurements are being made. The recommended wash-out volume is 1 liter (19), but smaller volumes may be necessary in restricted subjects. The alveolar sample volume should also be standardized; 500–750 ml should suffice for most methods of gas analysis.

Reproducibility of steady-state DL_{CO} measurements is primarily influenced by difficulties in the estimation of F_ECO and arterial CO_2 tensions particularly in patients with an increased V_D/V_T (8, 11).

TROUBLESHOOTING

Most of the causes of error in single-breath DL_{CO} measurements have been described in previous sections. Filley and coworkers reported that the steady-state DL_{CO} method is extremely sensitive to small analytical errors, particularly at rest (8). Opposite errors of 2% in F_ECO and 2 torr in $PaCO_2$ may cause as much as 40% error in the measured DL_{CO}. Other sources of error are variations in the breathing frequency and the dead space of the breathing valve.

CONTROVERSIAL ISSUES

Transfer Factor or Diffusion Capacity?

Countless controversies surrounding DL_{CO} measurements have created a great deal of confusion and undoubtedly have contributed to lack of uniformity, both in methodology and application, among various pulmonary laboratories. Even the traditional name itself "diffusing capacity" is deceptive in that it does not necessarily indicate "capacity" nor does it always follow that a patient with a reduced DL_{CO} suffers from a "diffusion" defect.

Methods and Instrumentation

Many of the controversies in these categories have been discussed in the text of the chapter. These include: Are there significant differences between DL_{CO} results when different types of analyzers are used (e.g., infrared versus gas chromatograph versus electrochemical cells)? Does automated equipment result in improved reproducibility and accuracy? Should V_A be obtained from the single-breath He or Ne dilution, or from multiple-breath dilution or wash-out techniques? How should breath-holding time be measured? When and how should we correct for CO back pressure in smokers? What is the most appropriate correction factor for hemoglobin? Should this be used to correct the measured value of DL_{CO} or the predicted value? What are the effects of acute and chronic residency at high altitudes on the DL_{CO} of normal subjects? Does the assumption that inspired test gas is saturated (ATPS) instead of dry (ATPD) lead to significant error (24)?

REFERENCES

1. Roughton FJW, Forster RE: Relative importance of diffusion and chemical reaction rates in determining rate of exchange of gases in the human lung, with special reference to true diffusing capacity of pulmonary membrane and volume of blood in the lung capillaries. *J. Appl Physiol* 11:290–302, 1957.
2. Forster RE, Roughton FJW, Cander L, et al.: Apparent pulmonary diffusing capacity for CO at varying alveolar O_2 tensions. *J Appl Physiol* 11:227–289, 1957.
3. Krumholz RA: Pulmonary membrane diffusing capacity and pulmonary capillary blood volume: An appraisal of their clinical usefulness. *Am Rev Respir Dis* 94:195–200, 1966.
4. Krogh M: The diffusion of gases through the lungs of man. *J Physiol (Lond)* 49:271–300, 1915.
5. Forster RE, Cohn JE, Briscoe WA, et al.: A modification of the Krogh carbon monoxide breath holding technique for estimating the diffusing capacity of the lung: A comparison with three other methods. *J Clin Invest* 34:1417–1426, 1955.
6. Ogilvie CM, Forster RE, Blackemore WS, et al.: A standardized breath holding technique for the clinical measurement of the diffusing capacity of the lung for carbon monoxide. *J Clin Invest* 36:1–17, 1957.
7. McGrath MW, Thomson ML: The effect of age, body size and lung volume change on alveolar-capillary permeability and diffusing capacity in man. *J. Physiol (Lond)* 146:572–582, 1959.
8. Filley GF, MacIntosh DJ, Wright GW: Carbon monoxide uptake and pulmonary diffusing capacity in normal subjects at rest and during exercise. *J Clin Invest* 33:530–539, 1954.
9. Cotes JE: *Lung Function,* ed 3. London, Blackwell Scientific Publications, 1975, chap 9, p 253.
10. Comroe JH: Retrospectroscope-pulmonary diffusing capacity for carbon monoxide (DL_{CO}). *Am Rev Respir Dis* 111:225–228, 1975.
11. Bates DV, Macklem PT, Christie RV: *Respiratory Function in Disease*. Philadelphia, WB Saunders Co, 1971, pp 93–94.

12. Morton JW, Ostensoe LG: A critical review of the single breath method of measuring the diffusing capacity of the lungs. *Dis Chest* 48:44–54, 1965.
13. Hamilton LH, Smith JR, Kory RC: The use of gas chromatography in the cardiopulmonary laboratory. *Am J Med Electron* 3:3–15, 1964.
14. Smith JR, Hamilton LH: DL_{CO} measurements with gas chromatography. *J Appl Physiol* 17:856–860, 1962.
15. Gaensler EA, Smith AA: Attachment for automated single breath diffusing capacity measurement. *Chest* 63:136–145, 1973.
16. DeGraff AC Jr, Romans W: Programmed valve sequencer and alveolar gas sampler for DL_{CO} measurements. *J Appl Physiol* 23:415–418, 1967.
17. Meade F, Saunders MJ, Hyett F, et al.: Automatic measurement of lung function. *Lancet* 2:573–575, 1965.
18. Kanner RE, Morris AH: *Clinical Pulmonary Function Testing*. Salt Lake City, Intermountain Thoracic Society, 1975, chap. IV, pp 11–12.
19. Ferris BG (principal investigator): Epidemiology standardization project, Part 2. *Am Rev Respir Dis* (appendix), July 1978.
20. Okubo T, Lenfant C: Calibration of gas chromatograph without standardized gas mixtures. *Respir Physiol* 4:255–259, 1968.
21. Burrows B, Kasik JE, Niden AH, et al.: Clinical usefulness of the single breath pulmonary diffusing capacity test. *Am Rev Respir Dis* 84:789–806, 1961.
22. Marks A, Cugell DW, Cadigan JB, et al.: Clinical determination of the diffusion capacity of the lungs. *Am J Med* 22:51–73, 1957.
23. Gelb, AF, Gold WM, Wright RR, et al.: Physiologic diagnosis of subclinical emphysema. *Am Rev Respir Dis* 107:50–63, 1973.
24. Crapo RO, Morris AH: Standardized single breath normal values for carbon monoxide diffusing capacity. *Am Rev Respir Dis* 123:185–189, 1981.
25. Dinakara P, Blumenthal WS, Johnston RF, et al.: The effect of anemia on pulmonary diffusing capacity with derivation of a correction equation. *Am Rev Respir Dis* 102:965–969, 1970.
26. Polgar G, Promadhat V: *Pulmonary Function Testing in Children*. Philadelphia, WB Saunders Co, 1971.
27. Bucci G, Cook CD, Barrie H: Studies of respiratory physiology in children. Part V. *J Pediatr* 58:820–828, 1961.
28. Weng TR, Levison H: Standards of pulmonary function in children. *Am Rev Respir Dis* 99:879–894, 1969.
29. Cadigan JB, Marks A, Ellicott MF, et al.: An analysis of factors affecting the measurement of pulmonary diffusing capacity by the single breath method. *J Clin Invest* 40:1495–1514, 1961.
30. Cinkotai FF, Thompson ML: Diurnal variation in pulmonary diffusing capacity for carbon monoxide. *J Appl Physiol* 21:539–542, 1966.
31. Smith TC, Rankin J: Pulmonary diffusing capacity and the capillary bed during Valsalva and Muller maneuvers. *J Appl Physiol* 27:826–833, 1969.
32. Clark EH, Woods RL, Hughes JMB: Effect of blood transfusion on the carbon monoxide transfer factor of the lung in man. *Clin Sci Mol Med* 54:627–631, 1978.
33. Daly JJ, Roe JW: Serial measurements of the pulmonary diffusing capacity for carbon monoxide in a group of men employed in industry. *Thorax* 17:298–301, 1962.
34. Forster RE, Fowler WS, Bates DV, et al.: The absorption of carbon monoxide by the lungs during breath holding. *J Clin Invest* 33:1135–1145, 1954.

Maximal Inspiratory and Expiratory Pressures

JACK L. CLAUSEN, M.D.

The measurement of maximal inspiratory pressure (MIP) is an important test of inspiratory muscle strength. Its primary usefulness is in the diagnosis and management of patients with neuromuscular disease or injuries involving the inspiratory muscles (diaphragms and accessory muscles) (1). MIP is also useful for evaluating patients whose strength of inspiration is reduced secondary to hyperinflation (as in emphysema) (2,3), severe chest wall deformities, or drugs (4). Measurements of MIP are commonly used to indicate when patients can be successfully weaned from ventilators (4). MIP is related to lung volume, being maximal at residual volume (RV) and close to zero at total lung capacity (TLC), and may be affected by changes in posture. Because the MIP value recorded is directly related to effort, effective instructions and patient compliance are essential for the test to be clinically useful.

Measurements of maximal expiratory pressures (MEP) are also used for the assessment of patients with neuromuscular disease. Because the MEP is an important factor for an effective cough, these measurements are often valuable in the evaluation of patients with impaired coughs and retained secretions.

Large reductions in expiratory muscle strength may produce elevations in RV and reductions in expiratory flow rates, which may be incorrectly interpreted as signs of obstructive airway disease. Since normal expiration is usually a passive event, if the inspiratory muscles are adequate, a reduced MEP is seldom a cause of respiratory failure unless secondary to complications of ineffective cough and retained secretions.

EQUIPMENT

1. Noseclip and rubber mouthpiece.
2. Three-way directional valve (Y or T, with approximately 2.5 cm diameter

PULMONARY FUNCTION TESTING
GUIDELINES AND CONTROVERSIES

ISBN 0-12-788125-5

outlets), with one outlet open to room air, the other sealed (rubber stopper) and containing a leak 1.0 mm in diameter and 15.0 mm in length (e.g., modified Hans Rudolf valve model 2100).

3. Either (1) a direct reading dial gauge, linear from -10 cm H_2O to at least -60 cm H_2O for MIP and 0 to at least $+100$ cm H_2O for MEP or, (2) an electronic pressure transducer and recorder, optimal range 0 to ± 250 cm H_2O. Accuracy: $\pm 2\%$ of full scale. The gauge or transducer is connected to the valve either directly or with tubing.

The 1.0×15.0 mm leak (we use a brass plug 15 mm in length with a 1-mm diameter hole) is important for preventing erroneously high readings resulting from the use of cheek muscles. Some patients with severe weakness of inspirtory muscles consciously (or unconsciously) use cheek muscles during maximal inspiratory efforts. The leak is large enough to allow air to fill the oral cavity, thereby reducing the effective force of the cheeks, but it is not large enough to result in changes in lung volume or reductions in the maximal pressures measured. A comfortable mouthpiece that minimizes leaks around the lips is essential. A mouthpiece with a flange that fits between the teeth and lips (scuba-type) is recommended.

QUALITY CONTROL

The accuracy of the pressure gauges should be assessed initially, at periodic intervals (e.g., every 3 months) and whenever erroneous measurements are suspected. A mercury manometer-type of blood pressure gauge is a convenient device for checking the accuracy of the high-pressure gauges.

PROCEDURES

MIP

1. Explain the procedure to the patient, emphasizing the importance of maximal effort.

2. Have the patient sit upright (note on report if the study is done in another posture).

3. With the three-way valve open to the atmosphere, connect the patient to the mouthpiece. Attach the nose clips, and check that the patient's lips are well sealed around the mouthpiece.

4. Instruct the patient to expire to RV. Turn the valve to the closed position (connected to the gauge or transducer) and instruct him to make a maximal

inspiratory effort sustained for at least 3 seconds (longer than 5 seconds is not necessary).

5. Record and maximum negative inspiratory pressure sustained *after* the initial 1-second period. Disregard the overshoots secondary to the inertia of the gauge needle or chest wall, or those pressures generated by facial muscles.

6. Have the patient rest, then repeat the test twice, recording all three values.

7. If the values observed are less than predicted, the understanding and cooperation of the patient should be reassessed. If there is an obvious spurious reason for his subnormal response, such as back or abdominal pain, or on inability to keep his lips tightly sealed around the mouthpiece, these factors should be noted on the report. Also important to document on the report are those cases in which the patient appears to be making a less than maximal effort during the test or seems to incompletely understand the instructions. The best method of both checking the performance of the MIP device and ensuring optimal understanding of the patient is for the technician to test his own MIP with the patient watching.

MEP

After connecting the patient to the mouthpiece and attaching the noseclips, have the patient inspire nearly to TLC. Close the three-way valve and record the maximal pressure observed during 2–3 seconds of maximal expiratory efforts (ignoring initial needle overshoot). Since this can be a very uncomfortable test due to the high pressures generated, for most clinical purposes it is usually only necessary to ascertain that the patient can generate a pressure of at least 100 cm H_2O. Once a pressure of 100 cm H_2O is obtained, greater efforts and repeat tests to define the true maximal expiratory pressure are seldom clinically necessary or useful.

CALCULATIONS

Take three measurements of MIP, and report the most negative value occurring *after* the first second (in centimeters H_2O). Report the most positive MEP, ignoring the transient maximum value.

NORMAL VALUES

The most useful predictive study for MIP at RV and MEP at TLC is the study of 60 males and 60 females (ages 20–86) by Black and Hyatt (5); the equations are given in Table 1.

Table 1 *Prediction Equations*

		LLN[b]
Males	MIP = 143 − 0.55A[a]	75
	MEP = 268 − 1.03A	140
Females	MIP = 104 − 0.51A	50
	MEP = 170 − 0.53A	95

[a] A equals age in years, valid for range 20–86. MIP and MEP are in centimeters H_2O.
[b] LLN is the approximate lower limit of normal, fifth percentile, independent of age.

The only currently available predicted values of MIP at FRC are from a study of 19 normals by Sharp et al. (3).

Testing at the University of California, San Diego, of the predictive values of the two previously mentioned studies for MIP confirmed their predictive validity; however, the MEP values predicted by Black and Hyatt are considerably higher than those observed in many apparently normal subjects: similarly, lower MEP values were observed by Gilbert et al. (6).

Expected Reproducibility

The reproducibility of both the MIP and MEP is highly dependent upon subject cooperation, but triplicate results within 20% are commonly obtained.

Troubleshooting

Erroneously low results are almost always due to poor patient cooperation or factors that physically limit a maximal effort (e.g., pain or a poor mouthpiece seal).

CONTROVERSIAL ISSUES

WHAT ARE VALID PREDICTIVE VALUES FOR MEP?

In some hospitalized patients without neuromuscular disease, extraordinary weakness, or hyperinflation, and in some normal subjects, MEP results are often not as high as those observed by Black and Hyatt (5) (6 and unpublished personal observations). Until additional experience is published that may resolve this minor issue, it is reasonable to accept lower limits of normal values for MEP to be 100 cm H_2O for men and 80 cm H_2O for women.

Should MIP Be Measured at RV or FRC?

Some physicians prefer to measure MIP at FRC for the following reasons: the MIP may then be more clinically applicable, because this is the lung volume at which tidal breathing normally occurs. Also, this is the lung volume at which MIP is measured in unconscious patients by airway occlusion during tidal breathing. However, one disadvantage of FRC measurements is that adequate normal predictive values have not been established at this volume.

REFERENCES

1. Black LF, Hyatt RE: Maximal static respiratory pressures in generalized neuromuscular disease. *Am Rev Respir Dis* 103:641-650, 1971.
2. Byrd RB, Hyatt RE: Maximal respiratory pressures in chronic obstructive lung disease. *Am Rev Respir Dis* 98:848-856, 1968.
3. Sharp JT, vanLith P, Nuchprayoon CV, et al.: The thorax in chronic obstructive lung disease. *Am J Med* 44:39-46, 1968.
4. Sahn SA, Lakshminarayan S: Bedside criteria for discontinuation of mechanical ventilation. *Chest* 63:1002-1005, 1973.
5. Black LF, Hyatt RE: Maximal respiratory pressures: Normal values and relationship to age and sex. *Am Rev Respir Dis* 99:696-702, 1969.
6. Gilbert R, Auchincloss JH Jr, Bleb S: Measurement of maximum inspiratory pressure during routine spirometry. *Lung* 155:23-32, 1978.

CHAPTER 18

Elastic Recoil and Compliance

ARTHUR DAWSON, M.D.

Lung compliance is a measure of the distensibility of the lungs and is defined as the change in lung volume per unit change in transpulmonary pressure (difference between mouth and pleural pressures). The compliance and elastic recoil of the lungs are measured by means of an esophageal balloon, which is swallowed and then positioned in the lower third of the esophagus, where pressure changes closely approximate pleural pressure changes (1). Static compliance is determined from plots of esophageal pressure versus volume at zero flow points. The recorded pressure is the most negative pressure to which the balloon is exposed. Most of the time, this will be at the tip of the balloon, but the point of minimal pressure will be displaced downward transiently by esophageal peristaltic waves. The 10-cm length of the esophageal balloon minimizes pressure changes due to esophageal contractions; however, the overall pressure may be shifted by increased esophageal tone, especially if there is too much air in the balloon. Dynamic compliance demonstrates the effects of respiratory frequency on lung compliance and is obtained from plots of esophageal pressure, volume, and flow. Measurements of compliance and elastic recoil are clinically used most often for the evaluation of patients with interstitial restrictive lung disease or emphysema. Patients with interstitial pulmonary disease may have increases in recoil and decreases in compliance. Conversely, decreases in recoil and increases in compliance are typical of patients with significant emphysema. The wide ranges of normal values for these parameters and the technical demands of the measurements limit their use. Their clinical usefulness in comparison with other more simple tests of lung function has not been established. Much of the following information is from Macklem's excellent methodology paper published by the National Heart and Lung Institute (2).

Many pulmonary physicians view measurement of lung elastic recoil as an

PULMONARY FUNCTION TESTING
GUIDELINES AND CONTROVERSIES

ISBN 0-12-788125-5

invasive and difficult procedure, suitable more for the research laboratory than for a clinical diagnostic test. It is true that swallowing an esophageal balloon is mildly unpleasant, but it is perfectly safe, and an experienced technician can usually assist even the most anxious patient to get the balloon in the correct position quickly and with minimal discomfort. Only a small amount of relatively inexpensive equipment is required: an esophageal balloon, a catheter, a pressure transducer, a spirometer, a mouth shutter (optional), and a two-channel strip chart recorder. In order to get accurate and reproducible results, however, it is important to pay careful attention to certain technical details. These may sound rather complex when they are described, but once understood they can be rapidly accomplished. Measurement of lung elastic recoil is, in my opinion, a valuable diagnostic test, which should be performed much more frequently than it is.

EQUIPMENT

Esophageal Balloon

The standard esophageal balloon is 10 cm long with a wall thickness of about 0.06 mm; although latex balloons can be made in the laboratory, satisfactory balloons are commercially available from Young Rubber Corporation, Enterprise Avenue, Trenton, New Jersey 08638. In my laboratory, we have for years used hand-dipped plastic balloons made from vinyl plastisol (3). These have slightly thicker walls than the thinnest rubber balloons, but they are very tough and durable, lasting through many tests and almost never developing leaks after insertion.

Catheter

The catheter should be #200 polyethylene tubing 100–140 cm in length. Multiple holes should be spirally arranged in the distal 9 cm contained within the balloon, which is sealed to the catheter with rubber cement. The seal can be reinforced with a few turns of tough thread. Some of the thinner rubber balloons may be adversely affected by rubber cement; these should be sealed to the catheter by wrapping tne proximal end of the balloon with very fine silk thread, which is then sealed with a small amount of Plioband glue. As an aid for positioning the balloon, the catheter should be marked 50 cm from its tip. Since ink marks tend to be erased, it is helpful to cement a few turns of thread around the catheter as a permanent marker. At the proximal end of the catheter, a short, thin-walled, metal cannula should be snugly inserted. This will connect to the positive port of the pressure transducer via a three-way plastic stopcock.

Pressure Transducer

Any of the commonly used pressure transducers capable of measuring differential air pressures up to 60 cm H_2O is satisfactory. The negative port of the transducer is connected via tubing and a two-way stopcock to the mouthpiece.

Pneumotachograph

If, in addition to static elastic recoil, measurements of dynamic compliance are to be made, a pneumotachograph will be required in order to identify points of zero flow. Alternatively, a spirometer with a flow output may be used.

Spirometer

Any spirometer with an electrical output may be used to provide the volume signal for the static volume-pressure curves. If a pneumotachograph is used, its signal may be electrically intergrated to determine volume.

QUALITY CONTROL

Determination of Optimal Balloon Air Volume

For pressure within the balloon to reflect accurately the esophageal pressure, only a minimal pressure gradient across the balloon wall can be tolerated. Lemen and associates (4) have described a simple method to determine the optimal volume of air for a given balloon-catheter system. The balloon is suspended upright in a beaker of water with the top (proximal end) at the surface. A few seconds are allowed for excess air to leave the balloon, then the stopcock is turned to occlude the catheter. The volume of air remaining, normally 0.2-0.5 ml, will result in no pressure difference across the balloon when it is in place in the esophagus. The volume can be measured after the balloon is in place by connecting a 2.0-ml glass syringe to the stopcock and having the patient perform a Valsalva maneuver. This volume should be reinjected into the balloon by injecting a larger volume (e.g., 2.0 ml) and removing the difference (e.g., 1.6 ml).

Balancing Frequency Response of Pneumotachograph and Esophageal Balloon

For measurements of dynamic compliance and related calculations, such as pulmonary resistance and work of breathing, it is essential that there be no phase lag between the esophageal pressure and pneumotachograph flow signals, since the esophageal pressures corresponding to zero flow must be accurately identified. Very large errors can result, especially at higher respiratory frequencies, if phase lags are uncorrected. Macklem (2) described a simple manner of balancing the two signals that requires a pump that can produce quasisinusoidal pressure waves at frequencies up to 15 Hz. This procedure is not necessary if only static compliance is to be measured.

PROCEDURE

Insertion and Positioning of the Balloon

Unless the patient has a very active gag reflex, there is no need to have the stomach empty prior to testing. The catheter (and evacuated balloon) is passed through the nostril and nasopharynx until its tip reaches the upper esophagus. Then with the aid of a few sips of water, it is advanced into the lower esophagus. Topical anesthesia of the nasal passages is strongly recommended, as the catheter in the nose tends to cause discomfort when a noseclip is applied. Anesthesia also reduces tearing and rhinorrhea, especially if lengthy studies are performed. We use two or three sprays of 4% cocaine in the nostril, administered with an atomizer; in addition, about 3 ml of viscous lidocaine is placed on the posterior tongue and swallowed.

Once the balloon has reached the lower esophagus, with the tip 45 cm or more from the nose, the catheter is connected to the pressure transducer, and the balloon is distended with 7–8 ml of air. The air volume is then adjusted to about 0.5 ml. When the esophageal pressure becomes more positive with inspiration, the balloon is in the stomach. As it is withdrawn and crosses the diaphragm into the esophagus, there is an abrupt reversal of the respiratory pressure swings, and inspiration produces a negative pressure. The balloon is withdrawn 10 cm further, so that its entire length lies in the esophagus. Slight adjustments of balloon position are then made to find a position where the end-expiratory pressure is most negative and the cardiogenic pressure pulsations are minimal. This is usually about 35–42 cm from the nares, depending mainly on the sitting height of the patient. A final test to assure proper positioning of the balloon is to look for a "tracheal artifact," defined as changes in esophageal pressure measurements during flexion or extension of the neck. If the balloon is too high, performance of the Mueller maneuver against a closed shutter will cause a drop in the pressure difference between the mouth and esophagus. The patient is instructed to pant at about 2 cycles/sec sufficient force to produce pressure swings of about 10 cm H_2O, while the mouth is occluded. During this maneuver, similar to panting in the body plethysmograph, the variations of transpulmonary pressure should be minimal. If large pressure swings occur, the balloon should be advanced slightly until they disappear. Once a final position of the balloon is determined, the catheter should be taped to the nose and the distance from the nostril to the tip of the catheter should be recorded.

Adjusting Air Volume

Since the pressure within the esophagus and balloon is subatmospheric, the balloon will tend to gain air volume when the tap is opened to atmospheric pressure. The patient empties the balloon while the tap is open to room air by performing a Valsalva maneuver, and a 3-ml syringe is connected to the tap while the Valsalva maneuver is maintained. The optimal volume of air, determined as described in the previous section, is injected into the balloon, and the stopcock is turned to connect the balloon to the transducer. It is not necessary to distend the balloon with 7–8 ml of air each time its volume is adjusted (4), but the air volume should be readjusted whenever the catheter is reconnected to the transducer.

Static Pressure–Volume Curves

While the patient breathes quietly, the pressure should drop with inspiration and rise with expiration. Occasional patients with severe obstructive lung disease may show positive end-expiratory pressures, but otherwise the pressure should remain negative throughout the respiratory cycle. Many patients develop periodic esophageal contractions during which the pressure is positive. It may be necessary to wait for a few minutes after the balloon is swallowed until these subside.

The patient is then connected to a suitable volume recording device, spirometer, or integrating pneumotachograph. The inspiration from which the recoil pressure at total lung capacity (TLC) is recorded should be preceded by a full inspiration in order to standardize the volume history of the lung. Recoil pressure at TLC is initially measured by instructing the patient to inspire fully and sustain his inspiratory effort for a few seconds. The maximal recoil pressure at TLC is generally taken as the initial pressure after flow ceases. Owing to "stress relaxation," this pressure tends to decay slightly as the inspiration is maintained. (See Controversial Issues.)

A series of static-deflation volume–pressure curves is then recorded by having the patient inspire fully, then expire slowly to near the residual volume while the mouthpiece is intermittently occluded for 1–2 seconds with the shutter. The recording of each of these static-deflation curves should be preceded by a full inspiration to standardize volume history.

At least three repeatable volume–pressure curves should be recorded. When several deflation curves are plotted, one may see one or more of them displaced from the others, generally toward more positive pressures. Such curves probably are associated with mild esophageal contraction and should be discarded. For clinical purposes, it usually is sufficient to measure only the deflation volume-pressure curve; if one is interested in evaluating hysteresis, then both inspiratory and expiratory curves should be recorded. Since all of the volume-pressure points must be recorded from a continuous stepwise inspiration from near residual volume to TLC followed by expiration to near residual volume, many patients will find it impossible to cease breathing for a sufficient length of time for the full inflation-deflation curve to be measured.

A few patients will consistently develop esophageal contractions whenever they attempt a full inspiration. In such subjects, the volume-pressure curve should be measured at several lung volumes in the range of 80% to 20% of the vital capacity, after which full inspiration is performed in order to determine the TLC volume. Recoil pressure at TLC can generally be estimated after several trials of full inspiration as the transpulmonary pressure immediately before the onset of esophageal contraction.

Dynamic Compliance

Dynamic compliance may be measured during quiet breathing by dividing inspiratory tidal volume by the pressure difference between points of zero flow. If the frequency dependence of dynamic compliance is to be assessed, then it is necessary to keep tidal volume and end-expiratory volume constant while the patient breathes at varying respiratory frequencies. Once the tidal and end-expiratory volumes are selected, the subject is instructed by displaying his lung volume on an oscilloscope with visual cues for TLC, functional residual capacity (FRC), and the tidal volume. He inspires to TLC, then expires to the desired FRC. Esophageal pressure and flow are recorded at the desired tidal volume and frequency for at least 10 breaths, after which the subject again inspires to TLC to be sure there has been no significant drift in the end-expiratory volume.

CALCULATIONS

Static Lung Compliance

C_{st} is the change in lung volume per unit change in transpulmonary pressure measured over the straight portion of the volume-pressure curve between FRC and FRC + 0.5 liter.

$$C_{st} = \Delta V/\Delta P_{st}$$

Its units are liters per centimeter H_2O. Specific compliance, C_{st}/FRC, may also be reported. Since inspiratory and expiratory compliance may differ, the measured parameter should be specified.

Coefficient of Retraction

This is used to express the maximal static recoil pressure of the lung relative to lung volume. The coefficient of retraction equals P_{st} at TLC divided by TLC. Much more information is gained from observation of the entire volume-pressure curve of the lung than by reporting of single parameters such as lung compliance. Therefore, the static pressure-volume curve should be plotted as transpulmonary pressure versus lung volume. It is also useful to plot lung volume not only as a percentage of the observed TLC, but also as a percentage of the predicted TLC.

NORMAL VALUES

Static Lung Compliance

The reported normal values for static lung compliance are quite variable. Some data from the pre-1970 literature are summarized in Reference 5. For normal adult males, the mean of expiratory compliance has been reported to be 0.262 (range, 0.147 to 0.375) (6). Begin and associates (7) report the static expiratory compliance for 64 normal adult subjects at 0.300 ± 0.081 (mean ± SD), with significantly higher values in older subjects and higher values for males than for females. They give the following regression equations for static expiratory compliance on age in years and height in centimeters. (C_{st} was measured between FRC and FRC + 0.7 liter.) For males,

$$C_{st} = 0.0024A + 0.00516H - 0.677$$

For females,

$$C_{st} = 0.0019A + 0.0039H - 0.471$$

Maximum Static Recoil Pressure

Normal values for this parameter also vary a good deal in the published reports. The figures in Table 1 are calculated from the individual data in 51 normal adults given by Knudson et al. (8). Although containing data from fewer subjects, the study by Turner et al. (9) is also a source for normal values for maximum static recoil and coefficient of retraction; in contrast with the data of Knudson, Turner's male subjects showed a definite decrease in maximum recoil pressure as age increased.

Table 1 *Normal Adult Values for Maximal Static Recoil Pressure*[a]

Sex	Age	Mean (in cm H_2O)	SD	Range
Males	< 50	34.5	9.3	21.5–48.0
Males	> 49	33.7	7.0	17.0–42.2
Females	< 50	33.7	7.2	21.0–48.0
Females	> 49	24.4	4.0	18.0–31.6

[a] Derived from Knudson et al. (8).

Coefficient of Retraction

The normal range for the coefficient of retraction was given as 4–8 cm H_2O/liter in a recent publication (10). We have calculated coefficients of retraction from the individual data of 51 normal adults reported by Knudson et al. (8). There was no significant correlation between the coefficient of retraction and age or height. The values for the coefficient or retraction given in Table 2 are taken from the Knudson data.

Static Volume–Pressure Curve

Several studies have reported normal values for static recoil pressure at different lung volumes, the latter expressed as a percentage of the observed total lung capacity (8,9,11,12), including some data for children and adolescents (12,13). When lung elastic recoil is measured in diseases that alter the total lung capacity, it may be misleading to report the pressures at a percentage of the observed TLC, and it is helpful, in addition, to report them as recoil pressure versus lung volume as a percentage of the *predicted* TLC. None of the published studies on normal recoil pressure has reported these parameters. To compute such data, we calculated the predicted TLC from the single regression equation given by Knudson et al. (8), which fits all of their subjects in the study cited below regardless of age or sex:

$$\text{TLC (liters)} = 0.12233\text{H} - 15.183$$

Table 2 *Normal Adult Values for the Coefficient of Retraction*

Sex	Mean	SD	Range
Males	5.36	1.42	2.41–8.16
Females	6.44	1.71	4.28–11.21

Table 3 *Normal Values for Static Pressure-Volume Curves*

Males < 50 years									
Upper limit	x	3.2	5.8	7.7	9.7	12.1	15.6	48.0	
	y	34.0	56.0	67.0	78.5	89.7	101.0	119.0	
Lower limit	x	7.5	9.2	12.0	14.7	19.1	25.0	44.0	
	y	38.5	48.1	62.0	72.4	80.9	87.3	89.8	
Males > 49 years									
Upper limit	x	2.7	3.5	6.3	9.5	12.3	16.7	32.0	42.2
	y	35.0	51.5	72.1	92.5	105.7	119.0	132.0	134.0
Lower limit	x	6.4	9.0	11.0	13.4	16.6	32.0	38.0	
	y	39.0	51.9	62.3	72.7	83.0	87.4	92.5	
Females < 50 years									
Upper limit	x	−0.4	2.5	4.2	6.6	9.2	13.3	21.0	33.5
	y	39.4	49.2	59.0	68.9	78.7	93.7	104.1	108.5
Lower limit	x	5.0	7.4	11.7	15.3	21.0	43.0	48.0	
	y	31.8	37.0	55.6	63.6	71.5	76.3	79.5	
Females > 49 years									
Upper limit	x	3.1	3.7	4.2	5.2	9.0	12.5	22.0	
	y	46.4	55.7	61.3	74.4	98.0	111.6	124.0	
Lower limit	x	5.4	7.3	9.5	11.8	21.0	25.0	30.0	
	y	31.4	36.2	55.2	66.3	78.5	85.6	93.7	

where H is the height in centimeters. Table 3 gives coordinates that were calculated from the data of Knudson et al. (8), which were obtained from 51 normal nonsmoking adults who had been screened for the absence of antitrypsin deficiency. They define the range of normal values for the static volume-pressure curve where x is the pressure in centimeters H_2O, and y the volume as %TLC predicted.

EXPECTED REPRODUCIBILITY

The reproducibility of measurements of lung elastic recoil pressures has not been systematically evaluated. Reproducibility will be much improved with meticulous attention to technique, especially correct position of the balloon in the esophagus and correct volume of air in the balloon. The reproducibility of tests from anxious, untrained, or dyspneic patients cannot be expected to equal that of normal volunteers recruited from healthy laboratory staff.

TROUBLESHOOTING

A summary of trouble shooting is given in Table 4.

Table 4 *Troubleshooting*

Problem	Possible cause	Solution
Shift in zero pressure	Drift in pressure recording equipment	Re-zero; if necessary, balance pressure amplifier
Rising end-expiratory recoil pressure	Increase in air volume in balloon	Empty balloon and add correct air volume
	External leak in catheter or fittings	Test system for leaks by seeing whether negative pressure is held. Repair leak. Check, especially the connections between catheter and metal adapter
	Change in balloon position (migrating down esophagus)	Reposition balloon and tape catheter securely to nose
Falling end-expiratory pressure	Decrease in balloon air volume	Empty balloon and add correct air volume
	Hole in balloon	Remove balloon and replace or terminate test
Positive pressures are not recorded correctly during forced expiration	Air volume in balloon too small and displaced entirely into catheter with positive pressure	Increase volume of air in balloon
Abnormally positive pressure when mouth shutter is closed	Mouth port of pressure transducer is open to atmosphere	Turn tap to correct position
Pressure "tops out" during maximal inspiration (likely in interstitial lung disease)	Pressure off scale	Decrease coarse gain on pressure amplifier
Failure to hold negative pressure with maximal inspiration	Slow change may be due to leak in balloon or connections	Check for leaks as described previously
	Rapid increase in pressure may be due to esophageal contraction	Repeat maneuver until satisfactory tracing obtained. Try giving patient extra viscous lidocaine
	Hiatal hernia	Note on report
Pressures appear damped	Catheter is kinked	Straighten catheter

CONTROVERSIAL ISSUES

The Static Recoil Pressure at TLC

Following a maximum inspiration to TLC, the recoil pressure, which is greatest immediately after flow ceases, tends to decay to a lower stable value, a phenomenon known as stress relaxation. The lower value may not be reached for 5–10 seconds and can be as much as 25% less than the initial recoil pressure. Successive maximum inspirations are followed by a progressive decrease in the maximum recoil pressure and by a diminution in the pressure decay due to stress relaxation. If the lung is inflated by a slow stepwise inspiration, little or no stress relaxation is observed after TLC is attained (14). Most recent investigators have followed the procedure recommended by Milic-Emili et al. (1) and have preceded measurements of recoil pressure with three maximum inhalations and recorded the TLC static pressure as the most negative pressure observed immediately after flow ceases. The three full inflations should minimize the effect of stress relaxation, but will not abolish it altogether. Some of the earlier standard sources for normal values have not followed this procedure or have not specified what point was taken as the maximum recoil pressure. Macklem recommends only a single inspiration to TLC, and stress relaxation would be more prominent if his procedure is followed (2). No doubt these variations in technique account for some of the considerable differences in reported normal values for maximal static recoil pressure and the coefficient of retraction.

It would seem that, for clinical purposes, recoil pressure should be measured in a manner reflecting the static mechanical properties of the lungs and in such a way as to get the best possible reproducibility. This would be best accomplished by preceding the measurement by three full inflations of the lungs and by recording the pressure when it reaches a stable value *after* stress relaxation is complete. However, since most of the available normal data for maximum recoil pressure all include a stress relaxation component, we would recommend recording both initial and final recoil pressures after inspiratory flow ceases. The effect of stress relaxation on static recoil pressure seems to be minimal at lung volumes below TLC.

REFERENCES

1. Milic-Emili J, Mead J, Turner JM, et al.: Improved technique for estimating pleural pressure from esophageal balloons. *J Appl Physiol* 19:207–211, 1964.
2. Macklem PT: *Procedures for Standardized Measurements of Lung Mechanics* (special publication). National Heart and Lung Institute, Division of Lung Diseases, November 1974; pp 1–7.
3. Crane MG, Hamilton DA, Affeldt JE: A plastic balloon for recording intraesophageal pressures. *J Appl Physiol* 8:585–586 (1956).

4. Lemen R, Benson M, Jones JG: Absolute pressure measurements with hand-dipped and manufactured esophageal balloons. *J Appl Physiol* 37:600–603, 1974.
5. Altman PL, Dittmer DS (eds): *Respiration and Circulation*. Bethesda, MD, Federation of American Societies for Experimental Biology, 1971, p 93.
6. Permutt S, Martin HB: Static pressure-volume characteristics of lungs in normal males. *J Appl Physiol* 15:819–825, 1960.
7. Begin R, Renzetti AD Jr, Bigler AH, et al.: Flow and age dependence of airway closure and dynamic compliance. *J Appl Physiol* 38:199–207, 1975.
8. Knudson RJ, Clark DF, Kennedy TC, et al.: Effect of aging alone on mechanical properties of the normal adult human lung. *J Appl Physiol* 43:1054–1062, 1977.
9. Turner JM, Mead J, Wohl ME: Elasticity of human lungs in relation to age. *J Appl Physiol* 25:664–671, 1968.
10. Fulmer JD, Roberts WC, von Gal ER, et al.: Morphologic-physiologic correlates of the severity of fibrosis and degree of cellularity in idiopathic pulmonary fibrosis. *J Clin Invest* 63:665–676, 1979.
11. Bode FR, Dosman J, Martin RR, et al.: Age and sex differences in lung elasticity, and in closing capacity in non-smokers. *J Appl Physiol* 41:129–35, 1976.
12. Yernault JC, Baran D, Englert M: Effect of growth and aging on the static mechanical lung properties. *Bull Eur Physiopathol Respir* 13:777–788, 1977.
13. Zapletal A, Paul T, Samanek M: Pulmonary elasticity in children and adolescents. *J Appl Physiol* 40:953–961, 1976.
14. Goldman HI, Becklake MR: Respiratory function tests: Normal values at median altitudes and the prediction of normal results. *Am Rev Tuberc Pulm Dis* 79:457–467, 1956.
15. Marshall R, Widdicombe JG: Stress relaxation of the human lung. *Clin Sci* 20:19–31, 1960.

CHAPTER 19

Bronchial Provocation Testing

JOE W. RAMSDELL, M.D.
DARRELL HAUER, B.S.
FREDERICK J. NACHTWEY, M.D.

Bronchial provocation testing identifies airway hyperractivity to a variety of agents. This may be useful in evaluating patients with symptoms suggestive of asthma but no evidence of airways obstruction upon routine pulmonary function testing. The technique may also be used to document bronchial hypersensitivity to specific work-related material or antigens in patients with histories suggestive of post-exposure bronchospasm or hypersensitivity pneumonitis. However, the main use of this technique continues to be as a research tool permitting the study of induced asthma or hypersensitivity pneumonitis in a controlled environment.

EQUIPMENT

Bronchial provocation testing requires a mechanism for delivering a reproducible amount of provocative material to the airways, and a method for monitoring the response. Various systems have been used for delivery of methacholine, histamine, or antigens. Most rely on a nebulizer from which the substance is aerosolized into the patient's mouth. As part of efforts to standardize bronchial inhalation challenge testing, it has been suggested that a specific aerosol delivery device, the dosimeter, may be used for administration of medications or antigens (1). The dosimeter consists of a breath-activated solenoid valve and a timing circuit that delivers a compressed gas at 20 psi to a DeVilbiss nebulizer (#42 or #646) for a specific, preselected time (generally 0.6 second), resulting in standard and reproducible aerosolization of the nebulizer contents. The guidelines for bronchial provocation testing published by the American Thoracic Society (ATS) suggested a variety of different methods for aerosol generation (2). A study by Ryan et al. that compared a dosimeter with a Wright nebulizer for the administra-

PULMONARY FUNCTION TESTING
GUIDELINES AND CONTROVERSIES

ISBN 0-12-788125-5

tion of histamine, reported no significant differences between the two methods for either the provocation concentration for reduction in FEV_1 by 20% or the reproducibility of results in 10 asthmatics (3). Although this study suggests that the less expensive Wright nebulizer could be substituted for the dosimeter, until more comparison studies are available, it is suggested that laboratories use the dosimeter system described in early efforts to standardize bronchial provocation testing (1).

Respiratory function may be monitored by any spirometry system that allows rapid and accurate determination of expiratory flows and volumes. In some situations, it is also desirable to obtain measurements of airways resistance and conductance.

There are certain aspects of provocative material preparation and delivery that are important for optimal test results. Methacholine chloride N.F. has strong hygroscopic properties necessitating desiccation if an accurate preparation based on weight is required. Methacholine crystals should be crushed, spread thinly on the surface of filter paper, and placed in a vacuum container. After desiccating, the methacholine should immediately be transferred to an appropriate weighing device (e.g., a Mettler balance), weighed, placed in a previously prepared volume of diluent, and thoroughly dissolved. Diluents that have been recommended for use include 0.5% NaCl + 0.275% $NaHCO_3$ + 0.4% phenol or 80% propylene glycol + 20% water (2). Studies that have adequately evaluated potential differences in results of bronchial provocation testing if different diluents are used are not available. In the absence of such studies, it is arbitrarily suggested that buffered saline-phenol be used as a diluent. Sterility should be assured by filtration through a 0.2-millipore filter into sterile vials. A stock solution of 50 mg/ml has a shelf life of 2 weeks if stored at 4° C. Appropriate dilutions are prepared from this stock solution as needed. Most laboratories using histamine prepare stock solutions of 10 mg/ml, which has a shelf life of one week at 4° C. The dilution schedules suggested for use (see Tables 1, 2, and 3) are those recommended by the committee on standardization appointed by the National Institute of Allergy and Infectious Diseases (1). The schedules for methacholine and histamine differ slightly from those recommended by the ATS (2); they offer an increased number of dilutions in the low range, where patients are often responsive. Dilutions of aqueous antigens are prepared from appropriate commercially available stock solutions and diluent. The estimated shelf life of the stock antigen preparation is 1 year (for concentrations of 1:20 or greater) and that of the dilutions 1 week, when each is stored at 4° C. The equipment and methodology necessary for evaluating the physiological response to the inhaled drugs or antigens do not differ from those used for clinical pulmonary function testing; available guidelines regarding selection of equipment and quality control should be selected and followed.

All labs undertaking bronchial provocation should have resuscitation equipment and appropriate drugs readily available.

PROCEDURE

The recommended standardized protocol for bronchial provocation testing includes a prechallenge evaluation of respiratory function (1). Patients with significant airways obstruction can be evaluated for reversibility of bronchospasm by testing airways response to sympathomimetic bronchodilators. Significant improvement acutely following bronchodilator administration is usually interpreted as evidence of bronchospasm and in most circumstances obviates the need for bronchial provocation testing. The correlation between a response to an inhaled bronchodilator and a response to inhaled methacholine in such patients has not been systematically evaluated. However, even patients with airways obstruction and no acute response to inhaled bronchodilators are very likely to have bronchial hyperreactivity to inhaled methacholine (4).

When undergoing bronchial provocation testing, patients should be free of any drugs with bronchodilating activity. Prior to testing, they should abstain from the use of (1) sympathomimetic drugs for at least 6 hours (8 hours for metaproterenol and 12 hours for terbutaline or salbutamol), (2) methylxanthines for at least 12 hours, and (3) sustained-release methylxanthines for at least 48 hours (2). Cromolyn sodium should be avoided for 48 hours prior to testing, especially if specific antigens are to be utilized (2). Corticosteroids will have little impact on the immediate response but may block a late response and should be discontinued for 12 hours prior to testing. Significant exercise and exposure to cold air should be avoided for at least 2 hours before testing. Smoking and ingestion of coffee, cola, or chocolate drinks should be discouraged for at least 6 hours prior to testing.

Following placement of noseclips and a determination of baseline respiratory function, the subject undergoes a series of five inhalations of the test material from a nebulizer driven by a dosimeter or a similar delivery control device. The subject is instructed to breathe out to the end of a normal tidal expiration, firmly grasp the mouthpiece of the nebulizer between the lips, press the dosimeter-activating button while inhaling slowly to total lung capacity (TLC) over 3–5 seconds, hold at or near TLC for 2–5 seconds, then expire normally. The first five breaths are of the diluent solution, to assess the presence of a nonspecific response. If no change is seen in respiratory function after 3 minutes, then the challenge begins, with inhalations of the lowest concentration of either methacholine or histamine. Respiratory function is evaluated 3 minutes following each inhalation. A positive response (defined in the section) at 3 minutes that is maintained at 6 minutes signifies a positive provocative study, and the test is terminated. Doses are increased according to the following schedules until a positive response is obtained or the maximum dose is reached. Suggested dilution increments for methacholine and histamine are listed in Tables 1 and 2.

The nature of the immediate positive response to bronchial provocation testing is fairly stereotyped, with a prompt (within 3–5 minutes) fall in expiratory flows

Table 1 *Dilution Schedule and Inhalation Units for Methacholine*[a]

Methacholine concentrations (mg/ml)	No. of breaths	Inhalation units per 5 breaths	Cumulative dose inhalation units
0.075	5	0.375	0.375
0.15	5	0.750	1.125
0.31	5	1.55	2.68
0.62	5	3.10	5.78
1.25	5	6.25	12.0
2.50	5	12.50	24.5
5.00	5	25.00	49.5
10.00	5	50.00	99.5
25.00	5	125.00	225.0

[a] Inhalation unit equals 1 inhalation of solution with 1 mg of drug per milliliter.

and increased airways resistance. Static lung volumes may or may not demonstrate a shift to a pattern of hyperinflation. The immediate changes in respiratory function resolve promptly following treatment with a bronchodilator or return to baseline over a 30- to 90-minute period if untreated.

The testing for antigenic hyperreactivity follows a similar sequence but with these changes: respiratory function is tested during an interval of at least 10 minutes between doses, and a response maintained for 20 minutes is significant. Following a positive immediate response, patients are closely followed for 24 hours in anticipation of a delayed response. This response, unique to antigen testing, is occasionally seen at 4–10 hours. It is more gradual in onset than the immediate response, less responsive to bronchodilators, and has the potential to evolve into sustained asthma (i.e., status asthmaticus) (5, 6). Followup should,

Table 2 *Dilution Schedule and Inhalation Units for Histamine*[a]

Histamine base concentrations (mg/ml)	No. of breaths	Inhalation units per 5 breaths	Cumulative dose inhalation units
0.03	5	0.15	0.15
0.06	5	0.30	0.45
0.12	5	0.60	1.05
0.25	5	1.25	2.30
0.50	5	2.50	4.80
1.00	5	5.00	9.80
2.50	5	12.50	22.30
5.00	5	25.00	47.30
10.00	5	50.00	97.30

[a] Inhalation unit equals 1 inhalation of solution with 1 mg of drug per milliliter.

Table 3 *Dilution Schedule and Inhalation Units for Antigens*

Antigen concentration	No. of breaths	Inhalation units per 5 breaths	Cumulative dose inhalation units
1:1,000,000	5	0.025	0.025
1:500,000	5	0.05	0.075
1:100,000	5	0.25	0.325
1:50,000	5	0.50	0.825
1:10,000	5	2.5	3.32
1:5,000	5	5.0	8.32
1:1,000	5	25.0	33.3
1:500	5	50.0	83.3

therefore, include hourly respiratory function testing for 8–12 hours after antigen administration to detect changes indicative of either bronchospasm or hypersensitivity pneumonitis (5–7). The initial concentrations of antigen used in antigenic bronchial provocation should be no higher than that which produced less than a 6- to 8-mm wheal on immediate hypersensitivity prick skin testing (2). A dosing schedule for antigens is listed in Table 3.

Other protocols have been utilized, usually involving serial inhalations of a fixed concentration of test antigen, with respiratory function testing after each inhalation or series of inhalations (8–12).

Evaluation of bronchial hyperreactivity or hypersensitivity pneumonitis to other substances, including occupationally related materials, is best individualized with an attempt made to duplicate the nature, duration, and level of exposure experienced by the subject. As in standardized testing, bronchodilators and other drugs that could have an impact on a positive response should be avoided (13). Individuals with occupational asthma also demonstrate hyperreactivity to methacholine (14).

Severe reactions are more common with antigens than with methacholine or histamine. For this reason, antigen testing should be reserved for laboratories with previous experience with antigens testing and the capability to follow patients for 24 hours. A physician experienced with the acute management of severe bronchospasm should be immediately available. It is desirable that the technician responsible for the testing be trained in cardiopulmonary resuscitation and in the recognition of the early symptoms of bronchospasm. The appropriate life support equipment and medications should always be readily available.

CALCULATION AND REPORTING OF RESULTS

Changes in respiratory function in response to bronchial provocation can be recognized by any of several physiological measurements of airways obstruction.

The most commonly used criterion has been a 20% decrement in forced expired volume at 1 second (FEV_1). Other parameters of expiratory flow have also been utilized as criteria, including a 25% fall in forced expiratory flow rates between 25% and 75% of vital capacity ($FEF_{25-75\%}$), a 25% fall in maximum expiratory flow at 50% of vital capacity ($FEF_{50\%}$), and a 25% fall in peak expiratory flows (FEF_{max}) (2, 12, 15, 16). Ideally, $FEF_{50\%}$ and $FEF_{25-75\%}$ should be corrected for changes in lung volume (see Chapter 17). Specific conductance (SG_{aw}) has been used, with a fall of 35% considered significant (15). Finally, measurements of hyperinflation, such as decrease in vital capacity (greater than 10%) and increase in functional residual capacity (greater than 25%), have been utilized (17). While SG_{aw} may be more sensitive for detecting bronchial hyperreactivity, measures of expiratory flow (FEV_1, $FEF_{25-75\%}$) may correlate better with a clinical diagnosis of asthma, because subjects with allergic rhinitis and no clinical evidence of asthma may have a significant fall in SG_{aw} in response to low doses of methacholine (15).

The reports of bronchial provocation testing results should specify the inhaled material tested, the cumulative inhalation dose at which a positive response occurred (provocative dose), the nature of the response when antigen material is tested (i.e., immediate or delayed response), the respiratory function parameter or parameters evaluated, and the magnitude of the change observed (as a percentage of the baseline).

The cumulative inhalation dose (CD) is the sum of the products of concentration multiplied by the number of breaths at that concentration: CD = (concentration A) × (5 breaths) + (concentration B) × (5 breaths) + (concentration C) × (5 breaths), etc. The term recommended for the expression of results consists of the provocative dose (PD), followed by the percentage of change and the parameter tested. This term is expressed in cumulative units over the time following exposure that the positive response occurred. For example, $PD_{35}SG_{aw} = X$ units/Y minutes, where X is the cumulative inhalation dose and Y the time at which a 35% fall in SG_{aw} was noted (1). Cumulative doses for the suggested dilution schedules are tabulated in Tables 1, 2, and 3.

NORMAL VALUES

Normal individuals will not show significant changes in respiratory function following completion of the testing sequence to maximum doses of five breaths of methacholine at 25 mg/ml or histamine at 10 mg/ml (1). Fewer than 5% of normal patients tested will show a fall in FEV_1 of greater than 20% in response in methacholine; in contrast, nearly 100% of "active" asthmatics show such changes, usually at low doses of methacholine or histamine (8, 12).

The need for careful observation and interpretation of a patient's complaints or symptoms following bronchial provocation is not eliminated by the documentation of the response of the various respiratory function tests. There are several subgroups of patients with allergic rhinitis or chronic obstructive airways disease who will demonstrate bronchial hyperreactivity by any or all of the criteria used to assess airways obstruction in methacholine or histamine testing (4, 8, 15). There is some evidence that patients with allergic rhinitis may show a fall in SG_{aw} while preserving expiratory flow rates in response to inhaled methacholine (15). However, this has not been a consistent finding (8). Patients with a remote history of asthma or chronic bronchitis show a 20–80% incidence of bronchial hyperreactivity (8, 12). Finally, patients with chronic obstructive airways disease that is not reversible on bronchodilator testing often show profound bronchial hyperreactivity to methacholine when FEV_1 and mid-lung flows are monitored (4).

Although relative sensitivity to methacholine and histamine may vary among individuals with bronchial hyperreactivity, the correlation of a positive response to one with a positive response to the other is quite good (18, 19).

TROUBLESHOOTING

Occasionally, erratic triggering of the dosimeter will occur. This usually indicates excessive moisture on the thermistor and can be rectified by exposing the thermistor to a low flow of compressed air for several seconds. Erratic triggering can often be prevented by holding the nebulizer horizontally (thermistor up) after introducing a solution.

As with any device utilized by a patient, care must be taken to insure cleanliness. Failure to adequately clean nebulizers may result in erroneous dose response curves. Also, if an unclean nebulizer that has been previously used to challenge with high doses of an antigen is subsequently utilized to determine a response to a diluent, a false positive may result.

Both TLC and FVC maneuvers can precipitate bronchospasm in some asthmatics, and this should be considered when performing and interpreting bronchial provocation tests.

REPRODUCIBILITY

The response to inhaled methacholine is felt to be quite reproducible over time, both in terms of sensitivity (i.e., provocative dose) and level of reduction in respiratory function. Studies using similar incremental approaches have shown that the response of 98% of subjects will vary by less than two dilutions during repeat testing (18). The reduction in respiratory function in response to methacholine shows excellent reproducibility with a correlation coefficient of 0.97–0.99 in several studies (11, 18, 20).

There are fewer studies on the reproducibility of histamine provocation testing. Ryan et al. noted the 95% confidence interval for repeat measurements of decrements of 20% in FEV_1 to be the observed value ±1 two-fold concentration difference (3). The response to serial antigen challenge is fairly reproducible, with approximately a 1 log variability in the PD_{35} for specific conductance (21).

Various factors have been shown to increase sensitivity to specific (i.e., methacholine, histamine, and antigenic) and nonspecific irritant provocative agents. These include recent viral infection, level of ambient allergens, and influenza immunization (22, 23). Such factors should, therefore, be considered when evaluating serial bronchial provocation studies.

CONTROVERSIES

Choice of Respiratory Function Parameters for Detecting Responses

Definitive data are not available for resolving the issue of which test is the best measure of respiratory function to use in bronchial provocation testing. FEV_1 or other parameters of expiratory flow are adequate in the majority of clinical situations (17). Although some investigators feel that measurements of airways resistance are important for the detection of responses in some subjects (2, 3), the specificity of this test parameter is reduced by the observation of large increases in airways resistance after bronchial challenge in significant numbers of "non-asthmatic" patients (15). Some individuals, probably with large airways spasm, may have minimal changes in expired flows with marked changes in airways resistance accompanied by symptoms during bronchial provocation testing. This fact should be considered if body plethysmography is not performed during the testing when a "normal" response to bronchial provocation is observed in individuals with episodic respiratory complaints.

Choice of Provocative Agent

The choice between methacholine and histamine appears to be arbitrary. Multiple investigations indicate that bronchial hyperreactivity to methacholine and histamine correlate well (8). Because experience with methacholine is more widespread, this is currently the preferred provocative material.

Distribution of Provocative Agents during Inhalation

Theoretically, the inspiratory flow rates and lung volumes at which inhalation of provocative materials occurs may alter the distribution pattern of the provocative material and, in turn, the bronchoprovocation response. In practice, these factors have not been observed to have a significant impact on either sensitivity or reactivity in most subjects (3).

Nonspecific Irritant Responses

The significance of bronchial hyperreactivity from "nonspecific" irritant responses is not well-defined. Many normal individuals will develop a decrease in SG_{aw} in response to such agents as cigarette smoke, SO_2, "smog," and citric acid. The incidence of bronchial hyperreactivity to methacholine or histamine in such individuals is not known. Also, both TLC maneuvers and forced expirations can induce bronchospasm in asthmatics (24, 25), which can complicate the evaluation of airways hyperreactivity to work-related materials or antigens. Other types of probable nonspecific responses in asthmatics include changes in respiratory function following inhalation of diluent or cold air. The response to cold air correlates so well with methacholine hyperreactivity that cold air may be as sensitive as methacholine or histamine for detecting airways hyperreactivity (26).

These nonspecific irritant responses reveal a patient's potential for developing airways obstruction and may be of clinical significance if symptoms correspond to periods of exposure. For this reason, instances of nonspecific irritant-induced bronchospasm require special care in testing (and interpretation of results).

Dosage Delivery Systems

A variety of systems for delivery of provocative materials will allow recognition of bronchial hyperreactivity (27). The theoretical advantage of a metered delivery system, such as the dosimeter, rests in the independence of total dose delivered to the rate of inspiration. A continuous flow nebulizer will deliver more test material over a slow inspiration than during a rapid inspiration. Since it may be difficult to control inspiratory rates in many patients, this makes standardization and reproducibility of test results difficult. In the one available study that compared a dosimeter with a neubulizer, however, there was no difference in reproducibility of bronchial provocation test results between the two methods (3).

REFERENCES

1. Chai H, Farr RS, Froehlich LA, et al.: Standardization of bronchial inhalation challenge procedures. *J Allergy Clin Immunol* 56:323–327, 1975.
2. Guidelines for bronchial inhalation challenges with pharmacologic and antigenic agents. American Thoracic Society News, Spring 1980, pp 11–19.
3. Ryan G, Dolovich MB, Roberts RS, et al.: Standardization of inhalation provocation tests; two techniques of aerosol generation and inhalation compared. *Am Rev Respir Dis* 123:195–199, 1981.

4. Nachtwey FJ, Ramsdell JW: Bronchial reactivity in chronic obstructive airways disease. *Am Rev Respir Dis,* suppl. 121:172 (1980).
5. Hargreave FE, Dolovich J, Robertson DG, et al.: The late asthmatic response. *Can Med Assoc J* 110:415-421, 1974.
6. Spector SL, Farr RS: Bronchial inhalation procedures in asthmatics. *Med Clin* North Am 58:71-84, 1974.
7. Fink JN: The use of bronchoprovocation in the diagnosis of hypersensitivity pneumonitis. *J Allergy Clin Immunol* 64:590-591, 1979.
8. Cockcroft DW, Killian DN, Mellon JJ, et al.: Bronchial reactivity to inhaled histamine: A method and clinical survey. *Clin Allergy* 7:235-243, 1977.
9. Felarca AB, Itkin IH: Studies with the quantitative-inhalation challenge technique. I. Curve of dose response to acetyl-beta-methylcholine in patients with asthma of known and unknown origin, hay fever subjects, and nonatopic volunteers. *J Allergy* 37:223-235, 1966.
10. Orehek J, Gayrard P, Smith AP, et al.: Airway response to carbachol in normal and asthmatic subjects. *Am Rev Respir Dis* 115:937-943, 1977.
11. Parker CD, Bilbo RE, Reed CE: Methacholine aerosol as test for bronchial asthma. *Arch Intern Med* 115:452-458, 1965.
12. Townley RG, Ryo UY, Kolotkin BM, et al.: Bronchial sensitivity to methacholine in current and former asthmatic and allergic rhinitis patients and control subjects. *J. Allergy Clin Immunol* 56: 429-442, 1975.
13. Slavin RG: Asthma in adults. III. Occupational asthma. *Hosp Pract* 13:133-146, 1978.
14. Lam S, Wong R, Yeung M: Nonspecific bronchial reactivity in occupational asthma. *J Allergy Clin Immunol* 63:28-34, 1979.
15. Fish JE, Rosenthal RR, Batra G, et al.: Airway responses to methacholine in allergic and nonallergic subjects. *Am Rev Respir Dis* 113:579-586, 1976.
16. Stanescu DC, Brasseur LA: Maximal expiratory flow rates and airway resistance following histamine aerosols in asthmatics. *Scand J Respir Dis* 54:333-340, 1973.
17. Haydu SP, Empey DW, Hughes DTD: Inhalation challenge tests in asthma: An assessment of spirometry, maximum expiratory flow rates and plethysmography in measuring the responses. *Clin Allergy* 4:371-378, 1974.
18. Spector SL, Farr RS: A comparison of methacholine and histamine inhalations in asthmatics. *J Allergy Clin Immunol* 56:308-316, 1975.
19. Laitinen LA: Histamine and methacholine challenge in the testing of bronchial reactivity. *Scand J Respir Dis,* suppl. 86:1-48, 1974.
20. Rubinfeld AR, Pain MCF: Relationship between bronchial reactivity, airway caliber and severity of asthma. *Am Rev Respir Dis* 115:381-387, 1977.
21. Rosenthal RR, Norman PS, Summer WR: Bronchoprovocation: Effect on priming and desensitization phenomenon in the lung. *J. Allergy Clin Immunol* 56:338-346, 1975.
22. Ouellette JJ, Reed CE: Increased response of asthmatic subjects to methacholine after influenza vaccine. *J Allergy* 36:558-563, 1965.
23. Rosenthal RR, Bleecker ER, Laube B, et al.: Effect of environmental antigen on cholinergic hyperreactivity. *Am Rev Respir Dis* 117 (Suppl, 2): 76, 1978.
24. Gayrard P, Orehek J, Grimaud C, et al.: Bronchoconstrictor effects of a deep inspiration in patients with asthma. *Am Rev Respir Dis* 111:433-439, 1975.
25. Orehek J, Gayrard P, Grimaud C, et al.: Effect of maximal respiratory maneuvers on bronchial sensitivity of asthmatic patients as compared to normal people. *Br Med J* 1:123-125, 1975.
26. Deal EC Jr, McFadden ER Jr, Ingram RH Jr, et al.: Airway responsiveness to cold air and hyperpnea in normal subjects and in those with hay fever and asthma. *Am Rev Respir Dis* 121:621-628, 1980.
27. Rosenthal RR (ed): Workshop proceedings on bronchoprovocation techniques for the evaluation of asthma. *J Allergy Clin Immunol* 64 (No. 6, pt 2), 561-692, 1979.

CHAPTER 20

Response to Bronchodilators

ANDREW L. RIES, M.D.

INTRODUCTION

The reversibility of airways obstruction can be assessed by measuring changes in pulmonary function after bronchodilator administration. Significant improvement after bronchodilator administration indicates that increased bronchomotor tone is contributing to airways obstruction; this finding may be useful in diagnosing asthma and suggests that bronchodilators would probably be beneficial in therapy. Worsening of pulmonary function may indicate paradoxical bronchospasm caused by bronchodilator medications.

Bronchodilator response testing is usually performed in patients with a clinical history suggesting reversible airways obstruction (e.g., intermittent breathlessness, wheezing, coughing), even when baseline flow rates are "normal," or in patients with evidence of expiratory obstruction on initial study. A negative bronchodilator response, however, does not necessarily indicate irreversibility. Such false negative responses occur for several basic reasons: (1) beneficial responses may require days or weeks of bronchodilator therapy (as might be expected with bronchospasm associated with mucous plugging or mucosal edema); (2) the physiological tests selected may not be as sensitive as the patient's own subjective improvement; (3) an objective response may be evident on tests other than the ones performed; (4) the medication may be delivered improperly; and (5) resistance to the drugs may develop during therapy.

EQUIPMENT

Although any drug can be evaluated for its effectiveness as a bronchodilator, testing for bronchodilator response is usually performed with any of the inhaled

PULMONARY FUNCTION TESTING
GUIDELINES AND CONTROVERSIES

ISBN 0-12-788125-5

sympathomimetics currently used clinically. These include isoproterenol, isoetharine, and metaproterenol administered in standard dosages. The drug can be delivered from a hand-held fluorocarbon-propellant canister, a rubber-bulb nebulizer, a compressed air nebulizer, or an ultrasonic nebulizer.

QUALITY CONTROL

The drug manufacturer's instructions on duration and conditions of storage should be noted and followed. Visually confirm that the device produces an inhalable aerosol.

PROCEDURE

When evaluating for reversibility of airways disease, bronchodilator medication should be discontinued prior to testing: 6 hours for inhaled sympathomimetics, 12 hours for short-acting oral theophylline preparations, and 24 hours for long-acting oral theophylline preparations. When testing the response to additional medication, patients should continue their normal medications. In both cases, the specific bronchodilators used and the time of the last doses should be recorded.

Baseline pulmonary function studies should be obtained following standard techniques; these tests will be repeated after bronchodilator administration. The studies most commonly used to assess bronchodilator response are the vital capacity (VC) and expiratory flow rates from spirometry and flow–volume loops. If resistance and conductance are to be measured in a body plethysmograph, these measurements should be performed prior to forced expiratory maneuvers. This will minimize the effects of maximal inspirations and forced expirations on subsequent measurements of airways resistance, thus minimizing the influence of induced bronchospasm on test results in asthmatics (1, 2).

During testing with commercially available canister-type inhalers, two bronchodilator inhalations 1 minute apart are generally adequate. Inhalation of the medication should occur during a slow inspiration from functional residual capacity (FRC) to total lung capacity (TLC) followed by breath-holding for several seconds. It is essential for valid testing that the aerosolized drug be optimally inhaled. Factors that ensure optimal inhalation include directing the aerosol spray into the larynx to minimize deposition in the mouth, administering the aerosol after airflow has begun, yet early enough in inspiration to ensure adequate airflow, and initiating a moderate inspiratory flow rate, one which is rapid enough to entrain and carry aerosolized particles, but not so fast that the particles impact on mucosal surfaces at sites where airflow changes direction. Coughing is often a sign that the aerosol has been delivered to the airways.

Repeat pulmonary function testing should be performed when at least 75% of the peak response to the drug is expected. Generally, testing should begin 10 minutes following isoproterenol administration and 20 minutes following metaproterenol or other longer-acting beta-agonists (3–5). Sensitivity of testing may be increased by relating changes in flow rates to specific lung volumes, since lung volumes in patients with hyperinflation may change appreciably after bronchodilators (e.g., maximum flow at 50% of prebronchodilator TLC or $FEF_{50\%}$ "isovolume"). Tests should be performed in the same sequence as in the baseline study. Additional testing up to 1–2 hours postbronchodilator may be necessary for optimal detection of paradoxical responses (6, 7).

Plethysmographic measurements of airways resistance and specific conductance (SG_{aw}) are more sensitive than the standard forced expiratory flow measurements in detecting patients with disease, but are less specific because of the larger responses to bronchodilators in normal subjects. The clinical usefulness of measurements of changes in absolute lung volumes, work of breathing, arterial blood gases, exercise tests, or expired flow rates following inhalation of different density gases has not been established.

CALCULATIONS

Postbronchodilator measurements should be compared with prebronchodilator values and reported along with the percentage of change from the baseline values. If it is desired to reference expiratory flow rate changes to specific lung volume, this is best accomplished by using measurements of lung volumes in a body plethysmograph. In most clinical situations, however, plethysmographic measurements are not employed. In this case, one assumes that TLC is unchanged and matches the pre- and postbronchodilator volume–time or flow–volume tracings at this point. The expired volume from the prebronchodilator TLC at which the particular flow rate occurs (e.g., $FEF_{50\%}$) is measured and subtracted from TLC on the postbronchodilator loop. The flow rate measured at this volume is the "isovolume" flow. The same approach can be used to generate an isovolume $FEF_{25-75\%}$ (8–10). Figure 1 illustrates this technique for flow–volume loops.

NORMAL RESPONSE

Defining the normal, nonasthmatic response to bronchodilator administration is difficult. Subjects with negative histories of asthma and no evidence of airways obstruction at the time of testing have generally been used in reference studies (10–16); however, the presence of obstructive airways disease in these subjects was not definitively excluded. The mean response of normal subjects to inhaled

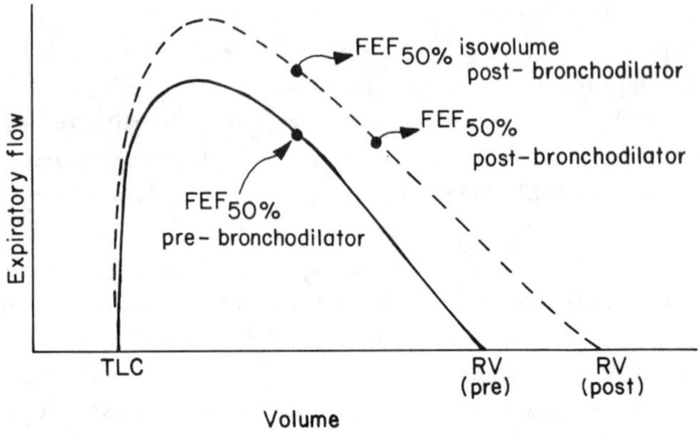

Fig. 1 *Flow-volume loops pre- and postbronchondilators with isovolume referencing at TLC. Note that the nonreferenced $FEF_{50\%}$ postbronchodilator is unchanged, whereas the $FEF_{50\%}$ isovolume shows significant improvement. ——, prebronchodilator; ----, postbronchodilator. RV is residual volume.*

bronchodilators in several studies is a 2–5% increase in FEV_1, an 8–16% increase in $FEF_{25-75\%}$, an approximately 10% increase in $FEF_{50\%}$, and a 24–58% increase in SG_{aw} (expressed as a percentage of improvement from baseline). Using the results of a large epidemiological study of subjects with normal flow rates and no consistent response to bronchodilators, Lorber et al. (10) defined the upper limits of normal values for response to bronchodilators as a 7% increase in FEV_1, a 17% increase in FEF_{50}%, and a 20% increase in $FEF_{50\%}$ isovolume. From a synthesis of these studies and clinical experience, we recommend that significant improvement in expiratory flow parameters be defined as follows:

1. FEV_1: an increase of at least 200 ml *and* 15% of baseline FEV_1.
2. $FEF_{50\%}$ or $FEF_{25-75\%}$ isovolume: a 30% increase.
3. $FEF_{50\%}$ or $FEF_{25-75\%}$: a 20% increase.

An increase in forced vital capacity (FVC) greater than 10% without significant changes in expiratory flows may reflect a bronchodilator response; however, increases in the ratio of FEV_1/FVC without significant increases in the absolute values for FEV_1 are not a reliable index of bronchodilator effects.

EXPECTED REPRODUCIBILITY

The reproducibility of measured bronchodilator responses in patients with "reactive airways disease" is not well defined. This is a complex problem, as many factors relating to a patient's clinical status may affect bronchodilator responses at a given time.

TROUBLESHOOTING

The most common reason for a "false negative" test is failure to effectively inspire the bronchodilator mist, either because of a poorly functioning aerosol device or incorrect inspiratory maneuvers.

CONTROVERSIAL ISSUES

Necessity for Tests Other than Spirometry

Spirometry or flow-volume loops are used most commonly in testing bronchodilator responses, and it is uncertain whether additional tests are necessary. It is well established that normal subjects may have large increases in SG_{aw} after administration of bronchodilators (11–16), indicating a significant amount of resting bronchogenic tone. This is similar to the response of many patients with asthma. Absent or small increases in forced expiratory parameters (e.g., FEV_1, $FEF_{25-75\%}$, or $FEF_{50\%}$) despite sizable decreases in airways resistance during panting maneuvers at FRC have been attributed to transient reductions in lung elastic recoil after large doses of isoproterenol (12), to dynamic compression of large airways causing lower than expected increases in forced expiratory flows (13), or to lack of change in small airways (15). The large magnitude of change in SG_{aw} in normal subjects makes the observation of similar changes in patients less useful in detecting a significant response. Although the available data suggest that plethysmographic measurements of lung volume may not increase the sensitivity of detection of responses to bronchodilators above that achieved with spirometric measurements, conclusive data to resolve this issue are not currently available.

The use of helium-oxygen curves may permit identification of the site of reversibility (peripheral versus central airways) (14, 17), but the clinical value of such observations is not established.

Superiority of Isovolume Referencing of Spirograms and Flow-Volume Loops

Several studies (e.g., 8, 9) have demonstrated that referencing changes in $FEF_{25-75\%}$ to the baseline TLC increased the detection of bronchodilator responsiveness in asthmatic patients. Lorber et al. (10) found that isovolume flow rates from flow-volume loops were better than nonreferenced flow rates in detecting reversible airways obstruction.

Inhalation of Bronchodilators

In this chapter, it is recommended that bronchodilators be inhaled from FRC rather than residual volume (RV). Theoretically, the inspired aerosol will be more evenly distributed to upper and lower lobes when inspired from FRC than from RV, where dependent airways may be closed or compressed. The study by Riley et al. (18) demonstrated significantly better responses when bronchodilators were inspired as a bolus at high (80% VC) compared to low (20% VC) lung volumes; however, inspiration from FRC was not tested. Many laboratories have patients inhale bronchodilators after expiration to RV; a definitive study to establish the superiority of inhalation from FRC is not available.

Defining a Significant Response to Bronchodilators

It has been suggested that a significant change in at least two out of three spirometric parameters (FVC, FEV_1, and $FEF_{25-75\%}$) should be seen before the response to bronchodilator is judged positive (19), but data to substantiate this recommendation were not presented. Other studies have suggested that certain single parameters (e.g., FEV_1, $FEF_{25-75\%}$, $FEF_{50\%}$ isovolume) are the best indicators of responsiveness to bronchodilators, but none evaluated the potential value of using multiple tests (9, 10, 20).

OPTIMAL DRUGS AND DOSES

A variety of drugs, doses, and time sequences for repeat testing have been used, but no one protocol has been shown to be optimal. Isoproterenol has the advantage of rapid onset and short duration. However, other inhaled sympathomimetics may be used, as long as the timing of repeat testing is adjusted to correspond with the peak drug activity period.

Contraindications for Administration of Bronchodilators

The absolute or relative contraindications for bronchodilator testing are not well established. Testing should generally be withheld from patients with unstable cardiovascular problems (e.g., angina, frequent premature ventricular contractions, recent myocardial infarction), unless specific approval is obtained from the patient's physician.

REFERENCES

1. Nadel JA, Tierney DF: Effect of a previous deep inspiration on airway resistance in man. *J Appl Physiol* 16:717-19, 1961.
2. Gayrard P, Orehek J, Grimaud C, Charpin J: Bronchoconstrictor effects of a deep inspiration in patients with asthma. *Am Rev Respir Dis* 111:433-439, 1975.

3. Sinclair JD: The response of asthmatics to bronchodilator aerosols. *NZ Med J* 65:524–527, 1966.
4. Freedman BJ, Meisner P, Hill GB: A comparison of the actions of different bronchodilators in asthma. *Thorax* 23:590–597, 1968.
5. Kennedy MCS, Thursby-Pelham DC: Some adrenergic drugs and atropine methonitrate given by inhalation for asthma: A comparative study. *Br Med J* 1:1018–1021, 1964.
6. Reisman RE: Asthma induced by adrenergic aerosols. *J Allergy* 46:162–77, 1970.
7. Trautlein J, Allegra J, Field J, et al.: Paradoxic bronchospasm after inhalation of isoproterenol. *Chest* 70:711–714, 1976.
8. Cockcroft DW, Berscheid BA: Volume adjustment of maximal midexpiratory flow: Importance of changes in total lung capacity. *Chest* 78:595–600, 1980.
9. Sherter CB, Connolly JJ, Schilder DP: The significance of volume-adjusting the maximal midexpiratory flow in assessing the response to a bronchodilator drug. *Chest* 73:568–571, 1978.
10. Lorber DB, Kaltenborn W, Burrows B: Responses to isoproterenol in a general population sample. *Am Rev Respir Dis* 118:855–861, 1978.
11. Watanabe S, Renzetti AD Jr, Begin R, et al.: Airway responsiveness to a bronchodilator aerosol: I. Normal human subjects. *Am Rev Respir Dis* 109:530–537, 1974.
12. McFadden ER Jr, Newton-Howes J, Pride NB: Acute effects of inhaled isoproterenol on the mechanical characteristics of the lungs in normal man. *J Clin Invest* 49:779–790, 1970.
13. Bouhuys A, van de Woestijne KP: Mechanical consequences of airway smooth muscle relaxation. *J Appl Physiol* 30:670–676, 1971.
14. Fairshter RD, Wilson AF: Response to inhaled metaproterenol and isoproterenol in asthmatic and normal subjects. *Chest* 78:44–50, 1980.
15. Stamm AM, Clausen JL, Tisi GM: Effect of aerosolized isoproterenol on resting myogenic tone in normals. *J Appl Physiol* 40:525–532, 1976.
16. Sobol BJ, Emirgil C, Waldie JR, et al.: The response to isoproterenol in normal subjects and subjects with asthma. *Am Rev Respir Dis* 109:290–292, 1974.
17. Ashutosh K, Mead G, Dickey JC, et al.: Density dependence of expiratory flow and bronchodilator response in asthma. *Chest* 77:68–75, 1980.
18. Riley DJ, Liu RT, Edelman NH: Enhanced responses to aerosolized bronchodilator therapy in asthma using respiratory maneuvers. *Chest* 76:501–507, 1979.
19. Report of the Committee on Emphysema. American College of Chest Physicians. Criteria for the assessment of reversibility in airways obstruction. *Chest* 65:552–553, 1974.
20. Light RW, Conrad SA, George RB: The one best test for evaluating the effects of bronchodilator therapy. *Chest* 72:512–516, 1977.

CHAPTER 21

Blood Gases

JOHN G. MOHLER, M.D.
CLARENCE R. COLLIER, M.D.
WILBUR BRANDT, M.S.
JOAN ABRAMSON, M.S., RCPT
GERDA VERKAIK, RCPT
STEVEN YATES, RCPT

Few laboratory measurements have as much clinical impact as the determinations of pH, and partial pressures of O_2 (PaO_2) and CO_2 ($PaCO_2$) from arterial blood. Arterial pH is measured to define the presence and magnitude of systemic acid–base disorders, and the $PaCO_2$ indicates whether these disorders are of respiratory or metabolic origin. The $PaCO_2$ is a very sensitive and specific indicator of the adequacy of ventilation. An elevated $PaCO_2$ always indicates that alveolar ventlation is inadequate, and a low $PaCO_2$ always indicates that alveolar ventilation is increased above normal levels, whether the increase is voluntary (as in the hyperventilation syndrome) or involuntary (as in compensated metabolic acidosis, aspirin overdose, and certain types of hypoxia).

Measurements of the PaO_2 serve as indicators of the adequacy of pulmonary oxygen exchange. A low arterial PO_2 may indicate either a low inspired oxygen tension, abnormal lung function, or the presence of a shunt. Measurements of PO_2 in mixed venous blood (PvO_2) indicate whether the delivery of oxgyen to the tissues is adequate for meeting metabolic needs.

The indications for blood-gas analyses are too numerous and diverse to be reviewed here. Basically, these measurements are indicated whenever it is suspected that problems with oxygenation, ventilation, or acid–base balance may be present.

Few quantitative laboratory tests have the extraordinary requirements for accuracy demanded of measurements of pH, PO_2, and PCO_2. Errors as small as 0.2 units in pH measurement, or 5 mm Hg in PO_2 and PCO_2 measurements, if they occur in certain critical ranges of measurement, may influence decisions regarding therapeutic intervention or oxygen therapy.

PULMONARY FUNCTION TESTING
GUIDELINES AND CONTROVERSIES

ISBN 0-12-788125-5

A complete review of the physiology of oxygen and carbon dioxide transport, a fascinating and complex subject, can be found in a number of textbooks and articles. Only those aspects essential to an understanding of the processes of measurement are briefly reviewed here.

The affinity of hemoglobin for oxygen may be altered by a number of chemical and physical variables, including pH, PCO_2, temperature, the presence of carboxyhemoglobin (COHb) or methemoglobin (met Hb), and the concentration of 2-3 diphosphoglycerate (2-3 DPG). The effects of any of these variables can be described graphically by plotting the percent oxygen saturation of hemoglobin ($\%HbO_2$) versus the PO_2 of the arterial blood (See Fig. 1). A shift of the curve to the right indicates decreased $Hb–O_2$ affinity and enhanced release of O_2 at the tissue level, while a shift to the left indicates the converse conditions. Causes of a right shift include decreased pH and increases in temperature, PCO_2, and 2-3 DPG. Causes of a left shift include increased pH, the presence of COHb and met Hb, and decreases in temperature, PCO_2, and 2-3 DPG.

Hemoglobin has a 200-fold greater affinity for CO than for O_2; thus, exposure to relatively low levels of inspired CO can result in significant numbers of Hb-binding sites being unavailable for oxygen transport. In methemoglobinemia, the iron in the Hb molecule is in the ferric (+++) form, which is unable to combine reversibly with (and thus transport) oxygen. In the presence of COHb, met Hb, or any other cause of abnormal $Hb–O_2$ affinity, the percent O_2 saturation calculated from measured PO_2 and total Hb may be inaccurate.

The measurement most commonly used to describe the affinity of Hb for oxygen quantitatively is the P_{50}, the partial pressure of O_2 at which 50% of the Hb is saturated with O_2 (temperature and pH are standardized at 37° C and 7.40). The normal P_{50} is 27; however, abnormal types of Hb may have altered affinities

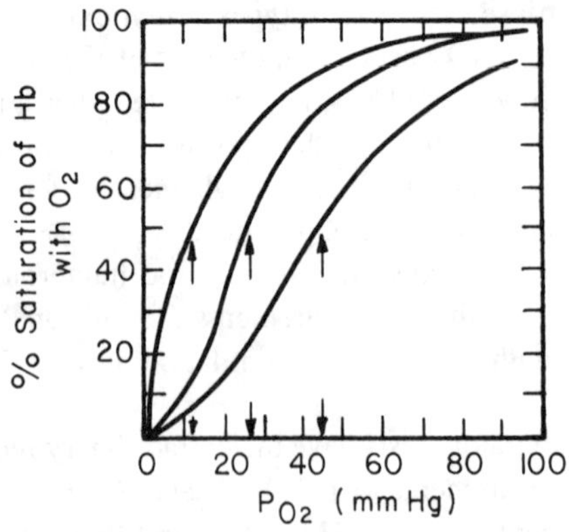

Fig. 1 *Oxyhemoglobin dissociation curves, shift to left, normal, and shift to right. Arrows mark P_{50}s.*

for O_2. For example, for Hb Chesapeake, the P_{50} is 19. As a consequence of shifts in the Hb-O_2 dissociation curve and the resulting changes in P_{50}, delivery of oxygen to the tissues may be either reduced or enhanced. Tissue O_2 delivery is also dependent on cardiac output, distribution of blood flow, Hb concentration, O_2 content, and PaO_2. P_{50} often changes in ways that seem to be compensatory when disturbances of these other delivery parameters occur. Although P_{50} measurements are often of interest, especially in the larger, research-oriented medical centers, their role in clinical decisions has yet to be defined, and they are currently seldom requested in the average hospital. P_{50} may be estimated "qualitatively" by comparing the *measured* oxygen saturation with that *calculated* from the standard dissociation curve. When Hb-O_2 affinity is evaluated in the presence of COHb or met Hb, the percent oxygen saturation should be referenced to the amount of Hb *available* for Hb-O_2 binding (= oxy- and deoxy-Hb) and not to the total amount of Hb present (= oxy-, deoxy-, Co-, and met Hb). (See Controversies.)

The *oxygen content* of blood represents the sum of the oxygen bound to hemoglobin and that dissolved in the plasma, and is most commonly measured to determine cardiac output by the Fick method. It can either be determined directly or estimated from careful measurements of the total Hb concentration, the percent oxyhemoglobin, and the PaO_2.

Despite the clinical and physiologic importance of blood-gas measurements, it has only been in the past 20 years that suitable instrumentation has been available for widespread measurements of PO_2 and PCO_2. The introduction of the Clark PO_2 electrode and the Stow-Severinghaus CO_2 electrode made possible rapid accurate measurements without the extraordinary levels of technical expertise required for the lengthy analyses by the classical techniques of Van Slyke and Haldane.

Introduction of these electrodes was followed by the development of instruments in which many of the technician's functions are now automated, including sample introduction, calculations, and even quality control. Although such automation is impressive, it is important to appreciate that the most important components of the units, the Clark and Stow-Severinghaus electrodes, are basically unchanged. It is even more important to appreciate that an understanding of the principles of operation, quality control, and troubleshooting is as vital to proper operation of automated units as it was to that of the older manual systems.

In this chapter we consider the five measurements most often made in blood-gas laboratories: pH, PO_2, PCO_2, percent oxyhemoglobin, and O_2 content. Because measurement of P_{50} may become more widespread in the future, it is also discussed. Because of the diversity of instrumentation currently available for making these measurements, and the differences among these instruments in operating and performance characteristics, specific details on each instrument are not reviewed. Instead, general principles of operation and quality control are presented. For more specific details, the reader will need to review information available from manufacturers and other published evaluations of equipment.

INSTRUMENTATION

pH

The pH of blood can be measured with a special electrode comprised of two half-cells. One, the measurement half-cell, has a special glass membrane that is permeable only to H^+ ions; the other is a stable reference electrode, most commonly a mercury calomel half-cell. A KCl salt bridge connects the electrode and reference half-cells. The electrical potential of the H^+ ions that pass through the membrane and into the electrode chamber is a logarithmic function of the concentration of H^+ ions. The selective permeability of the special glass membrane to H^+ ions may be altered over the course of time, either by the development of cracks, or by the deposition of protein on the membrane.

PCO_2

The measurement of the partial pressure of CO_2 in blood is most commonly made using a Stow-Severinghaus electrode. This is a standard pH glass electrode bathed in a $NaHCO_3$ buffer solution, which is separated from the blood sample by a special membrane that is permeable only to CO_2. Diffusion of CO_2 from the blood into the buffer solution produces equilibrium of the partial pressure of CO_2; the result is a proportional change in the H^+ concentration of the buffer solution, which is measured by the pH electrode. The diffusion characteristics of the membrane can markedly affect the response time of the electrode and thus the accuracy of CO_2 measurements.

PO_2

The partial pressure of oxygen in blood is most commonly measured using the Clark electrode, which consists of a platinum cathode and a Ag–AgCl anode, with a polarizing voltage of 0.5–0.6 volts and completion of the electrical curcuit by a KCl electrolyte bridge. Deposition of protein on the platinum electrode is prevented by a special membrane that permits the free passage of O_2. Oxygen diffuses through the cathode electrolyte solution to the platinum electrode surface where it is reduced, altering the conductivity of the electrolyte solution. This causes a change in current between the cathode and the anode, which is proportional to the partial pressure of oxygen in the blood sample. The consumption of oxygen by the electrode may cause gradients of oxygen tension near the cathode that may differ for gases, aqueous buffers, and blood. These gradients may (at least in part) be responsible for the differences in current output from the O_2 electrode which may be observed when PO_2s are measured in gases and then in blood samples of the same PO_2. The magnitude of the factor (the blood-gas factor) is dependent upon several variables including the membrane thickness, the material used for the membrane, the diameter of the cathode, and the pressure flow characteristics of the sample near the cathode. The development of the microelectrode (approximately 25 μm in diameter), which is used in most new analyzers, has reduced the O_2 consumption by the electrode, the magnitude of the blood-gas factor, and the need for complex methods of stirring the samples near the cathode.

The output of the Clark electrode can be significantly altered by exposure to low concentrations of halothane (a commonly used anesthetic agent) (1). The clinical significance of this observation, however, is determined by the frequency with which blood samples containing halothane are analyzed.

In addition to the Clark and Stow-Severinghaus electrodes, the partial pressures of O_2 and CO_2 in blood can also be measured with a mass spectrometer or gas chromatograph, when they are equipped with special gas-permeable membranes. However, the costs of instrumentation and problems with clogging of the sampling system limit the usefulness of such systems for routine blood-gas analyses; hence these systems are not discussed further.

O_2 Saturation of Hemoglobin

The early observation that arterial blood is a different color than venous blood is the basis for the spectrophotometric method of measuring the percent of oxyhemoglobin. The two-wavelength method, described by Hufner in 1900, measures the amount of oxyhemoglobin relative to the amount of deoxy-, or "reduced" hemoglobin. This method has the significant disadvantage of overestimating the percent of oxyhemoglobin of the total hemoglobin when COHb and met Hb are present. A similar two-wavelength method can be used for the measurement of COHb.

Three-wavelength systems can make simultaneous measurements of reduced, oxy-, and carboxyhemoglobin (2). A four-wavelength instrument recently developed by Instrumentation Laboratories, the IL 282, also measures methemoglobin. After the blood is injected into the instrument, it is hemolyzed by the automated addition of a standard volume of hemolysate. The light from a thallium neon hollow cathode is measured at 535, 585.2, 594.5, and 626.6 nm, using interference filters mounted on a motor-driven filter wheel. A logarithmic amplifier receives currents from the sample and reference cells at each wavelength and generates an output voltage equivalent to absorbance. The absorbance of a "zeroing" solution at each wavelength is subtracted, then the four resulting absorbance values are substituted in four equations that relate the concentration of each species of hemoglobin to the characteristic absorption of light at each frequency.

Although the accuracy of measurements with this instrument is unaffected by differing levels of oxyhemoglobin or carboxyhemoglobin, levels of methemoglobin above 10% may cause errors in oxy- and carboxyhemoglobin determination (3). Other substances in the blood that absorb light at the specified wavelengths may also interfere with the accuracy of the results. Such substances include methylene blue, Evans blue, and sulfhemoglobin. The absorption characteristics of nonhuman or abnormal human hemoglobins may differ from those of normal human hemoglobin, thereby requiring different equations (3).

O_2 Content

Van Slyke Technique

The total oxygen content of blood samples is classically measured by the technique of Van Slyke and Neill in which O_2 is liberated by the addition of ferricyanide solution to a known amount of blood in a closed, constant-volume container; the amount of O_2 is determined by precisely measuring the decrease in pressure after the chemical absorption of O_2 (4). The more recent micro-Van Slyke method offers the advantages of smaller sample size and decreased time of analysis (5).

Although the Van Slyke technique can be very accurate and precise (6–9), it requires painstaking technical skills, and about 20 minutes are needed for each determination.

Galvanic Cell Method

For routine measurement of O_2 content, a galvanic cell is more suitable than the Van Slyke technique. The only instrument of this type which is in current wide use is the Lex-O_2-Con, developed by Lexington Industries. A special precision syringe with a Chaney adapter is used to inject a 20-μliter sample of blood into the instrument where scrubber gases (97% N_2, 2% H_2, and 1% CO) passing over a catalyst remove the O_2 from the blood and transfer it to a galvanic fuel cell. This cell develops a current proportional to the amount of O_2 delivered to it. Integration of the current output is used to calculate the total O_2. The addition of CO to the scrubber gas hastens the scrubbing process by markedly reducing the rate of hemoglobin reassociation with oxygen. The unit is calibrated by the injection of 20 μliters of room air; the use of the same syringe with the Chaney adapter for both calibration and sample introduction minimizes errors due to volume differences between syringes. The accuracy and precision of this unit have been reported to be as good as those of the Van Slyke technique (7–9). Sample analysis time is about 6 minutes.

QUALITY CONTROL

In the design of an optimal quality control program for blood-gas measurements, the need for accuracy, precision, and 24-hour availability conflicts with the need for reasonable quality control costs and the limitations of sensitive and relatively unstable instrumentation. Of the variety of options for quality control, each has significant disadvantages.

Limits of Acceptability for Quality Control Determination

Absolute recommendations for the quality control of blood-gas measurements are not currently feasible, because of inherent differences in the performance characteristics of different analyzers, differences in quality control methodologies, differences in clinical needs for accuracy and precision, and a lack of consensus of opinion on the feasibility of tonometry of blood in all clinical laboratories. Instead, each laboratory must define its own target values (expected values) and acceptable limits of precision based on the instrumentation and methodology used, and verified under conditions in which the techniques of analysis are known to be satisfactory. If, in the course of routine measurements, a quality control determination falls outside of these laboratory-specific limits of acceptability ("out-of-control"), then the performance of the analyzer should be corrected by appropriate calibration or troubleshooting procedures. Correction of the problem should then be verified by a repeat quality control determination before the analyzer is used for additional clinical measurements.

The limits of acceptability most commonly used are the mean ±2 standard deviations (SD), preferably derived from 20 or more determinations. The bias introduced by extreme outlying values is avoided by recalculating the mean and SD after outliers greater than 3.0 SD from the original mean are excluded. A variety of statistical techniques are used for more sensitive detection of out-of-control situations and include the use of t-test comparisons of the means of multiple determinations, trend analyses, or the recognition of a critical number of consecutive results above or below the expected value (10). In order to comply with guidelines of the Joint Commission for Accreditation of Hospitals (JCAH) (as well as many states' regulations), there must be careful documentation of all quality control procedures and corrective actions.

pH ELECTRODES

2-Point Calibration

Routine calibrations should include the use of two buffer solutions that span a significant portion of the pH range measured in clinical samples. Most commonly used are phosphate buffer solutions, one with a pH of 7.384, and one with a pH of 6.840. These buffer solutions should be checked initially and weekly against buffer solutions referenced to National Bureau of Standard (NBS) buffer solutions. Storage bottles must be kept capped except during sample transfer in order to avoid the deleterious effects of CO_2 absorption or contamination with bacteria or fungi. Two-point calibrations should be done every 4 hours, or whenever calibration settings are altered.

1-Point Calibration

One-point checks of pH calibration should be done before each blood gas determination or series of determinations (as required by state regulations in California), or every 20 minutes, or whenever the pH result of a sample is suspected to be erroneous.

Commercially available alternatives to the standard phosphate buffer solutions for routine quality control include buffer solutions equilibrated with gas in sealed glass vials for which the target (expected) value for pH has been established in reference to NBS standard buffer solutions.

One potential disadvantage of aqueous buffer solutions is that they may not detect alteration in electrode performance secondary to deposition of protein on the membrane (11). This problem may be suspected if significant prolongations in the response time of the electrode are noted. Many automated instruments minimize this problem with automated membrane-flushing systems. Frozen standard serum that has been tonometered with a standard CO_2 concentration and analyzed for pH by multiple determinations, has been reported to be more useful than aqueous buffers for detecting persistent protein contamination of the membrane (12). However, the use of tonometered serum as a high-frequency, routine quality control agent cannot be recommended until more evidence is available that the considerable extra work required is justified by the observed frequency of protein contamination (see Controversies). Contamination may be avoided by flushing the pH electrode with a protein-cleaning solution at a frequency not less than once every tenth blood sample. Also, normal saline rather than distilled water should be used if the electrode needs to be flushed after analysis of blood.

The glass membranes in pH electrodes deteriorate over time or when exposed to pH values outside those encountered clinically. Therefore, the electrodes should be stored in a pH 7.40 buffer solution and changed at the frequency recommended by the manufacturer.

PO_2 Electrodes

In contrast with the pH electrode, which is linear, relatively stable, and easy to calibrate, the PO_2 electrode presents special problems.

Blood-Gas Factor

The response of the Clark-type O_2 electrode may be up to 25% lower when measuring blood than when measuring gas of the same PO_2 (the ‘‘blood-gas factor'') (13). In more contemporary models of blood-gas analyzers, the blood-gas factors are usually much smaller; in three systems tested, the range was 1.2–5.79% (14). Analyzers with similar electrode diameters and membranes may have different blood-gas factors (14) and for a given analyzer, the blood-gas factor may vary depending on the characteristics of the blood sample (15). Differences in electrode output between aqueous buffer solutions and blood, which are both tonometered with the same gas, also occur (15, 16). Although the blood-gas factor is usually attributed to O_2 gradients that develop as a result of O_2 consumption by the electrode, recent evidence suggests that other factors, such as contamination of the sample with either calibrating gas or flushing solutions may also be important (16).

If gas or tonometered buffer solutions are used for calibration, the magnitude of the blood-gas or blood-buffer factor should be determined initially for each instrument; if it is of sufficient magnitude, measurements should be corrected by this factor.

Careful tonometry techniques are essential for correct determination of blood-gas/buffer factors at several pressures. Because these factors may not be linearly related to PO_2, they should be defined at appropriate intervals over the range of measurement of clinical interest (e.g., PO_2 values of 40, 70, 100, 150).

Some automated instruments use a programmed algorithm to correct for the blood-gas factor; at least one model allows the user to dial in the blood-gas factor used in the automated computations. In either case, the validity of the corrections should be confirmed initially. It should also be appreciated that if the blood-gas factor changes, the automatic calculation may be erroneous.

Tonometry of Blood

Because of the unique oxygen-binding characteristics of hemoglobin and the complex viscosity characteristics of normal fresh blood, tonometry of whole blood remains the optimal method for assessing the accuracy and precision of PO_2 measurements. Although usually adequate for quality control of pH and PCO_2 measurements, none of the currently available commercial solutions sealed in glass vials (aqueous buffer solutions, or those containing denatured red blood cells or hemoglobin) are, to date, able to satisfy PO_2 quality control requirements as well as tonometered blood. Blood tonometry does, however, require increased budget, space, and time allocations (for purchase, storage, operation, and maintenance of equipment); it also increases the employee's exposure to possible infection with hepatitis and does not eliminate the necessity for purchasing pH calibration buffer solutions. Because of these disadvantages, many laboratories have not found blood tonometry to be a feasible method of quality control.

As part of the initial evaluation of equipment, tonometry should be done at three different levels of PO_2 and PCO_2; thereafter, it should be performed at a minumum of two levels after each change in electrodes, and routinely at least once a day.

The blood used for tonometry should be less than 24 hours old and obtained from patients without hepatitis; it should also not exhibit significant hemolysis, high (> 20,000) white blood cell counts, or high lipid levels. Bubble tonometers may have the advantage of simplicity and lower initial cost and capabilities for simultaneous preparation of multiple samples of different gas tensions. Foaming of the sample is a problem with some units. It has been recommended that bubbles should be relatively large (2–7 mm), because small bubbles cause elevations in gas tension above target values secondary to compressive surface tension effects (17). Thin-film tonometry (18) offers the advantages of causing minimal foaming and using smaller amounts of calibrating gases.

The gas used for tonometry should be humidified at the temperature of the tonometer prior to introduction into the tonometry chamber. Gas flow rates and sample mixing times should be in accordance with the manufacturer's instructions or the best available recommendations. Too rapid a gas flow rate may cool or dehydrate the blood sample. The tonometry chamber should be at the same temperature as the blood-gas analyzer (usually 37.0° C).

Correct sample transfer techniques are crucial for optimal tonometry results. The syringe should be purged with tonometer gas 3–5 times before loading blood, then 0.2–0.5 ml of blood should be drawn into the syringe and expelled to ensure that no bubbles are within the syringe. The pressure used to transfer the sample from the tonometer to the syringe should be minimal to avoid formation of bubbles. The sample should be transferred rapidly to the blood-gas analyzer in order to minimize sample cooling and gas diffusion. Target values for tonometered blood should be corrected for water vapor pressure at the temperature and barometric pressure of the tonometer.

Despite optimal techniques, precise recovery of target values for PO_2s greater than 150 mm Hg may be difficult. In the range of PO_2s of 20–150 mm Hg, recovered values should be within 5 mm Hg of target values.

To prevent bacterial contamination, all parts of the tonometer in contact with fluid, including the humidification chamber, should be disinfected routinely. Some laboratories add small amounts of antibiotics to the tonometer sample to prevent bacterial growth and its associated effects on the pH and PO_2 of the tonometered solution. Concentrations of 0.5 μg of bacitracin and 0.01 μg per ml of neomycin per milliliter of blood have been found to be effective.

Laboratories that do not include tonometry of blood as a quality control procedure should split blood samples with a laboratory that does tonometry to compare results.

Aqueous Buffer Solutions

The use of commercially available ''pre-tonometered'' aqueous buffer solutions packaged in sealed glass vials eliminates the time and technical demands required for preparing a tonometered sample and reduces the risk of hepatitis. If used properly such materials are very useful for assessing the accuracy of pH and PCO_2 measurements. However, the blood-gas or blood-buffer PO_2 differences that are observed with many instruments necessitate the additional use of tonometered blood as a part of an optimal quality control program. Interlaboratory comparison programs in which virtually identical vials of aqueous buffers from the same production lot are analyzed using a number of different blood-gas analyzers have shown that, in the clinical range for PO_2, intermodel differences can be quite large (e.g., a mean PO_2 value of 73 for model A, and a mean PO_2 of 52 for model B) for aqueous buffers; much smaller differences are observed measuring tonometered blood (e.g., a mean PO_2 of 65 for model A, mean PO_2 of 63 for model B). Thus, when manufacturers of some quality control products specify the expected ranges of measurements for each lot of materials, the ranges for PO_2 are often so wide (e.g., 51–74) as to be of limited usefulness for adequate quality control.

Laboratories may overcome the disadvantages of these wide ranges by defining an expected mean value and range for each lot of buffer based on multiple determinations ($n \geqslant 20$) using a single satisfactorily functioning instrument. In these circumstances, the range may be quite narrow (e.g., 95% of values falling between 61 and 66), thereby increasing the usefulness of these products. Routine quality control determinations that fall outside of these limits indicate that analyzer performance has changed. The magnitude of the change that might be expected with blood, however, cannot always be ascertained from the results, as the buffers may be more (or less) sensitive than blood to changes in instrument performance.

The manufacturers' instructions regarding the shaking of the vial and the equilibration temperature immediately prior to opening the vial should be followed closely. Caution should be taken not to wrap one's fingers around the vial during shaking because this increases the vial temperature, thereby altering the partial pressure of gas in solution. Equilibration of the vial at temperatures outside of the recommended range may necessitate the use of a correction factor.

Solutions of Hemoglobin and Buffer or Denatured Red Cells Suspended in Buffer

These materials are currently commercially available in pre-tonometered sealed glass vials. Although their behavior in blood-gas analyzers should theoretically approximate the behavior of fresh whole blood more closely than that of the aqueous buffer solutions, significant differences have been observed between PO_2 measurements made using these solutions and fresh whole blood tonometered to the same oxygen tension; hence, for optimal quality control, occasional checks with tonometered blood are still necessary. These materials may be more sensitive than aqueous buffer solutions to equilibration temperatures immediately prior to the opening of the vial (often a water bath is required); thus, manufacturers' instructions must be carefully followed.

Fluorocarbon Emulsions

These newly developed materials offer the advantage of possessing an oxygen capacity and affinity that may more closely approximate those of blood than do those of aqueous buffer solutions, and thus they may represent a significant contribution to quality control programs of the future.

Gas Calibration

Because of the drift characteristics of oxygen electrode-amplifier systems, there is a need for frequent (and convenient) calibration checks. Tonometered blood cannot meet this need because of the technical demands and inconvenience of sample preparation. Although some types of analyzers have built-in systems using automatically tonometered buffers to meet this need, the majority of analyzers incorporate systems that deliver calibration gases to the electrodes for convenient and rapid setting and checking of calibrations. In such systems, the calibration gases should be heated and humidified to the temperature of the analyzer (usually 37° C) before passing the electrodes. The need for a blood-gas correction factor must be determined for each instrument as previously discussed.

CO_2 ELECTRODES

The problems associated with calibration and quality control of the CO_2 electrode, while not as simple as those seen with the pH electrode, are not as complex as those encountered with the O_2 electrode. With the exception of the issues discussed in the following, the recommendations presented for the O_2 electrode are applicable to the CO_2 electrode and are not repeated.

One important difference between the CO_2 and O_2 electrodes is that most investigators have concluded that blood-gas or blood-buffer correction factors are not needed with CO_2 electrodes. An important exception to this conclusion was that contained in the report by Bateman of the need for correction factors for the calibration of the CO_2 electrodes, which his group tested with both gases and tonometered buffer solutions (15). Because of this report, it is recommended that the accuracy of measurements of PCO_2 in blood be confirmed by tonometry before uncorrected gas or buffer calibrations are used routinely. It will be found, however, that most analyzers will not need a correction for CO_2 measurements.

A second important difference is that in contrast with the problems encountered with the use of aqueous buffers for quality control of O_2 measurements, the commercial quality control materials currently available show minimal interinstrument differences in PCO_2 measurements. These products appear to be as useful as tonometered blood for quality control of PCO_2. However, because of the current need to use tonometered blood for quality assurance of O_2 measurements, it is easy to incorporate tonometry of CO_2 as part of an optimal quality control program.

Frequency of Calibration and Reference Controls for PO_2 and CO_2 Electrodes

One-point checks of calibrations (most commonly using the gas or tonometered buffer systems built into most analyzers) should be done before each blood gas determination or series of measurements (not less than once every 20 minutes). The necessity of calibration checks before each clinical measurement is controversial; objective data supporting or disproving the need for this recommendation is not available (see Controversies).

Two-point calibrations using liquid quality control solutions should be done at least every 8 hours and whenever readjustment of the 1-point calibration exceeds 3.0 mm Hg for PO_2 or 2.00 mm Hg for CO_2.

For optimal quality control, calibration should be verified with tonometered blood at two different levels of gas tensions at least once every 8 hours and whenever the electrodes are reassembled or replaced. These recommendations differ from the current guidelines of the California State Department of Health Services, which indicate that use of third-point calibration gases are satisfactory reference controls.

Calibration Ranges

Regardless of the materials used for calibration, the instrument should be calibrated over the span of values measured clinically. Although the linearity of the outputs should be checked initially by calibration checks using at least three values within the clinical range (0–150 for PO_2, 0–60 for PCO_2), the linearity of most analyzers is such that only two-point calibration checks are necessary for routine quality control in these ranges.

For laboratories needing to make accurate measurements of PO_2 above 150 mm Hg, the linearity in this upper range of PO_2s needs to be assessed. While some instruments automatically correct electrode outputs for alinearity at higher PO_2, the validity of this correction should be confirmed during the initial evaluation. Other manufacturers recommend recalibration of the instruments using gases in the range in which blood is to be measured. The accuracy of high PO_2 measurements in some instruments can be improved by flushing the intake with a gas of high PO_2 immediately prior to the introduction of a sample.

Analyzer Temperature

The PO_2 of blood (in the range of 70–100 mm Hg), rises 7% for each degree centigrade increase in temperature; for PCO_2, the increase is 4% per degree, and for pH, 0.0146 units per degree. In addition, the output of the Clark-type electrode itself increases 3% per degree. Thus, it is extremely important that the temperature of the sample and electrode be closely regulated (19). Almost all blood-gas instruments currently in use provide for automatic regulation of the sample and electrode temperature, usually maintaining a temperature of 37° C.

If not limited by the design of the analyzer, the accuracy of this temperature setting should be checked with a precision thermometer (one that has been checked against an NBS standard) initially and whenever problems with temperature regulation are suspected. Most currently available commercial quality control materials are not as sensitive to temperature variations as is blood; one (triethanolamine acetate in a bicarbonate and acetate buffer) is more sensitive.

It is essential to document the composition of gas mixtures used for gas calibrations and tonometry. The standard recommendation for accomplishing this critical step in quality control is to analyze the gas composition by the Scholander technique (20). Realistically, however, because of the widespread use of modern gas analyzers, very few blood-gas or clinical chemistry laboratories have maintained the technical expertise necessary for accurate measurements by the Scholander technique. The problem is compounded by the anecdotal reports from some clinical and physiological laboratories that the reported composition of certified tanks of gas mixtures from commercial sources cannot always be trusted. It is clear that objective data on the reliability of commercial sources of reference-quality gas mixtures would be useful before formulating costly recommendations for quality assurance of reference gases for the thousands of blood-gas laboratories in this country. However, acknowledging the current absence of such data, the following guidelines are offered:

1. Purchase of at least two tanks of gravimetrically filled gas mixtures, each containing two different levels of CO_2 and O_2 within the range measured clinically.
2. Verify the composition of the gas mixtures by sending the tank to a laboratory with demonstrated expertise in the Scholander technique. If such measurements are not available, independent alternative measurement methods (calibrated mass spectrophotometry and gas chromatography) should be used.
3. Use these tanks exclusively as long-term reference standards against which the composition of less costly tanks of standard gas mixtures (used for tonometry and gas calibration) can be checked (i.e., measure the concentrations of both mixtures by mass spectrometry, gas chromatography, or as a last resort, by O_2 and CO_2 electrodes of demonstrated linearity).

4. Overlap analyses of full and near-empty standard gas mixtures for routine confirmation of gas composition. Check every tenth tank (not less often than every 3 months) against the gravimetric reference tanks.

5. Laboratories unable to meet the preceding recommendations should confirm the accuracy of their calibrating procedures by comparisons of their analyses of tonometered blood with those of a laboratory that uses gravimetric reference gases.

O_2Hb, COHb, Met Hb, and Total Hb

Optimal reference standards for the spectrophotometric measurements of the different forms of hemoglobin are not currently available for routine use in clinical blood-gas laboratories. Commercially available solutions of hemoglobin or viscosity adjusted dyes are promising, but definitive conclusions about their efficacy as reference standards await more thorough evaluation. When necessary, the accuracy of O_2Hb measurements can be assessed from Van Slyke measurements of O_2 content and capacity using fresh whole blood (assumed to have a normal P_{50}). COHb measurements can be compared with measurements of CO by infrared or gas chromatography techniques (2). Met Hb measurements can be checked with the spectrometric method of Rodkey and O'Neal (21). The standard reference technique for total hemoglobin determinations is the *cyanmethemoglobin* method (22).

For routine quality control of spectrophotometer measurements of hemoglobin species, the manufacturers' recommendations should be followed. In the IL 282, the spectrophotometric measurements of percent of O_2Hb, percent COHb, and percent met Hb are made relative to the measurement of total hemoglobin. In this instrument, the only user-adjustable calibration is the value of total hemoglobin that is calibrated against a whole blood sample whose total Hb content has been determined by the cyanmethemoglobin method (assayed in triplicate and the mean value used for the calibration's target value). Many laboratories substitute commercially available calibration dyes or solutions of hemoglobin for the cyanmethemoglobin method; published comparisons of the efficacy of these materials with standard reference methods are, however, currently not available.

For accurate results, it is essential that hemolysis is complete, that there are no air bubbles in the cuvette, and that the temperature of the cuvette is accurately controlled. According to one report (3), accurate measurement of total hemoglobin requires a full 5 minutes of vigorous mixing of the syringe using twisting rotation prior to sample injection. Mixing may be improved by placing a washer inside the syringe.

O_2 CONTENT

Reference Method

The Van Slyke method is the best available reference method for confirming the accuracy of O_2 content measurements using galvanic cells. However, the high level of expertise required for accurate results with this technique realistically precludes its use in most clinical chemistry and blood-gas laboratories.

Routine Quality Control

Periodic (e.g., weekly) assessments of accuracy can be done using fresh whole blood tonometered with 100% O_2, and establishing an acceptable range of accuracy for the O_2-binding capacity of normal hemoglobin. The fuel cell should be recharged and replaced in accordance with the manufacturers' instructions or best available recommendations. According to one report on the Lex-O_2-Con Unit (23), the cell should be recharged every 6 months in normal use, every 2 months with heavy use (30–50 measurements a day), when the measurements take longer than 4 minutes to reach equilibrium, or when the mean measurement of oxygen-binding capacity falls below acceptable limits. As is the case for hemoglobin measurements, blood samples must be very well mixed prior to delivery to the instrument.

The routine calibration recommended by the manufacturer of the Lex-O_2-Con galvanic cell instrument is the injection of a known volume of room air. Since sample volume must be carefully controlled, it is important that the syringe used for this calibration procedure is the same as that used for injecting blood samples.

INTERLABORATORY COMPARISONS AND PROFICIENCY TESTING

A valuable confirmation of the validity of a laboratory's calibration and measurement procedures is to split samples and compare results with other laboratories. A community-based program utilizing weekly distribution of tonometered blood samples has been operated by the University of Washington in Seattle since 1971 (24). Similar programs have been established by the University of Southern California Medical Center and other groups.

As a result of national surveys that indicated an unacceptably high prevalence of erroneous results of clinical chemistry and bacteriologic testing, the 1967 Federal Clinical Laboratory Improvements Act included requirements for enrollment of licensed clinical laboratories in proficiency testing programs. State and federal regulatory agencies were given the responsibility for choosing the procedures for which proficiency testing would be mandated. Regulatory agencies also have the power to suspend licensure of laboratories that do not achieve satisfactory levels of performance in proficiency testing programs.

Until recently, proficiency testing was required only for certain tests done in clinical chemistry and bacteriology laboratories. In the past 3 years, both state and federal regulatory agencies have stated that, in the near future, enrollment in proficiency testing programs might be required of laboratories performing blood-gas measurements (25).

Proficiency testing involves the distribution of suitable uniform samples for testing the accuracy of the analyses in question, the tabulation of results submitted by each laboratory, and the subsequent grading of each laboratory's results (26). Because the limits of acceptability for results of testing are often based (at least partially) on the results of all participating laboratories, proficiency testing could be considered a large-scale interlaboratory comparison program.

The analyses of PO_2 and PCO_2 pose unique challenges in finding materials suitable for proficiency testing. The use of tonometered blood is obviously not feasible for statewide or national testing. In 1979, the California Thoracic Society (CTS) (27) and the College of American Pathologists (28) independently established proficiency testing programs using aqueous buffer solutions, pre-tonometered and sealed in glass vials suitable for shipping. The data collected from these programs and research done by the reference laboratories of the CTS program indicate that it is feasible to do proficiency testing for pH and PCO_2 using aqueous buffer solutions, but, for reasons discussed previously, aqueous buffer solutions are not suitable for proficiency testing of PO_2 measurements. However, it is possible, and in fact likely, that improved quality control products suitable for wide-scale proficiency testing of PO_2 measurements will be available in the near future.

The future of proficiency testing for blood-gas measurements is difficult to predict. The current position of many regulatory agencies is that, because of the problems with assessment of the accuracy of PO_2 measurements, proficiency testing (or interlaboratory comparison) programs are primarily educational adjuncts to appropriate internal quality control programs.

Two fundamental questions remain to be answered: Is there a need for proficiency testing of blood-gas measurements? If so, will proficiency testing programs result in improvements in the accuracy and precision of blood-gas measurement? It is very clear from the experience of the CTS program that such programs are very useful for improving communication among professionals responsible for clinical blood-gas measurements, manufacturers of blood-gas instrumentation and quality control products, and regulatory agencies. These programs can also contribute significantly to our understanding of blood-gas instrumentation and quality control procedures.

PROCEDURES

Collection of Sample

Unique precautions must be employed during the collection of blood samples for determination of blood-gas parameters so that contamination with room air, or leakage or diffusion of gases from the sample is minimized. Clean, sterile glass syringes with close-fitting plungers are the best means of sample transfer as they allow easy inspection and removal of large air bubbles, permit minimal contamination or loss of gases, and freely fill from arterial pressures. The high cost of purchase, cleaning, and sterilization of glass syringes, their susceptibility to breakage, and their appeal to the drug addicts who steal them has prompted the widespread use of disposable plastic syringes. Some plastic syringes, however, will permit significant contamination or loss of gases (29); especially if a sample has high PO_2, a low hemoglobin concentration, or is stored for a long period of time prior to analysis (29–31). Recently, special preheparinized plastic syringes have been introduced, which have special venting systems allowing easy filling of the syringe with normal arterial pressures.

The syringe is usually pretreated with heparin to prevent clotting. Excess amounts of heparin solutions can adversely affect the accuracy of blood-gas measurements (30), therefore, the syringe should be flushed with heparin solution (1000 units/ml) and the excess volume ejected out prior to blood sampling (see Controversies). The use of dry or lyophilized heparin obviates the problem of dilution by heparin solution but may not be as effective in preventing clot formation. For analyzers able to measure small samples, glass capillary tubes can also be used for sample collection if careful attention is directed towards minimizing contamination or gas loss.

Methods of Sampling: Optimal Sites of Sampling

The use of very small diameter needles (25 gauge) (32) will minimize trauma to the artery; however, because of the restriction of sample flow, more expertise is required for successful arterial sampling than is the case with the larger, more commonly used needles (20–23 gauge). Nevertheless, this expertise is well worth developing (32), for in addition to improved patient comfort, the need for local anesthetics is usually obviated, and the time required for postpuncture arterial compression is reduced. Regardless of the puncture technique that is chosen, the need for rapid punctures with minimal patient discomfort is paramount.

In infants, small (25–26 gauge) scalp vein needles are often used for collecting arterial samples. In adults and occasionally in infants, indwelling arterial catheters are useful when multiple samples must be drawn; blood may be sampled rapidly, and the acute physiologic consequences (hyperventilation or breath holding) of pain and anxiety often associated with "single stick" blood sampling are usually absent. However, complications are more common with indwelling catheters, particularly if they are left in place for prolonged periods. (For further discussion of arterial catheterization, see Chapter 25 on hemodynamic monitoring.) "Arterialized" capillary blood samples can be used as substitutes for arterial blood when one must minimize iatrogenic blood losses or when problems preclude arterial sampling. (For details see Chapter 26 on pediatrics).

The preferred site for arterial sampling in adults is the radial artery. The brachial artery is the second choice. The femoral artery should be used only as a last resort because of the risk of undetected postpuncture bleeding. In infants, the temporal artery is commonly used for arterial samples.

Drawing the Arterial Sample

A suggested step-by-step procedure for drawing arterial samples is as follows:

1. Check the syringe for free movement of the syringe plunger.
2. If the patient is on anticoagulant therapy, has a bleeding disorder, or has reduced levels of platelets (less than 50,000), it is usually best to confer with the patient's physician prior to sampling. If the need for an arterial puncture is confirmed, it should be done with the smallest possible needle, using only a single puncture attempt at each site, with prolonged arterial compression after puncture attempts, and follow-up observations to confirm the absence of postpuncture bleeding.
3. The use of gloves when drawing blood from patients with hepatitis positive blood is highly recommended.
4. In order to reassure the patient, the procedure is explained.
5. The artery is palpated and the puncture site inspected. Punctures should not be made through infected skin or other skin lesions. If the radial artery is the sampling site, the adequacy of the collateral flow through the ulnar artery should be confirmed by the Allen test (see Chapter 25 on hemodynamic monitoring).
6. The site should be cleaned with alcohol or another appropriate disinfectant.
7. The use of a local anesthetic is optional; if used, the patient should first be asked about drug allergies. The anesthetic is best injected in the dermis, and then into the subcutaneous tissue above the artery and finally on either side of the artery. Always check by aspiration that the needle is not *in* the blood vessel. Caution must be exercised during injection to avoid injury to the artery, which may result in prolonged spasm. After injection, sufficient time must be allowed for the anesthetic effect to take place before puncture.
8. The artery is generally secured with two fingers about 3 cm apart, taking care not to occlude flow. With the beveled surface facing up, the needle is

inserted parallel to the course of the artery at an angle with the skin surface of about 45°.

9. The artery should be entered slowly with close observation of the syringe immediately above the needle hub for evidence of blood flow. Should the needle pass through both walls, pull back slowly, again watching for flow or arterial pulsations before attempting a second puncture.

10. When the lumen is entered, blood should flow freely into the syringe, moving the syringe plunger.

11. When an adequate sample volume has been obtained (usually 2–5 ml), withdraw the syringe and needle and, using a sterile gauze, immediately apply firm pressure at the entry site for at least 1 full minute (many laboratories suggest 2–3 minutes). With the other hand expel any large air bubles from the syringe and gently roll it a couple of times to ensure adequate mixing of heparin.

12. Remove needle from syringe and cap it (or insert tip of needle into rubber stopper or another appropriate guard device), and immerse sample in ice slush. Verify the accuracy of the patient's name on the sample label.

13. After release of puncture site pressure, observe the site for evidence of bleeding for 2–5 minutes. Reapply pressure for 3 minutes or longer if bleeding reoccurs.

Sample Storage

Obviously, it is preferable to analyze the blood as soon as possible after withdrawal. However, if glass syringes (or syringes appropriate for blood-gas use) with close-fitting plungers are used, and the PO_2 of the blood sample is below 150, storage in ice for up to 2 hours will cause minimal changes in gas tensions (33).

Samples stored at room temperature may have appreciable changes in gas tensions if analyses are delayed. Hess et al. (34) demonstrated an 8% drop in PO_2 when blood from control subjects was stored at room temperature for 65 minutes prior to analysis, and virtually no decrease when the blood was stored on ice. In patients with markedly elevated white blood cell or platelet counts, the decrease in PO_2 was more than 25% when the samples were held for 65 minutes at room temperature. For samples with high PO_2 (> 150), the decrease in PO_2 during sample storage may be very rapid (33); for those samples where the accuracy of the PO_2 is important (e.g., shunt calculations), it is imperative that samples be stored at 0° C in glass syringes with close-fitting plungers, and analyzed as soon as possible after withdrawal.

Blood-Gas Analysis of Sample

Blood should be injected or aspirated into the analyzer following the manufacturer's instructions carefully. With some analyzers, maximal accuracy may be achieved by the "double-push" technique whereby readings are taken from a second sample which is injected soon after the first sample (15). Analysis of a second aliquot of the sample on a second instrument is a very effective method of quality assurance. If the results differ significantly (PO_2 and PCO_2 differences greater than 3 mm Hg, pH > 0.03 units difference) each instrument should be recalibrated prior to reanalysis of the sample.

Hemoglobin Saturation

There are instances when samples for oxyhemoglobin or carboxyhemoglobin analyses require special handling. For instance, special procedures must be used when COHb analysis is requested on postmortem blood, which may contain significant amounts of methemoglobin (35). Also, blood samples from patients with aberrent forms of hemoglobin, such as sickle cell anemia, may require extra hemolyzing diluent in order for complete hemolysis to be achieved.

Measuring P_{50}

To measure P_{50} by the standard method, the blood sample is tonometered at three oxygen concentrations spanning the linear portion of the HbO_2 dissociation curve near 50% saturation (3%, 3.5%, and 4% O_2 are typical); the PCO_2 in the tonometry gases is kept constant at 40 mm Hg. After careful measurements of pH, PO_2, and %HbO_2, the PO_2s are corrected to a standard pH of 7.40 (see Calculations) and plotted versus the %HBO_2 on a graph. The P_{50} is calculated from the slope of the plotted points.

Recently, it has been shown (36, 37) that the P_{50} can be calculated (without tonometry) from routine measurements of blood gases and %HbO_2 from a single sample of blood. (See Calculations.) The method is most accurate when the %Hb O_2 of the sample is near 50%, but results are usually within 2 mm Hg of standard P_{50} measurements when the saturation is between 20% and 90% (37), the range within which venous saturations usually occur.

CALCULATIONS

Relationship of pH to $[H^+]$

pH equals -$\log_{10} a_{H+}$ where a is the relative molal activity.

Use of Pressure Terms

PO_2 and PCO_2 are usually expressed in millimeters of mercury or torr. In Europe, where the use of the international system of units is becoming more common, gas pressures are expressed in kiloPascals (kPa) (1 mm Hg = 0.133 kPa).

Temperature Corrections

If the results of pH, PO_2, and PCO_2 measurements are to be corrected to the patient's body temperature (see Controversies), the following equations are recommended, assuming an analyzer temperature of 37° C:

$$\Delta T = T_{(C)} - 37 = 5/9\ (T_{(°F)} - 98.6)$$

$$\text{pH corrected} = \text{pH measured} - \Delta T\ (0.0146 - 0.0065\ (7.4 - \text{pH measured}))$$

Note that this equation was originally derived for use with analyzers at 38°C (38).

$$PCO_2 \text{ corrected} = (PCO_2 \text{ measured})\ (10^{0.019\Delta T}) \qquad \text{(ref 38)}$$

$$PO_2 \text{ corrected} = (PO_2 \text{ measured})(e^{y})$$

where

$$y = (0.058\ (\ (0.243\ PO_2 \text{ measured}/100)^{3.88} + 1)^{-1} + 0.013)\ (\Delta T) \qquad \text{(ref 39)}$$

For a PO_2 below 100, an adequate simplified equation is

$$PO_2 \text{ corrected} = (PO_2 \text{ measured})\ (10^{0.031\Delta T}) \qquad \text{(ref 38)}$$

$[HCO_3^-]_p$

For calculation of HCO_3^- in plasma from measurements of pH and PCO_2 (at 37° C):

$$[HCO_3^-]_p = 10^{y}$$

where

$$y = \text{pH} + \log_{10} PCO_2 - 7.604 \qquad \text{(ref 40)}$$

The apparent pK′ of 7.604 includes a pH electrode correction of 0.01

% O_2Hb

$$\%O_2Hb = (100)\ (O_2Hb)/(\text{Red Hb} + O_2Hb + COHb + \text{met Hb})$$

where Red Hb is reduced hemoglobin; O_2Hb is oxyhemoglobin; COHb is carboxyhemoglobin; and met Hb is methemoglobin; hemoglobin components are expressed in gm% (gm/100 ml). Note that if COHb and/or met Hb are not measured, this should be stated on the report.

O_2 Content

For calculation of volume percent O_2 (O_2 content) from measurements of hemoglobin, percent O_2Hb (see $\%O_2Hb$), and PO_2:

$$\text{vol}\%O_2 = (1.39)(\text{total hemoglobin in gm }\%)(\%O_2Hb/100) + 0.0031\ PO_2\ (\text{mm Hg})$$

Estimated $\%HbO_2$

For estimating percent O_2Hb from measurements of pH, PO_2, and PCO_2 (assuming a normal P_{50} and negligible amounts of COHb and met Hb), the following equation can be used (see Controversies):

$$\%O_2Hb = 100Y/(Y + 23{,}400) \qquad \text{(ref 39)}$$

where $Y = (PO_2')^3 + 150\ PO_2'$, and where PO_2' is the PO_2 measured at 37° C and corrected by the following calculation to the value expected at pH = 7.40 and PCO_2 = 40.

PO_2 at Standard Conditions

PO_2 at a pH of 7.40 and a PCO_2 of 40 is calculated in the following manner:

$$PO_2' = (PO_2\ \text{measured})\ (e^y) \qquad \text{(ref 39)} \qquad \text{(Eq. 1)}$$

where

$$y = (\ (PO_2\ \text{measured}/26.7)^{0.184} + 0.003\ BE_b - 2.2)(7.40 - \text{pH measured})$$

where BE_b is the base excess of blood (see the following).

Base Excess of Blood

$$BE_b = K_b\ \{[HCO_3^-]_p - 24 + \beta_b[(pH)_m - 7.4]\}$$

where

$$\beta_b = 7.7 + 1.43\ \text{Hb (gm \%)} \qquad \text{and} \qquad K_b = 1 - 0.0143\ \text{Hb (gm \%)} \qquad \text{(ref 41)}$$

assuming (gm% Hb) = (mmole/liter Hb) (0.6206). β_b is the nonbicarbonate buffer value of the blood ($d[HCO_3^-]_p/dpH$) and K_b corrects for inhomogeneity of buffer value between cells and plasma.

Base Excess of Extracellular Fluid

$$BE_{ECF} = K_{ECF}\ [[HCO_3^-]p - 24 + \beta_{ECF}\ ((pH)_m - 7.4)]$$

where

$$\beta_{ECF} = 3.7 + 0.53\ Hb \qquad \text{and} \qquad K_{ECF} = 1 - 0.0143\ Hb/3 \qquad \text{(ref 42)}$$

β_{ECF} is the experimentally determined nonbicarbonate buffer value of ECF ($d[HCO_3^-]_p/dpH$) and K_{ECF} corrects for the inhomogeneity of buffer value between RBC and the rest of the ECF fluid. K_{ECF} is usually a small correction (0.93) and can be ignored. BE_{ECF} is also termed the in vivo base excess. The buffering power of the ECF is approximately one-third that of the blood, because the interstitial fluid has a limited contribution to buffering and serves mainly to dilute the buffering power of the blood. The BE_{ECF} represents the strong base or acid that must be theoretically added to the ECF to bring the pH to 7.4 after the PCO_2 has been adjusted to 40. Siggaard-Andersen now changes the sign and calls it the titratable acidity of the ECF.

Calculation of P_{50} without Tonometry

The following calculations were derived from the work of Collier (36). Other sources of equations are indicated. The P_{50} can be calculated from a single blood analysis of pH, PO_2, PCO_2, and $\%O_2$ Hb with high accuracy if the O_2 Sat is near 50%, but an acceptable degree of accuracy can be obtained if the O_2 Sat is between 20% and 90%.

CO Not Present

The computation of P_{50} is simple if no CO is present in the blood and can be done in three steps:

1. Calculate PO_2' from Eq. 1.
2. Calculate the PO_2 corresponding to the measured O_2 Sat on the standard curve Ps (ref 39)

$$Ps = e^y \qquad \text{(Eq. 2)}$$

where

$$y = 0.385 \ln \frac{S}{(100 - S)} - (0.72S)^{-1} + 3.32 - \frac{(S/100)^6}{6}$$

3. Calculate P_{50}

$$P_{50} = 26.7\ (PO_2')/Ps$$

CO Present

The presence of CO in blood necessitates some new definitions:

$$SO_2A = \frac{100\ [HbO_2]}{[HbO_2] + [\text{Red Hb}]}$$

and

$$SO_2T = \frac{100\ [HbO_2]}{[HbO_2] + [\text{Red Hb}] + [HbCO]}$$

SO_2A represents the percent of saturation of the available O_2 binding sites, and SO_2T represents the percent of saturation of the total binding sites. If SCO represents the %HbCO present, then:

$$SO_2T = SO_2A(1 - (SCO/100))$$

The P_{50} in the presence of CO is calculated on the basis of $SO_2A = 50\%$. The P_{50} at $SO_2A = 50\%$ in the presence of CO is calculated in four steps:

1. Calculate PO_2' from Eq. 1.
2. Calculate T_{50}, the P_{50} of a standard curve in the presence of CO:

$$T_{50} = \frac{100 - SCO}{100 + SCO} f\left(50 + \frac{SCO}{2}\right)$$

where the function f is the functional operation performed in Eq. 2 and the independent variable $[50 + (SCO/2)]$ can be equated with S in that equation. T_{50} can also be calculated by a more simple equation if $SCO < 40\%$ (ref 43):

$$T_{50} = 26.7 \left(\frac{100 - SCO}{100 + SCO}\right)^{0.634}$$

or by an even simpler one if SCO is less than 20%:

$$T_{50} = 26.7 - 0.3\ SCO$$

3. Calculate PO_2 on the standard curve for a saturation of the sum of SO_2T and SCO:

$$P_{SCO} = \frac{SO_2T}{\Sigma} f(\Sigma)$$

where Σ equals SO_2T plus SCO and f is the function of Eq. 2.

4. Calculate P_{50} in presence of CO:

$$P_{50}(CO) = T_{50}\,\frac{PO_2'}{P_{SCO}}$$

The CO-free P_{50} can be calculated by:

$$P_{50}\ (\text{CO-free}) = 26.7\ (PO_2'/P_{SCO})$$

In Vivo P_{50}

The in vivo P_{50} means the P_{50} computed at the patient's temperature and at the PCO_2, pH, and SCO existing in the blood sample. It can be calculated as follows:

$$P_{50}\ (\text{in vivo}) = (T_{50})\ (PO_2)c/P_{SCO})$$

$(PO_2)c$ is the PO_2 at the subject's body temperature, calculated by the most appropriate equation. T_{50} is calculated using the most appropriate of the three equations given. P_{SCO} is calculated by manipulating the P_{50} (CO-free) equation above.

P_{50} in the Presence of Methemoglobinemia

There is insufficient data at present to make these corrections.

TROUBLESHOOTING

Because each model of blood-gas analyzer, spectrophotometer, and galvanic cell gas analyzer is relatively unique, suggestions for troubleshooting are very specific for a particular instrument; hence, that subject is not reviewed here. The reader is referred to the excellent discussions on troubleshooting that are included in the instructions from most manufacturers of instruments or quality control materials.

NORMAL VALUES

pH

Normal values for pH at sea level are generally assumed to be within the range 7.35–7.45. The number of healthy, nonsmoking subjects studied to substantiate the validity of these limits is, however, scanty.

PCO_2

The definition of the normal range for arterial PCO_2 is complicated by the fact that in some studies of normals, investigators automatically excluded data from subjects with PCO_2s less than 35, because these low PCO_2s were attributed to acute hyperventilation. In none of the studies was $PaCO_2$ significantly correlated with age. In a study of 80 normal subjects (smokers were not excluded), Mellemgaard (44) reported a mean $PaCO_2$ ±1 SD of 38.4 ± 2.9 (calculated range for 95% of subjects was 32.6–44.2). Filley's (45) study of 19 normal males produced a mean ±2 SD of 38.8 ± 3.16 and a range of 32–44. Minty (46) calculated a range of 95% of normal subjects of 30–45.8 from the results of seven published studies that used indwelling catheters for sources of blood (which presumably would eliminate the hyperventilation sometimes associated with single-stick arterial sampling). Clinicians most often define the normal range for $PaCO_2$ as 35–45. In an American Thoracic Society Workshop on regulation of ventilation (47), the range of normalcy was defined as 36–44. Whether PCO_2s that are between 30 and 35 occur in relaxed normal subjects or are always indicative of hyperventilation is an unresolved controversy.

Acute and chronic changes in PCO_2 are known to occur in subjects who move to high altitudes, but the magnitude of changes and possible correlations with age are not well defined. In one study comparing residents living at sea level in Lima, Peru, with Peruvians residing at 4500-m elevations, the mean PCO_2s were 39 and 30, respectively (48). In the Intermountain Manual on pulmonary function testing (49), the normal range for PCO_2 in Salt Lake City (elevation 1340–1520 m) was reported to be 30–40; in Denver (elevation 1580 m), the range was reported to be 34–48.

PO_2

Studies that have defined normal values for PO_2 have been complicated by a number of factors, including the failure to exclude smokers, differing altitudes of residency of study subjects and differences in posture during blood sampling. In a study of 80 subjects (smokers not excluded) ages 15–75 seated at an inclination of 75°, Mellemgaard (44) reported a prediction equation of $PO_2 = 104.2 - 0.27 \times$ age (in years). From the published plot of results, the SD around the regression line is approximately 6.0. Sorbini (50) studied 152 normals (smokers were excluded) ages 14–84 who lived at an elevation of about 500 m; subjects were supine during blood sampling. After correcting the data so it would represent the expected PO_2 at sea level, he established a prediction equation of $PaO_2 = 109 - 0.43 \times$ age (in years). The SD was ±4.10. This age regression is larger than that reported by Mellemgaard (44) and others. This disparity may be due to differences in the populations studied, or, more likely, to airway compression or closure in older subjects breathing in the supine posture. For both Sorbini's and Mellemgaard's data, for a subject aged 70, the lower limit of normal would be approximately 72.

As is the case with $PaCO_2$, the normal values for PaO_2 from high altitude residents are not well defined. In the previously mentioned comparison of Peruvians living at sea level and 4500 m elevation (48), the mean PaO_2s were reported to be 87 and 45, respectively. In Salt Lake City (elevation 1340–1520 m), the normal range for PO_2 was reported as 68–85 (age range not specified); for Denver (elevation 1580 m), the range was 65–75 (age range again not specified) (49).

Arterial O_2 Saturation

Because of the paucity of appropriate studies that directly measured O_2 saturation in normal subjects, ranges of normalcy must be predicted from assumptions of normal P_{50} and published age-related prediction equations for PaO_2. Assuming a pH of 7.40 and a lower limit of normal 72 for PaO_2 at age 70, the predicted lower limit for O_2 saturation at this age would be 95%.

Arterial O_2 Content

Similarly, because of the absence of appropriate studies, ranges of normalcy for O_2 content can only be estimated from prediction equations for PaO_2, assumptions of normal pH and P_{50} and knowledge of the normal range for hemoglobin appropriate for a subject's age, sex, and possibly race. The normal range usually cited is 15–23 vol%.

Carboxyhemoglobin

Normal values are not precisely defined and are directly related to exogenous CO pollution secondary to general atmospheric levels of CO or smoking habits. The upper limit of normal for nonsmokers is about 1.5%, and for smokers, up to 10%.

Methemoglobin

The upper limit of normal is 1.5%.

Total Hemoglobin

The normal range for males is 13.5–18.0 gm/100 ml; for females 12.0–16.0 gm/100 ml.

P_{50}

The most commonly used predicted normal value for P_{50} is 27. Studies that have adequately defined the range of normalcy and possible relation to age, body

Table 1 *Reproducibility of ABG Measurements by Different Methods*

Parameter	Method	Range of repeated measurements	Comments
pH	pH Electrode	±0.02	
PO_2	Clark electrode	±3.0 mm Hg	20–150 mm Hg
PCO_2	Severinghaus-type electrode	±3.0 mm Hg	20–60 mm Hg
Total Hb	Spectrophotometer	±0.2 gm/100 ml	
$\%O_2Hb$	Spectrophotometer	±1.0%	
%COHb	Spectrophotometer	±1.0%	
%Met Hb	Spectrophotometer	±1.0%	
O_2 Content	Galvanic cell	±0.5 vol%	
O_2 Content	Van Slyke	±0.6 vol%	Expertise required
P_{50}	O_2 electrode, spectrophotometer, tonometer	±2.0 mm Hg	

size, sex, or race are not available. In the Peruvian comparison of residents at sea level and 4500 m, the P_{50}s were 27.2 and 24.7, respectively (48).

REPRODUCIBILITY

The ranges given in Table 1 (±2 SD) for repeated measurements from the same sample of blood are what might be expected to be achieved in a clinical blood gas laboratory.

CONTROVERSIES

Correcting ABG Parameters to Patient's Temperature

An example of the magnitude of corrections for a patient with hypothermia and a body temperature of 30° C is given in Table 2. Whether or not blood-gas results

Table 2 *Effect of Temperature Change on Blood-Gas Parameters*

Temperature	pH	PO_2	PCO_2	O_2 Sat	HCO_3
37° C (analyzer temp)	7.32	74	44	92.6	21.6
30° C (patient temp)	7.44	43	29	92.6	21.6

should be corrected to the patient's temperature is a very controversial issue. The most compelling argument in favor of doing so is that partial pressure is a thermodynamic measurement, and the results should represent a condition in the patient rather than the values in the analyzer at 37° C. One of the principal arguments against temperature correction is that we currently have limited understanding of the significance of abnormal pH, PO_2, or PCO_2 results in cases of extreme hypo- or hyperthermia (e.g., what are the hazards of a PO_2 of 40 at the patient's temperature of 28° C? Does a PCO_2 of 50 indicate respiratory insufficiency if the patient's temperature is 41° C?) Another argument against temperature correction is that when a patient's temperature is changing, temperature correction makes the interpretation of serial blood gases difficult. Also, many patients' temperatures are either not reported or reported from measurements made hours before the blood was drawn. For a broader perspective, the reader is referred to an intriguing discussion by Rahn et al. (51) of the evolution of the relationship between body temperature, pH, and blood gases as measured in various species.

The Necessity of Two Blood-Gas Analyzers

Currently, a fully automated blood-gas analyzer can cost more than $20,000, hence some laboratories have only one instrument. Even with the most modern instruments, however, the "down-time" after changes of electrode membranes may be as long as 4 hours (52). The occasional clinical need for a "stat" analysis at a time of instrument malfunction or servicing necessitates a second stand-by unit in some laboratories. Another argument in support of having two operational analyzers available is that the analyses of blood with a second instrument (either on every sample, every third sample, or whenever the accuracy of the results is suspect) is an excellent addition to a quality control program. As is the case with most controversies, resolution awaits the availability of objective data on the frequency of equipment malfunction and the effectiveness of second instrument analyses for detecting errors.

Tonometry of Blood for Quality Control Programs

There is considerable difference of opinion as to whether or not tonometry of blood should be an essential part of quality control programs in all blood-gas laboratories. Some argue that the stringent requirements for technical expertise and for tonometry performance are too costly for some laboratories, and that if such laboratories did rely on tonometry of blood, the clinical measurements might be less accurate than if other more simple methods of quality control were used. Others argue that such conclusions are based on experience gained with use of older more cumbersome models of tonometers, and that the new tonometers available *are* appropriate for routine use in all blood-gas laboratories, and no more demanding of technical expertise than a blood-gas analyzer (18). Objective data to resolve this controversy is not currently available.

The Best Material for Quality Control of Blood-Gas Analyzers

Although tonometry is currently considered the best method of quality control, improvements in commercially available quality control products are likely. Whether or not such new products will replace the need for tonometers will need to be determined on the basis of objective studies of the product's reproducibility and its sensitivity and specificity to analyzer malfunction.

Blood-Gas Analyzers for Hospitals with Limited Access to Factory Service

For hospitals in isolated rural areas or some foreign countries, the availability and costs of equipment service are a key consideration in selection of equipment. The problem is complicated by the fact that such hospitals often do not have highly trained technicians available. The automated quality control and troubleshooting features of some of the more sophisticated analyzers currently available would seem to be attractive features for such hospitals. However, the complexity of such equipment often necessitates a visit by a factory-trained service technician if malfunction does occur. Data documenting the long-term service needs of various types of analyzers are needed for objective resolution of this controversy.

Reporting Calculated O_2 Saturation and O_2 Content Values

Calculations of O_2 saturation and O_2 content from measurements of PO_2 and hemoglobin will obviously be in error if the assumptions of a normal P_{50} and absence of COHb and met Hb are not valid. If calculated values are reported, it should be stated on the report that the numbers are estimates based on the above-mentioned assumptions.

Differences Between Calculated HCO_3 and Measured HCO_3

Calculated HCO_3 is determined from PCO_2 and pH. The blood-gas samples are usually arterial blood, are kept anaerobic and cool, and are usually analyzed soon after withdrawal. The clinical laboratory samples are usually venous, may not be anaerobic, and often are analyzed hours after sample withdrawal. In the auto-analyzers used in most clinical chemistry labs, the plasma is acidified and the CO_2 evolved is measured. While the plasma sample is in the sample cups there may be a loss of CO_2. In addition, since this methodology assumes a normal pH, there may be some errors in HCO_3 determination in patients with abnormal blood pH.

Saving Samples for 4–6 Hours

Some laboratories require that all blood-gas samples be saved in ice for 4–6 hours after analyses so that in case the results are questioned, the samples can be reanalyzed. An alternative approach for reassuring clinicians of the accuracy of measurements is to have a policy that for all bloods with significantly abnormal results (e.g., a PO_2 of 35 or a PCO_2 of 20) or results that are dramatically different from previous results from the same patient, the technician should repeat the analysis on a second instrument and write on the report "abnormal results confirmed on second analyzer."

Errors Secondary to Dilution with Heparin

Although correction factors have been published for correcting blood-gas measurements for the dilution effects of heparin and saline, they are seldom used in clinical practice. The most practical solution is to keep the proportion of heparin to less than 0.1 ml for 5 ml of blood, or use dry or lyophilized heparin.

Frequency of Calibrations of the O_2 and CO_2 and pH Electrodes

Some authorities recommend checking calibrations before each blood-gas determination (11). Regulations of California's State Department of Health Services require 1-point calibration checks before each determination "or series of determinations." Some automated analyzers make 1-point calibration checks every 20 minutes. There is a paucity of published objective information from which recommendations regarding this controversy can be derived. Many of the instrument malfunctions that can cause erroneous measurements (change in sample or electrode temperature, gas bubble under membrane, torn or loose membrane, or protein contamination) can occur suddenly, suggesting that calibration checks should be done before each clinical measurement regardless of the stability of the electrode output under normal conditions. An alternative procedure is the measurement of each sample on two different analyzers; in this situation, calibration checks can be done in accordance with the drift characteristics of the instruments (e.g., every 20–30 minutes).

ELECTRODE OUTPUT REPRESENTING THE "TRUE" GAS OR H^+ CONCENTRATION

Mapleson et al. (53) have demonstrated that a 100% response of the O_2 electrode can take as long as 10 minutes. The response time can vary with the PO_2, the particular electrodes used, and, for a given electrode, may even vary from day to day (53). Some investigators have established response times from calibration readings at comparable gas concentration made prior to measurements of samples (15). Most automated instruments use the electrode output at a predetermined time before the full response is achieved and correct this output by extrapolation to estimate the full response output. Improvements in electrode and automated sample delivery systems have generally reduced the response times of electrodes; whether or not the variability of response times among electrodes has been improved has not been objectively established.

P_{50} EXPRESSED AS PERCENT OF THE TOTAL HEMOGLOBIN AND AS PERCENT OF HEMOGLOBIN AVAILABLE FOR O_2 BINDING

Most sources defining the P_{50} do not specify whether to reference the percentage of saturation to the total hemoglobin or to the hemoglobin *available* for oxygen binding. Many feel it is preferable to express the saturation as the percentage of hemoglobin *available* for O_2 binding because this will result in a more meaningful description of the affinity of hemoglobin for oxygen in the presence of large amounts of COHb and met Hb. Until the definition is standardized, reports should specify which definition is used.

REFERENCES

1. Maekewa T, Okuda Y, McDowall DG: Effect of low concentrations of halothane on the oxygen electrode. *Br J Anaesth* 52:585-587, 1980.
2. Maas AHJ, Hamelink ML, and DeLeeuw RJM: An evaluation of the spectrophotometric determination of HbO_2, $HbCO_2$ and Hb in blood with the Co-Oximeter IL 182. *Clin Chim Acta* 29:303-309, 1970.
3. Dennis RC, Valeri CR: Measuring percent oxygen saturation of hemoglobin, percent carboxyhemoglobin and methemoglobin, and concentrations of total hemoglobin and oxygen in blood of man, dog and baboon. *Clin Chem* 26:1304-1308, 1980.
4. Van Slyke DD, Neill JM: The determination of gases in blood and other solutions by vacuum extraction and manometric measurement. *J Biol Chem* 61:523-584, 1924.
5. Brix O: A modified Van Slyke apparatus. *J Appl Physiol* 50:1093-1097, 1981.
6. Gregory IC: Assessment of Van Slyke manometric measurements of oxygen content. *J Appl Physiol* 34:715-717, 1973.
7. Kusumi F, Butts WC, Ruff WL: Superior analytical performance by electrolytic cell analysis of oxygen content. *J Appl Physiol* 35:299-300, 1973.

8. Valeri CR, Zaroulis CG, Marchionni L, et al.: A simple method for measuring oxygen content in blood. *J Lab Clin Med* 79:1035–1040, 1972.
9. Butts WC, Kenny MA, McCoubrey PG: Rapid method for measurement of oxygen in human blood. *Clin Chem* 19:1196–1197, 1973.
10. Westgard JO, Falk H, Groth Torgny: Influence of a between-run component of variation, choice of control limits, and shape of error distribution on the performance characteristics of rules for internal quality control. *Clin Chem* 25:394–400, 1979.
11. Adams AP, Morgan-Hughes JO, Sykes MK: pH and blood-gas analysis, methods of measurement and sources of error using electrode systems. *Anaesthesia* 22:575–597, 1967.
12. Bird BD, Henderson FA: The use of serum as a control in acid-base determination. *Br J Anaesth* 43:592–594, 1971.
13. Rhodes PG, Moser KM: Sources of error in oxygen tension measurement. *J Appl Physiol* 21:729–734, 1966.
14. Bird BD, Williams J, Whitman JG: The blood gas factor: a comparison of three different oxygen electrodes. *Br J Anaesth* 46:249–252, 1974.
15. Bateman NT, Musch TI, Smith, CA, et al.: Problems with the gas-calibrated PCO_2 electrode. *Respir Physiol* 41:217–226, 1980.
16. Hansen JE, Stone ME, Ong ST, et al.: Comparison of blood gas measurements between tonometered quality control materials, plasma, and blood. Abstract, *Am Rev Respir Dis* 123:92, 1981.
17. Cotes, JE: *Lung Function Assessment and Application in Medicine,* ed 4. London, Blackwell Scientific Publications, 1979.
18. Chalmers C, Bird BD, Whitwam JG: Evaluation of a new thin film tonometer. *Br J Anaesth* 46:253–259, 1974.
19. Bainton CR, Severinghaus JW: Modification of the radiometer BMS-3 electrode to improve thermal stability. *Anesthesiology* 33:548–550, 1970.
20. Scholander PF: Analyzer for accurate estimation of respiratory gases in one-half cubic centimeter samples. *J Biol Chem* 167:235–250, 1947.
21. Rodkey FL, O'Neal JD: Effects of carboxyhemoglobin on the determination of methemoglobin in blood. *Biochem Med* 9:261–270, 1974.
22. VanKampen EJ, Zijlstra WG: Standardization of hemoglobinometry II. The hemoglobincyanide method. *Clin Chim Acta* 6:538–544, 1961.
23. Clerbaux TH, Frans A, Detry JM, et al.: Drift in the oxygen content measured with the Lex-O_2-Con: Long-term assessment. *J Lab Clin Med* 87:717–719, 1976.
24. Delaney CJ, Leary ET, Raisys VA, et al.: Proficiency testing for blood gas quality control. *Clin Chem* 22:1675–1684, 1976.
25. Clausen JL: Proficiency testing for arterial blood gas measurements. *American Thoracic Society News* pp. 6–7, Spring 1981.
26. Rej R, Vanderlinde RE: Proficiency testing in acid-base analyses: An interlaboratory evaluation. *Clin Chim Acta* 49:161–167, 1973.
27. Clausen JL, Hansen JE, Misuraca L, et al.: Interlaboratory comparisons of blood gas measurements. Abstract, *Am Rev Respir Dis* 123:104, 1981.
28. Itano M: CAP blood gas survey—First years experience. *Am J Clin Pathol* 74:535–541, 1980.
29. Abramson J, Verkaik G, Mohler JG: Blood gas stability in terumo plastic and glass syringes. *Respir Care* 23:63–64, 1978.
30. Cissik JH, Salustro J, Patton OL, et al.: The effects of sodium heparin on arterial blood gas analysis. *Cardiovas Pul (CVP)* 5:17–35, 1977.
31. Scott PV, Horton JN, Mapelson WW: Leakage of oxygen from blood and water samples stored in plastic and glass syringes. *Br Med J* 3:512–516, 1971.
32. Sabin S, Taylor JR, Kaplan AI: Clinical experience using a small-guage needle for arterial puncture. *Chest* 69:437–439, 1976.

33. Eldrige F, Fretwell LK: Change in oxygen tension of shed blood at various temperatures. *J Appl Physiol* 20:790-792, 1965.
34. Hess CE, Nichols AB, Hunt WB, et al.: Pseudohypoxemia secondary to leukemia and thrombocytosis. *N Engl J Med* 301:361-363, 1979.
35. Freirich AW, Landau D: Carbon monoxide determination in post mortem clotted blood. *J Forensic Sci* 16:112-119, 1971.
36. Collier CR: Oxygen affinity of human blood in presence of carbon monoxide. *J Appl Physiol* 40:487-490, 1976.
37. Aberman A, Cavanilles JM, Weil MH, et al.: Blood P_{50} calculated from a single measurement of pH, PO_2 and SO_2. *J Appl Physiol* 38:171-176, 1975.
38. Severinghaus JW: Blood gas calculator. *J Appl Physiol* 21:1108-1116, 1966.
39. Severinghous JW: Simple accurate equation for human blood O_2 dissociation computation. *J Appl Physiol* 46:599-602, 1979.
40. Maas AHJ, Van Heijst ANP, Visser BF: The determination of the true equilibrium constant and the practical equilibrium coefficient for the first ionization of carbon acid in solutions of sodium bicarbonate, cerebrospinal fluid, plasma, and serum at 25° and 38°. *Clin Chim Acta* 33:325-343, 1971.
41. Siggaard-Anderson O: *The Acid-Base Status of the Blood,* (ed 4). Baltimore, Williams and Wilkins, 1974 p. 51.
42. Brown EB Jr, Attebery BA: In vivo and in vitro carbon dioxide dissociation in Altman PL and Dittmer DS (eds): *Respiration and Circulation.* Bethesda, Maryland, Federation Amer Soc Exp Biol, 1971.
43. Ledwith JW: Determining P_{50} in the presence of carboxyhemoglobin. *J Appl Physiol* 44:317-321, 1978.
44. Mellemgaard K: The alveolar-arterial oxygen difference: Its size and components in normal man. *Acta Physiol Scand* 67:10-20, 1966.
45. Filley GF, Gregoire F, Wright GW: Alveolar and arterial oxygen tensions and the significance of the alveolar-arterial oxygen tension difference in normal men *J Clin Invest* 33:517-529, 1954.
46. Minty BD, Nunn JF: Regional quality control survey of blood-gas analysis. *Ann Clin Bio chem* 14:245-253, 1977.
47. Conference report: Workshop on assessment of respiratory control in humans: VII measurements of the responsiveness of the respiratory apparatus in disease, Turino GM (chairman). *Am Rev Respir Dis* 115:883-887, 1977.
48. Benson OO: *Physics and Medicine of the Atmosphere and Space,* Benson OO (ed). New York, Wiley, 1960, pp. 352-369.
49. *Clinical Pulmonary Function Testing,* Kammer RE and Harris AH (eds). Salt Lake City, Utah, Intermountain Thoracic Society, 1975, P II-15, II-16.
50. Sorbini CA, Grassi V, Solinas E, et al.: Arterial oxygen tension in relation to age in healthy subjects. *Respiration* 25:3-13, 1968.
51. Rahn H, Reeves RB, Howell BJ: Hydrogen ion regulation, temperature, and evolution. *Am Rev Respir Dis* 112:165-172, 1975.
52. Rubin P, Bradbury S, Prowse K: Comparative study of automatic blood-gas analyzers and their use in analyzing arterial and capillary samples. *Br Med J* 1:156-158, 1979.
53. Mapleson WW, Horton JN, Ng WS, et al.: The response pattern of polarographic oxygen electrodes and its influence on linearity and hysteresis. *Med Biol Eng* 8:585-593, 1970.

CHAPTER 22

Exercise Testing

JAMES E. HANSEN, M.D.

Several recent reports (1–5) discuss the importance and techniques of exercise testing. Exercise testing is useful in the evaluation of dyspnea, ventilatory response, disability evaluation, the determination of need for and efficacy of oxygen supplementation, and the quantitation of cardiovascular and pulmonary dysfunction. In addition, serial evaluations may be helpful in assessing the results of therapeutic interventions.

The exercise protocol selected depends upon the available personnel, equipment, space resources, and the number and type of patients undergoing exercise evaluation. A few accurate, simple measurements are more valuable than multiple ones of doubtful accuracy. Of the many possible combinations of resources, several strategies for equipping a laboratory are suggested in this chapter.

EQUIPMENT

System without Equipment

Important observations, measurements, and useful clinical judgments can be made without sophisticated equipment. All that is required is the patient and a stairwell, hallway, or course. Observation of the walking patient's breathing and speaking pattern, along with measurement of the pulse rate, distance covered, and time required are sufficient data for basic analysis. The 12-minute walking distance test, in which the patient is instructed to walk as much distance as he or she can in 12 minutes, is one popular approach (6).

ISBN 0-12-788125-5

Simplified System

This system allows measurement of heart rate (HR), electrocardiogram (EKG), inspired or expired volume per minute ($\dot{V}_I$ or $\dot{V}_E$), tidal volume (V_T), respiratory frequency (f), and estimate of work rate. Required equipment includes the following:

1. *EKG with chest electrodes.* Two EKG electrodes may be placed at the anterior axillary lines in the fourth and fifth intercostal spaces with the ground electrode on the forehead or over one of the vertebral spinous processes.
2. *Dry-gas meter.* The Parkinson-Cowan dry-gas meter has a low resistance to flow, is reliable to approximately 1% of volume, and can be adapted to recording by use of a photoelectric cell registering pointer movement. Corrosion and leaks eventually develop from condensed exhaled water vapor; therefore, placement on the inspired side and/or regular calibrations are desirable.
3. *Cycle ergometer (mechanical, or electromechanical) or treadmill.* The Monark mechanical cycle, braked by a strap and weight whose position is controlled by the operator, is portable, reliable, and inexpensive, but pedaling frequency must be carefully controlled using a metronome to obtain accurate power (work rate). Electromechanical cycles allow variation in pedaling frequency and somewhat finer adjustment of power. The speed of the treadmill should be adjustable from 1.5 to 10 kph and grade from 0 to 30%. Side platforms and handrail are important.
4. *Other equipment including humidifier, tubing, values, stopwatch and metronome.* Lloyd, Koegel, or modified Otis-McKerrow valves are all of low resistance and satisfactorily separate inspired from expired air during exercise. The dead spaces of these valves are 46, 64, and 115 ml, respectively. A valve with less dead space is preferable for patients with smaller ventilatory capacity. For studies using gas from cylinders, e.g., oxygen during exercise, a device to partially humidify inspired gas is desirable. A flat chamber (20 by 40 by 10 cm) can be fabricated of Plexiglas with large bore inlet and outlet on the top above the water level.

Manually Operated System with Analysis of Mixed Expired Gas

In addition to the measurements derived from the system already described, the following system allows measurement of oxygen uptake ($\dot{V}_{O_2}$), carbon dioxide output ($\dot{V}_{CO_2}$), ventilatory equivalents for oxygen and carbon dioxide ($\dot{V}_E/\dot{V}_{O_2}$ and $\dot{V}_E/\dot{V}_{CO_2}$), oxygen pulse (millileters of oxygen uptake per heart beat), and efficiency of work at several levels of exercise. Equipment required in addition to that of the simplified system is:

1. Plastic Douglas-type bags, neoprene meterological balloons, or mixing chamber (fabricate), and 100-ml glass syringes with three-way stopcocks.
2. Tissot spirometer.
3. CO_2 analyzer, mass spectrometer, or Scholander or Haldane apparatus.
4. O_2 analyzer, mass spectrometer, or Scholander or Haldane apparatus.
5. A multichannel recorder is highly desirable.

Several plastic balloons or bags are necessary for direct collection of expired gas. They should be rinsed with expired gas before use and checked for leaks and rate of loss of CO_2 if analyses of gas concentration must be delayed. Gas samples from the bags or balloons can be stored for many hours in oiled 100-ml glass syringes with three-way stopcocks (stored plunger up until analysis so that the weight of the plunger places the gas content under pressure) (7). Properly performed analyses of gas samples using a Scholander or Haldane apparatus give the highest possible accuracy, but are time-consuming. A Tissot spirometer with volume of 120 liters is ideal for the measurement of volume of bag contents and calibration of other volume and flow devices. Alternatively, expired gas can be directed through a mixing chamber (2) from which mixed expired gas is continuously sampled by gas analyzers. A mixing chamber can be fabricated from Plexiglas. It should have a volume of approximately 7 liters, baffles to facilitate mixing, and large bore inlet and outlet. The washout characteristics of mixing chambers may give erroneous results if mixed expired gas concentrations are rapidly changing (i.e., with increments in work rate every minute).

The mass spectrometer allows rapid analysis of CO_2 and O_2 as well as other gases. Zirconium fuel cells, some polarographic oxygen analyzers, and some infrared CO_2 analyzers are satisfactory for rapid gas analysis.

A multichannel recorder is highly desirable for calibration of equipment, integration of flow to volume, and recording of flow, volume, gas concentrations, and EKG or heart rate (with cardiotachometer).

Automated or Semiautomated System

Systems can be purchased commercially or fabricated (8, 9), which allow repetitive measures of flow or volume, gas concentrations, calculations from these values, and graphical or tabular displays.

In addition to yielding measurements as accurate and reproducible as those obtained from manual systems, a breath-by-breath system also allows measurement of end tidal CO_2 and O_2 ($P_{ET}CO_2$ and $P_{ET}O_2$), peak flow, and expiratory flow pattern. Breath-by-breath analyses may allow one to follow the changes of rapidly incremental exercise more accurately than mixing chamber analyses. Additional equipment required is (1) Fleisch pneumotachograph and differential pressure transducer (or other flow or volume device), and (2) calculator or computer with four-channel analog to digital (AD) converter and printer.

A four-channel AD converter can accept flow, O_2 and CO_2 concentrations, and heart rate signals. These signals may be transmitted to a desktop calculator or computer for temporary storage and later calculation. A cathode ray tube (CRT) allows the collected data to be displayed during the test. The data may be calculated breath-by-breath, or averaged over several breaths. A printer is needed for data output, and a graphics plotter is useful. An automated system with a calculator/computer and printer/plotter markedly reduces hand measurements and calculations and eliminates the need for a multichannel recorder.

Other Additions

Additional resources that may be required for use of the systems described in the preceding include the following:

1. indwelling arterial cannula or catheter for sampling blood, with transducer for systemic blood pressure measurement;
2. nasal prongs, gas regulator, and a source of oxygen;
3. Swan-Ganz pulmonary artery catheter with transducer;
4. ear-oximeter; and
5. multiple lead EKGs.

An arterial line allows blood-gas and blood pressure measurements. This allows measurement of arterial carbon dioxide and oxygen tension ($PaCO_2$ and PaO_2), arterial oxygen saturation (SaO_2), pH, arterial oxygen content (CaO_2), bicarbonate (HCO_3^-), and lactate, and to calculate, with some systems, alveolar-arterial oxygen difference [$P(A\text{-}a)O_2$], and physiologic dead space (V_D). As arterial punctures during exercise are difficult, an indwelling catheter with stopcock and slow or intermittent heparin infusion at a concentration of 1000 units per 100 ml diluent should be used.

Although seldom used in clinical testing, Swan-Ganz catheters allow measurement of mixed venous blood, pulmonary artery pressures, cardiac output, and stroke volume. In addition, peripheral arterial oxygen saturation can be monitored with an ear oximeter. Serial multiple lead EKGs can be obtained.

QUALITY CONTROL

Power

Cycles should be calibrated using manufacturers recommendations. With a mechanical cycle, pedaling frequency must be controlled using a metronome.

With an electromechanical cycle (10), the pedaling frequency may vary from 40 to 80 cycles/min without significant change in power. Calibrate treadmill grade by geometry (height divided by horizontal distance) and speed by measuring the length of the belt and counting the number of cycles per minute.

Volume and Flow Rates

For accurate volume calculations, one must make measurements for complete ventilatory cycles rather than for exact predetermined periods. This is especially true with brief collection periods or low ventilatory frequencies.

A water-sealed spirometer, preferably large, is the standard for volume measurements; used in association with a stopwatch or timing device, it becomes a standard for flow measurements. If a 1-, 3-, or 4-liter syringe is used for calibration, it should be checked against the spirometer. Because a dry-gas meter may develop leaks, it should be checked weekly. A vacuum cleaner with rheostat control and a variable constriction is a useful device for obtaining a wide range of flow rates.

Bags and balloons should be checked for leaks. Bags and balloons should also be checked for rate of diffusion of carbon dioxide by filling with a known gas (mixed expired gas is satisfactory), drawing oiled 100-ml syringe samples at intervals, and measuring the serial samples for progressive decline in CO_2.

A Fleisch pneumotachograph transducer signal is dependent not only on flow rate, but also the temperature and viscosity of the measured gas. (See Chapter 9 for a more detailed discussion of these factors.) Cooling the expired gas to room temperature by passing it over water before passing it through the pneumotachograph decreases error by allowing calibration of the unheated pneumotachograph at room temperature. Room air and mixed expired gas have viscosities within 2%, but calibration factors need to be changed if a high oxygen concentration (high viscosity) is used. The pneumotachograph is usually linear over the lower 2/5 of its rated maximum flow rate, but above that flow rate, turbulence causes an increasing error. This alinearity is corrected electronically by some manufacturers. With initial use, it is wise to check the pneumotachograph and transducer over a wide range of flow rates, using the Tissot spirometer, vacuum cleaner, and stopwatch. If the pneumotachograph and transducer are used to determine volume by intergration of flow, they should be checked daily with a 1-, 3-, or 4-liter syringe at high and low flow rates to determine calibration factors and assure reasonable linearity (full range within 2%).

Gas Analyzers

Gas analyzers must be calibrated with gases of known concentration. Since the analyses furnished by suppliers are *not* consistently reliable, cylinder calibrating gases are best analyzed for CO_2 and O_2 by Scholander or Haldane technique. Mass spectrometer analysis of calibrating gases is appropriate only if the mass spectrometer itself has been calibrated. If the patient is to breathe room air during exercise testing, the gas analyzers should be calibrated so that dry room air measures 20.93% O_2 and 0–0.1% CO_2; otherwise, additional calculations are necessary to correctly measure O_2 uptake and CO_2 output. As most analyzers are pressure-dependent and therefore flow-dependent, it is essential that the resistance to flow be similar during times of calibration and measurement. Gas can be delivered to the O_2 or the CO_2 analyzer heads through a drying agent unless breath-by-breath analysis, which requires rapid responses, is used. If a drying agent is not used, it is imperative to know the exact water content of the gas delivered to the infrared CO_2 and polarographic or fuel cell O_2 analyzers as they treat water vapor as inert gas. For example, if an oxygen analyzer samples a 24° C gas saturated with water (PH_2O = 23 mm Hg) and records a fractional concentration of oxygen (FO_2) of 0.160, the FO_2 of the dry gas would really be 0.155 [$(760-23)/760 \times 0.160 = 0.155$]. If a Perkin-Elmer mass spectrometer (which ignores water vapor) is used, it can be calibrated with room air by turning the H_2O dial to zero and then the fixed gas dial until O_2 reads 20.9–21.0%.

If a mixing chamber is used, there is a "delay" in rinsing based on expired volume rather than time. The delay is exponential and should be measured for the chamber to see when 98% or 99% of the new value is reached. The expired gas concentrations need to be aligned correctly with the expired volumes they represent.

For breath-by-breath analysis, the transport time from the mouthpiece to the gas analyzer heads, and the rise time of the analyzers after receipt of a square wave signal must be known so that expired gas concentrations can be paired with exhaled volumes. Most gas analyzer readings initially change rapidly in response to a change in gas concentrations and then more slowly as they get closer to an asymptote. We found empirically in our system that if we plotted milliseconds of time versus analyzer reading, the correct time for calculating delay occurred when 50% of the *area* had been reached (8). As the rise time characteristics of the analyzer change with use, it is wise to check this characteristic daily or several times weekly.

Integrated Measurement

Initially, the values obtained from integration of flow and expired gas concentration should be compared with the values calculated from simultaneous Douglas bag collections, both at rest and at several levels of exercise. In this way, errors in calculation or gas analyzer response or pneumotachograph response may be detected. The respiratory exchange ratio (R) value is a relatively sensitive measure of the gas analyzers' accuracy and the appropriateness of the equations and corrections for moisture and temperature. A resting R value of a fasting relaxed individual will nearly always be between 0.70 and 0.85. In a healthy individual, the R value will always rise above 1.00 with exhausting incremental exercise. A normal person walking at the same speed and grade or overcoming the same resistance on a cycle ergometer should have a $\dot{V}_{O_2}$ within 20% of the predicted value for this level of work from other laboratories. An individual's $\dot{V}_{O_2}$ should be within 10% of his or her mean value on repetitive measures. Values outside this range suggest errors in measurement of delays, power, ventilation, and/or gas concentrations.

TESTING PROCEDURES

PRELIMINARY EVALUATION

Preliminary evaluation of the patient includes history and physical, EKG to exclude unsuspected or evolving cardiac disease, and, usually, routine pulmonary function studies, including lung volumes, flow rates, maximal voluntary ventilation, carbon monoxide diffusing capacity (DL_{CO}), and, often, arterial blood gas analysis and response of flow rates to inhaled bronchodilator. The choice of exercise testing procedures will depend on the equipment available and the need for diagnosis, quantitation of illness or infirmity, or evaluation of response to treatment.

The patient needs to become familiar with the equipment before resting measurements are taken and actual testing begins. Cycle seat height should be adjusted so that the subject's legs are almost completely extended at the bottom of the downstroke. The patient should practice cycling at the correct rate with a low resistance load. If a treadmill is used, the patient needs to practice getting on the moving belt and walking without supporting his weight on the guard rails. Several trials of starting and stopping on the treadmill may be necessary before the patient feels confident and comfortable. At cessation of exercise, the treadmill should be slowed gradually rather than stopped abruptly. During one of the preliminary trials, the patient should breathe with a mouthpiece and noseclip in place.

If a patient is too weak, dyspneic, or uncoordinated to ride a cycle ergometer or walk on a treadmill, walking slowly down the hall arm-in-arm with a physician and an assistant over a known distance may be the only feasible exercise.

Criteria for cessation of exercise, which are recommended by Jones et al. (2) and our laboratory, include angina, light-headedness, sudden pallor or cyanosis, increased ventricular premature contractions or other significant rhythm disturbances, progressive ST segment depression, decrease in systolic blood pressure greater than 20 mm Hg, or a rise in systolic blood pressure to a value greater than

280 mm Hg. With predetermined or suspected heart disease, it may be wise to limit maximal heart rate in some patients to 85% of maximal predicted (see equation for maximal heart rate in Other Maximum Predicted Values). Emergency drugs, intravenous sets, syringes, oxygen, manual resuscitation bag, and accessories for intubation should be on hand, with rapid access (less than 2 minutes) to a cardiac defibrillator.

Arterial Catheterization

If pulmonary vascular disease or interstitial lung disease is suspected, arterial catheterization is especially desirable to quantitate the V_D/V_T and $P(A\text{-}a)O_2$ at rest and during exercise. An arterial catheter or oximeter is necessary if one needs to evaluate the need for or value of oxygen supplementation by measuring PaO_2 at rest or during exercise. If an arterial blood specimen is obtained by arterial needle stick immediately after exercise ceases, the PO_2 and PCO_2 measured are not equivalent to the levels of PO_2 and PCO_2 that existed during exercise. An arterial catheter can be inserted in a brachial artery by the Seldinger (11) technique or by inserting a teflon Becton-Dickenson ''long dwell'' catheter over a needle directly into a brachial or radial artery.

With the modified Seldinger technique, the arm is extended fully at the elbow, the skin is shaved, cleansed, and draped, and the brachial artery pulsation identified in the antecubital fossa and upper arm. The skin and periarterial areas at the contemplated puncture site are infiltrated with local anesthesia. A Cournand or Riley needle with sharp obturator is inserted into the brachial artery at a 45° angle so that there is a free flow of arterial blood through the lumen. Sometimes the artery is punctured through the inner wall on insertion of the needle, therefore, the needle should always be withdrawn slowly with the inner obturator removed. When the needle tip is in the lumen of the artery, it should be advanced approximately a centimeter, while maintaining a free flow of blood. Usually the hub of the needle will need to be depressed to free the needle point from the inner arterial wall. An assistant or the operator can temporarily occlude the brachial artery in the upper arm until a nylon monofilament or flexible metal guideline is inserted into the needle hub. The line is inserted into the brachial artery past the needle tip; the needle is withdrawn; the plastic cannula, whose tip fits smoothly over the guideline is inserted several centimeters up the arterial lumen; the guideline is withdrawn; and the catheter is connected (via an adapter if necessary) to a three-way stopcock in an accessible position. Blood samples can be withdrawn when desired from the stopcock, discarding and replacing a small volume of heparinized solution on each occasion. The catheter can be connected to a sterile pressure transducer for continuous blood pressure measurement and its patency maintained with a pressurized slow drip of heparinized solution.

When it is necessary to measure pulmonary artery pressure or obtain mixed venous samples, a Swan-Ganz catheter can be inserted via one of the arm veins.

Estimation of Mixed Venous CO_2 Content and Cardiac Output

For several decades, rebreathing techniques have been utilized to estimate mixed venous carbon dioxide pressure at rest. More recently, Jones and his colleagues (2) have described rebreathing equipment and techniques for use during exercise; gases with high O_2 and low *or* high CO_2 concentrations are rebreathed. Extrapolation from estimated mixed venous CO_2 pressure to mixed venous CO_2 content, combined with measured arterial CO_2 content and CO_2 output, using the Fick equation, allows estimation of cardiac output (2).

Exercise Protocols

If steady-state measurements are desired, then the patient should be at a constant level of rest or activity for 4 minutes, with expired gas volumes and concentrations measured for the last 30-60 seconds. Blood gas specimens and gases should be collected over complete ventilatory cycles. As a usual minimum, measurements should be made at three levels: breathing room air at rest, during low-grade exercise, and during more stressful exercise.

If equipment is available for rapid and accurate serial measures during incremental exercise, the exercise level can be incremented by a fixed amount (on a treadmill, in percent grade or speed; on a bicycle, in watts) every minute until the patient is exhausted. The exercise load should be incremented rapidly enough for the patient to reach exhaustion in 6–10 minutes. The highest $\dot{V}_E$, $\dot{V}_{O_2}$, and HR recorded are considered the $\dot{V}_E$ max, $\dot{V}_{O_2}$ max, and HR max. Experience will assist one in judging the proper increment. With rapid incremental exercise, the patient will recover quickly and the study can be repeated in 30–45 minutes, with oxygen breathing, if desired.

Exercise-Induced Bronchospasm

If exercise-induced bronchospasm is suspected, measurements of FEV_1, peak flow, or specific airway conductance (SG_{aw}) should be made just before exercise and at 2-5 minute intervals for 20-30 minutes beginning promptly after the cessation of maximal exercise.

Oxygen Administration

In patients with significant hypoxemia on room air, it is possible to partially assess the advantages of reducing hypoxemia and possible hazards of ventilatory suppression by removing the mouthpiece and administering oxygen by nasal prongs, at several flow rates during rest or exercise with concurrent measurements of oximetry, arterial blood gases, or in rare instances, pulmonary artery pressures.

It is impossible to measure $\dot{V}_{O_2}$ accurately while administering oxygen by prongs. With fixed inspired concentrations of O_2, the error in $\dot{V}_{O_2}$ measurement tends to increase as the fractional concentration of inspired oxygen (F_IO_2) increases, although the measures of $\dot{V}_E$ and $\dot{V}_{CO_2}$ remain accurate.

One can evaluate several other parameters if the patient breathes 100% oxygen:

1. The percentage of right-to-left shunt after nearly complete nitrogen washout.
2. The effect of suppressing ventilation in those individuals who are limited in their exercise by dyspnea.
3. Carotid body function by measuring change in ventilation at 15–30 seconds after onset of oxygen breathing. (High PaO_2 markedly reduces input to the respiratory center from the carotid body.)

CALCULATIONS

Gas Volumes

In all calculations, the fractional concentration of N_2 (FN_2) is considered to include all of the inert gases, i.e., nitrogen plus rare gases. In all calculations involving FCO_2, or FO_2, FCO_2 plus FO_2 plus FN_2 equals 1.0000, as if FH_2O were zero. Scholander and Haldane analysis values can be used directly. With other analyzers, values displayed or recorded need to be adjusted so that dry-gas fractions total 1.000. Volume values should also be adjusted for volumes removed for O_2 or CO_2 analyses. I recommend including the valve dead space in calculating $\dot{V}_E$ and V_T but excluding the valve dead space in calculating $\dot{V}_E/\dot{V}_{O_2}$, $\dot{V}_E/\dot{V}_{CO_2}$ and V_D/V_T.

$$V(BTPS) = V(ATPS) \times \frac{(273 + 37) \times (PB - PH_2O \text{ at t})}{(273 + t) \times (PB - 47)}$$

where t is ambient temperature in degrees centigrade, BTPS is body temperature and pressure, saturated, ATPS is ambient temperature and pressure, saturated with water vapor, and PB is barometric pressure.

At a temperature t of 10–40° C,

$$PH_2O = 10 - 0.3952t + 0.03775t^2$$

$$V(STPD) = V(ATPS) \times (PB\text{-}PH_2O \text{ at t})/760(1+0.00367t) \qquad (7)$$

where STPD is standard temperature and pressure, dry.

$$\dot{V}_E = \dot{V}_I \times F_IN_2/F_EN_2$$

$$V_T = \dot{V}_E/f$$

where f is frequency of respirations per minute.

$$\dot{V}_{CO_2}(STPD) = \dot{V}_E(STPD) \times (F_ECO_2 - 0.0004)$$

where F_ICO_2 is 0.0004

$$\dot{V}_{O_2}(STPD) = \dot{V}_E(STPD) \times [0.265(1 - F_EO_2 - F_ECO_2) - F_EO_2]$$

where F_IO_2 is 0.2093

$$R = \dot{V}_{CO_2}/\dot{V}_{O_2},$$

where R is respiratory exchange ratio.

Ventilatory equivalents are defined as

$$\frac{\dot{V}_E(BTPS)}{\dot{V}_{CO_2}(STPD)} \text{ or } \frac{\dot{V}_E(BTPS)}{\dot{V}_{O_2}(STPD)}$$

Power and Efficiency

$$1 \text{ W} = 1 \text{ joule/sec} = 0.0143 \text{ kcal/min} = 6.12 \text{ kilopond-meter/min}$$

$$1 \text{ MET} \approx 3.5 \text{ ml } O_2/\text{kg/min}$$

$$1 \text{ kcal/min} = 200\text{–}210 \text{ ml } O_2/\text{min}$$

at average efficiency.

Efficiency (%) on cycle is 0.3T/(Y − Z), where T is power in watts near anaerobic threshold, Y is $\dot{V}_{O_2}$ in liters per minute at T watts and Z is $\dot{V}_{O_2}$ in liters per minute at 0 watts (derived from data in reference 4).

$$O_2 \text{ pulse} = \frac{\dot{V}_{O_2} \text{ in ml/min}}{\text{HR in beats/min}} = \dot{V}_{O_2} \text{ in ml/beat}$$

Gas Pressures

$$PAO_2 = P_IO_2 - \{PaCO_2 \times [F_IO_2 + (1 - F_IO_2)/R]\}$$

where $PaCO_2$ equals $PACO_2$

Physiologic Dead Space

$$P_ECO_2 = F_ECO_2 \times (PB - 47)$$

$$V_D \text{ of patient} = \left[V_T \times \frac{(PaCO_2 - P_ECO_2)}{(PaCO_2 - P_ICO_2)} \right] - V_D \text{ of valve}$$

$$\frac{V_D}{V_T} \text{ of patient} = \left[\frac{(PaCO_2 - P_ECO_2)}{(PaCO_2 - P_ICO_2)} \right] - \left(\frac{V_D \text{ of valve.}}{V_T - V_D \text{ of valve}} \right)$$

Sample Values and Calculations

The subject is a male, 45 years old, with a weight of 70 kg and height of 170 cm. PB is 750. Room air is inspired. Room temperature is 22° C. PH_2O at 22° C is 20 mm Hg. PH_2O at 37° C is 47 mm Hg. Valve dead space is 64 ml. Expired gas volume measurements made at room temperature, saturated. Subject exercised on cycle ergometer until exhaustion. Data collected is given in Table 1 and calculated values in Table 2.

Table 1 *Measured Values*

	Rest	0 Watts	90 Watts	210 Watts
Volume collected (liters)	8.6	14.3	17.1	50.3
Time collected (sec)	64	61	30	33
Complete breaths	13	14	9	21
Heart rate	76	90	142	179
F_ECO_2	0.035	0.039	0.040	0.033
F_EO_2	0.167	0.164	0.163	0.179
PaO_2 (mm Hg)	92	90	92	101
$PaCO_2$ (mm Hg)	39	39	38	30
pHa	7.41	7.39	7.40	7.30

Calculations:

$$\dot{V}_E \text{ (BTPS)} = 8.6 \times \frac{60 \times (273 + 37) \times (750 - 20)}{64 \times (273 + 22) \times (750 - 47)} = 8.8 \qquad \text{(Eq. 1)}$$

$$\dot{V}_E \text{ (STPD)} = 8.6 \times \frac{60 \times 730}{64 \times 760 \times (1 + 0.00367 \times 22)} = 7.17 \qquad \text{(Eq. 2)}$$

$$\dot{V}_{CO_2} = 7.17 \times (0.035 - 0.0004) = 0.248 \qquad \text{(Eq. 3)}$$

$$\dot{V}_{O_2} = 7.17 \times [0.265(1 - 0.167 - 0.035) - 0.167] = 0.319 \qquad \text{(Eq. 4)}$$

$$R = 0.248/0.319 = 0.78 \qquad \text{(Eq. 5)}$$

$$f = 13 \times 60/64 = 12.2 \qquad \text{(Eq. 6)}$$

$$V_T, \text{ (in liters)} = 8.8/12.2 = 0.72 \qquad \text{(Eq. 7)}$$

$\dot{V}_E$ at BTPS excluding valve dead space is given by

$$\dot{V}_E = 8.8 - (0.064 \times 12.2) = 8.02 \quad \text{(Eq. 8)}$$

$$\dot{V}_E/\dot{V}_{CO_2} = 8.0/0.25 = 32 \quad \text{(Eq. 9)}$$

$$\dot{V}_E/\dot{V}_{O_2} = 8.0/0.32 = 25 \quad \text{(Eq. 10)}$$

$$V_D/V_T = \frac{[39 - (703 \times 0.035)]}{[39 - (703 \times 0.0004)]} - \left[\frac{0.064}{0.72 - 0.064}\right] = 0.27 \quad \text{(Eq. 11)}$$

$$PAO_2 = 703 \times 0.2093 - 39\left[0.2093 + \frac{(1 - 0.2093)}{0.78}\right] = 99.3 \quad \text{(Eq. 12)}$$

$$P(A - a)O_2 = 99 - 92 = 7 \quad \text{(Eq. 13)}$$

$$O_2 \text{ pulse (ml/beat)} = 0.319 \times 1000/76 = 4.2 \quad \text{(Eq. 14)}$$

Efficiency, in percent, from 0 to 90 watts, is given by

$$0.3 \times 90/(1.48 - 0.59) = 30.3 \quad \text{(Eq. 15)}$$

Table 2 *Calculated Values*

	Rest[a]	0 W	90 W	210 W
$\dot{V}_E$, BTPS (liters/min)	8.8 (1)	15.3	37.3	99.2
$\dot{V}_E$, STPD (liters/min)	7.2 (2)	12.5	30.4	84.6
$\dot{V}_{CO_2}$, STPD (liters/min)	0.25 (3)	0.48	1.21	2.79
$\dot{V}_{C_2}$, STPD (liters/min)	0.32 (4)	0.59	1.48	2.52
R	0.78 (5)	0.81	0.82	1.11
f, breaths/min	12.2 (6)	13.8	18	38.2
V_T, BTPS (liters)	0.72 (7)	1.11	2.07	2.60
$\dot{V}_E$, BTPS (liters/min)				
Excluding valve	8.0 (8)	14.4	36.1	96.8
$\dot{V}_E/\dot{V}_{CO_2}$, BTPS/STPD	32.0 (9)	30.0	29.9	34.6
$\dot{V}_E/\dot{V}_{O_2}$, BTPS/STPD	25.0 (10)	24.4	24.4	38.4
V_D/V_T	0.28 (11)	0.24	0.23	0.20
PAO_2 (mm Hg)	99 (12)	101	102	120
$P(A\text{-}a)O_2$ (mm Hg)	7 (13)	11	10	19
O_2 pulse (ml/beat)	4.2 (14)	6.5	11.3	14.1
Efficiency (%), in the range of 0–90 W, is 30				

[a] Numbers in parentheses refer to equation numbers.

NORMAL PREDICTED VALUES

Resting Values

$$P(A\text{-}a)O_2 \text{ (in mm Hg)} = 10 + 0.43\,(y - 20),$$

where y is age in years. Standard deviation (SD) is 4.1 (where $pCO_2 = 40$, and $R = 0.8$), [derived from data of Sorbini et al. (12) and experience at UCLA].

$$V_D/V_T < 0.40,$$

excluding the dead space of the valve.

$$V_D\ (\text{ml}) = 0.859Y + 1.32H + 0.264\ V_T - 905/f - 179,$$

where Y is age in years, H is height in centimeters, V_T is tidal volume in millileters, and f is breathing frequency per minute. SD is 28 ml (13).

Values Near the Anaerobic Threshold

The anaerobic threshold is defined as the level of $\dot{V}O_2$ just below that at which metabolic acidosis and the associated changes in gas exehange occur. With incremental exercise testing, the changes are a stable $\dot{V}_E/\dot{V}_{CO_2}$ or $P_{ET}CO_2$ accompanied by a rising $\dot{V}_E/\dot{V}_{O_2}$ or $P_{ET}O_2$ (4). The lower limit of normal for a typical adult is a $\dot{V}_{O_2}$ of 1 liter/min for males, and 0.8 liter/min for females; these values would represent the typical O_2 requirements of a normal subject walking at 4–5 km/hr on a level surface (14).

$\dot{V}_E/\dot{V}_{CO_2}$ (BTPS/STPD) equals 28–30 at sea level (4, 14, 15).

$\dot{V}_E/\dot{V}_{O_2}$ (BTPS/STPD) equals 23–27 at sea level (4, 14, 15).

$\dot{V}_E/\dot{V}_{O_2}$ (mean ± SD) at $\dot{V}_{O_2}$ of 1.0 liter/min = 24.2 ± 3.7, 24.8 ± 4.8, 26.8 ± 4.2, 27.9 ± 4.2 for men 20–40 years, men > 40 yrs, women 20–40 years, and women > 40 years, respectively [A.D. Dawson, personal communication March 1980, from data of S.G. Spiro (3)].

HR (mean ± SD) at $\dot{V}_{O_2}$ of 1.0 liter/min = 107.5 ± 11.4, 106.2 ± 14.7, 137.2 ± 17.1 and 136.7 ± 21.3 for men 20–40 years, men > 40 years, women 20–40 years, and women > 40 years respectively [A.D. Dawson, personal communication, March 1980, from data of S.G. Spiro (3)].

Oxygen pulse at $\dot{V}_{O_2}$ of 1.0 liter/min can be calculated from previous paragraph.

$$V_D/V_T = 0.12 \text{ to } 0.24\ (15).$$

$$V_D\ (\text{ml}) = 1.01\ Y + 0.985H - 0.45\dot{V}_{CO_2} + 21.76\dot{V}_E - 5.69f - 27.7$$

where Y is age in years, H is height in centimeters. $\dot{V}_{CO_2}$ is in milliliters per minute, $\dot{V}_E$ is in liters per minute, f is in breaths per minute, and SD equals 52 ml (16).

Treadmill

$\dot{V}_{O_2}$ in liters per minute STPD is given by:

$$\dot{V}_{O_2} = 0.0035B\ \{2.3 + 0.32\ (V - 5)^{1.65} + G[0.2 + 0.07\ (V - 2.5)]\},$$

where B is body weight in kilograms, V is velocity in kilometers per hour, and G is grade in percent. (assumes $\dot{V}_{O_2}$ of 0.2 liter/min equals 1 kcal/min energy.) Valid with velocity over 4 km/hr (17).

$\dot{V}_{O_2}$ in liters per minute STPD is given by:

$$\dot{V}_{O_2} = \left[\frac{H(1.766V^{0.176} - 1.445) \times 2.2B(0.328V^2 - 2.45V + 9.66)}{(0.0136H - 0.9525) \times 10^5}\right] + 0.0189VG$$

Valid for men 160–185 cm and 60–90 kg at velocity of 1.6–5.3 km/hr (18).

$V_{O_2}max$ in liters per minute is

$$\dot{V}_{O_2}max = 0.001B\ (68.3 - 11.9Z - 0.413Y)$$

for a sedentary adult, where B is body weight in kilograms, Z is 1 if male, and 2 if female, and Y is age in years (18).

$$\dot{V}_{O_2}max \text{ in ml/kg/min} = 68.3 - 11.9Z - 0.413Y \quad (19).$$

Cycle Ergometer

$\dot{V}_{O_2}$ in liters per minute STPD is

$$\dot{V}_{O_2} = 0.001\ (5.8B + 151) + 0.0101W,$$

where B is body weight in kilograms and W is watts work rate (4). On a cycle ergometer, it is suggested that the $\dot{V}_{O_2}max$ values be 90% of the treadmill values of Bruce (19).

Other Maximum Predicted Values

Maximum heart rate in beats per minute is 210 − 0.65Y where Y is age in years (2).

Maximum oxygen pulse in milliliters per beat is

$$\frac{\dot{V}_{O_2}max \text{ in ml/min}}{\text{HR max in beats/min}}$$

$$\dot{V}_E max/MVV\ (\%) = 50\text{–}70$$

At sea level, $P(A-a)O_2$ normally does not increase more than 10 mm Hg over resting values (20).

Maximum f in breaths per minute is 40–45.

EXPECTED REPRODUCIBILITY

Equipment

Volume and flow measurements should be reproducible within 2%. Duplicate O_2 and CO_2 analyses by Scholander or Haldane methods should agree within

0.04%. Oxygen and carbon dioxide analysis by other analyzers should be reproducible within 0.1%. Small errors in F_ECO_2 or F_EO_2 may cause large errors in $\dot{V}_{CO_2}$, $\dot{V}_{O_2}$, R, or ventilatory equivalents. For example, an increase in F_EO_2 from 0.141 to 0.143 with concomitant increase in F_ECO_2 from 0.061 to 0.063 will cause measured R to increase from 0.866 to 0.935 and measured $\dot{V}O_2$ to decrease 4.4%. The same increase in F_EO_2 with a concomitant decrease in F_ECO_2 from 0.061 to 0.059 will cause R to decrease from 0.866 to 0.862 and measured $\dot{V}_{O_2}$ to decrease by 2.7%. Small errors in PaO_2, or $PaCO_2$, or R will cause proportional errors in $\dot{V}_E$, $\dot{V}_{CO_2}$ and $\dot{V}_{O_2}$.

Biological Reproducibility

Total variability was measured in 11 consecutive patients exercised twice, 2–10 days apart. The average difference in $\dot{V}_E$ at 10 W, 60 W, and maximum exercise were 11%, 11%, and 8%, and in $\dot{V}_{O_2}$ were 12%, 8%, and 8%, respectively (D.Y. Sue and J. E. Hansen, unpublished, January 1980).

TROUBLESHOOTING AND COMMON ERRORS

Table 3 lists common errors in exercise testing due to improper equipment, technique, or calculations, and their solutions.

Table 3 *Common Errors and Possible Causes and Solutions*

Possible causes	Possible solutions
1. $\dot{V}_E$ inaccurate	
Leaks in bag or balloon	Repair or replace.
Leak in dry-gas meter	Calibrate and repair.
Pneumotachograph (PTG)	Clean and dry PTG.
PTG alinear at high flow due to cooling or turbulence	Cool gas before passing through cool PTG. Precede PTG by smooth tube equal to diameter of PTG with length 3 or more times diameter. Linearize electronically. Increase PTG size.
Calculation error	Check timing, temperature, humidity, calibration; include pump flow factors.
2. $\dot{V}_{CO_2}$ inaccurate	
Error in $\dot{V}_E$ measure	See Section 1.
Diffusion of CO_2 through bag or balloon	Avoid delay in analysis.
Calibration gases inaccurate	Analyze calibrating gases by Scholander or Haldane technique.
Scholander or Haldane analysis inaccurate	Does room air equal 20.89–20.93% O_2 and 0.03–0.06% CO_2?
CO_2 analyzer not linear	Calibrate at several points; check manual; clean head.

Table 3 *Common Errors and Possible Causes and Solutions—Continued*

Possible causes	Possible Solutions
CO_2 analyzer error	Resistance and flow must be similar during calibration measurement
Calculation error	Use correct water vapor and conversion factors
3. $\dot{V}_{O_2}$ inaccurate or R inappropriate	
Error in $\dot{V}_E$ or FCO_2 measure	See Sections 1 and 2.
O_2 analyzer not linear	Calibrate at several points.
O_2 analyzer error	Check manual; clean head; resistance and flow must be similar during calibration and measurement.
Calculation error	Equation is based on dry-gas measures; eg., $FO_2 + FN_2 + FCO_2 = 1.0000$.
4. $\dot{V}O_2$ too low or high for work performed	
$\dot{V}_{O_2}$ inaccurate	See Sections 1, 2, 3.
Cycle incorrectly calibrated	Recalibrate; resistance not zero at "zero load" pedaling.
Treadmill speed or grade incorrect	Express grade in %, not degrees; check speed and belt length and belt tension.
No error	Patient has low efficiency (high $\dot{V}_{O_2}$ required for given amount of work).
5. EKG tracings poor or cardiotachometer inaccurate	
QRS complex too small	Change lead placement or increase gain.
Poor skin preparation	Correct or replace electrode.
Pulse rate erroneous despite good EKG signal	Recalibrate.
6. $\dot{V}O_2$ and HR not linearly related	
Error in $\dot{V}_{O_2}$ measure	See Sections 3, 4 and 5.
Mixing chamber used	Use longer flushing period or only steady state measures.
Caused by disease	
7. Arterial catheter draws poorly or BP tracing dampens	
Tip against vessel and wall	Rotate catheter or withdraw a few millimeters.
Clots in catheter	Aspirate catheter; keep catheter filled with heparinized fluid.
8. VD/VT erroneously elevated at rest	
Calculation error	Consider V_D of valve.

CONTROVERSIAL ISSUES

The Clinical Usefulness of Exercise Testing

Although exercise testing may be valuable in patients with respiratory, cardiovascular, or neuromuscular disease, the clinical usefulness of measuring the multitude of parameters that can be measured during exercise is somewhat controversial and will not be considered here. As a generalization, it is clear at this time that quantitative assessment of exercise performance is clinically useful for diagnostic purposes, assessments of impairment, disability evaluations, and for following responses to therapy; which particular parameters are most useful remains an unresolved issue.

TREADMILL VERSUS CYCLE

Safety and Ease of Exercise

Some clinicians prefer a treadmill and others a cycle ergometer. From the patient's viewpoint, most consider walking to be more natural than cycle riding. All patients require a brief orientation and training session to learn to get on the moving treadmill belt safely. With a mouthpiece in place, the patients may have difficulty signaling when they are exhausted and wish to stop walking or running on the treadmill. Thus a signal code should be prearranged. Many treadmills do not have slow enough speeds to accommodate dyspneic patients. On the other hand, after a few minutes of practice and adjustment of seat height (and strapping of the most uncoordinated subjects' feet to the pedals), most individuals are able to pedal. Some are unable or unwilling to pedal at 60 rpm. On a cycle one has the advantage of stopping at will, but the disadvantage of seat discomfort after riding for long time periods.

Quantitation and Calibration

For quantitation of work rate, cycle riding is preferred over the treadmill. Walking and running efficiency improve measurably after one uses a treadmill once or twice. Efficiency also varies with the grade and speed and causes variability in results. At higher work rates it may be necessary to increase both speed and grade to exhaust some patients, thus making it very difficult to evenly increment the work rate. However, calibration of treadmill speed and grade can be checked easily. For the cycle, there is little or no increase in efficiency of pedaling with training, and work rates can be incremented rapidly and predictably. With mechanical cycles, the patient must pedal at a constant rate, usually 50–60 cycles/minute, whereas with an electromechanical cycle, the work rate will be within 5% at a given setting even though the pedaling frequency may vary from 40 to 80 cycles/min. Calibration of a cycle may be time-consuming or require special instrumentation. Maximum oxygen uptake is usually about 10% lower on a cycle ergometer than on a treadmill.

Catheter Use

When using arterial or venous catheters for blood sampling, pressure measurements, or during infusions, the cycle is preferred over the treadmill. On the cycle, the site of withdrawal is relatively fixed, and stopcock and syringe manipulation is much easier. Also, the position of the heart relative to the transducer is more constant with the cycle than with the treadmill.

Other Considerations

The costs of an electromechanical cycle or study treadmill are equivalent (approximately $5000) whereas a reliable mechanical cycle costs less than $1000. Treadmills require more horizontal and vertical space, are noisier, heavier, bulkier, and more difficult to move or transport. For rehabiliation programs, either a treadmill or a measured walking course is desirable.

Steady-State versus Incremental Exercise

Steady-state exercise can be performed with simpler equipment than incremental exercise. It also allows the estimation of cardiac output by rebreathing techniques. Steady-state exercise, however, needs to be repeated at several levels of work, each of 4–6 minutes duration if one wishes to estimate the anaerobic threshold or maximum oxygen uptake. In contrast, with work rate incremented every minute until exhaustion or cessation of exercise, a single 6–10 minute incremental exercise bout (preferably on a cycle) gives the same information in a shorter period of time. Incremental exercise to exhaustion is less tiring than several bouts of steady-state exercise at different work rates to exhaustion. With incremental exercise, recovery is quicker, and the test can be repeated again with a variable such as oxygen breathing added if desired.

The distance or duration of walking at a submaximal pace is a specific type of steady-state exercise often used as a measure of improvement in rehabilitation programs. The distance or duration can improve strikingly with only minimal improvement in the anaerobic threshold or $\dot{V}_{O_2}max$.

Invasive versus Noninvasive Measures

The least invasive procedure necessary for clinical diagnosis or management is always preferable. End tidal O_2 and CO_2 values closely approximate calculated mean alveolar values at rest and during exercise in normal subjects, but differences increase with disease states or abnormal breathing patterns. Rebreathing maneuvers during steady-state exercise combined with arterial blood analyses allow estimation of cardiac output without mixed venous samples, but require some training and recovery time and cause dyspnea. Oximetry is especially useful in gauging the effect of supplemental oxygen. Without additional arterial values, it does not allow measurement of V_D or $P(A{-}a)O_2$. Arterial blood obtained by arterial stick immediately after cessation of exercise does not measure the values present during exercise and is not recommended for the measurement of $P(A-a)O_2$. The anaerobic threshold can probably be estimated from expired gas values during incremental exercise with an accuracy equivalent to arterial lactate or bicarbonate levels.

Basic Systems versus Component Systems versus Commercial Preassembled Complete Systems

A basic system that measures only ventilation and heart rate provides enough information to meet many clinical needs; for labs unfamiliar with the technical demands of more complex measurements, such a system has the very important advantage of increasing the likelihood that the measurements will be accurate. Using such a system as a first step allows the technical and medical personnel to gain a better understanding of the advantages and limitations of exercise testing without the expense and potential confusion that oftens arises when overly sophisticated testing is attempted.

If a laboratory elects to measure expired gas concentrations and the parameters that can be derived from this data as part of their exercise testing, the choice of whether to assemble a system from components or purchase a preassembled complete system is an important decision. Assembling a system from components enables one to use equipment a laboratory may already have, allows greater flexibility for changes in the future, and often is less expensive; the expertise and time required, however, is often considerable. Packaged complete exercise systems offer the obvious advantage of requiring minimal development time and are often engineered to maximize ease of operation and reduction of data. However, they are often quite expensive, not necessarily more accurate than component systems, and usually offer less flexibility, if it is desired to use gas analyzers for purposes other than exercise testing. As with any other type of automated testing system, data that confirms the accuracy of the measurements made by the system should be available prior to clinical use; rigorous quality control procedures are as important as with manual systems. Most desirable in microprocessors or computer systems are units that allow for programming changes should they be needed in the future.

REFERENCES

1. Jones NL: Exercise testing in pulmonary evaluation. *N Engl J Med* 293:541–544, 647–650, 1975.
2. Jones NL, Campbell EJM, Edwards RHT, et al.: *Clinical Exercise Testing*. Philadelphia, WB Saunders Co, 1975.
3. Spiro SG: Exercise testing in clinical medicine. *Br J Dis Chest* 71:145–172, 1977.
4. Wasserman K, Whipp BJ: Exercise physiology in health and disease. *Am Rev Respir Dis* 112:219–249, 1975.

5. Wasserman K: Breathing during exercise. *N Engl J Med* 298:780–785, 1978.
6. McGavin CR, Gupta SP, McHardy GFR: Twelve minute walking test for assessing disability in chronic bronchitis. *Br Med J* 1:822–823, 1976.
7. Consolazio CF, Johnson F, Pecora L: *Physiological Measurements of Metabolic Functions in Man*. New York, McGraw-Hill, 1963.
8. Sue DY, Hansen JE, Blais M, et al.: Measurement and analysis of gas exchange during exercise using a programmable calculator. *J Appl Physiol* 49:456–461, 1980.
9. Wilmore JH, Costill DL: Semiautomated approach to the assessment of oxygen uptake during exercise. *J Appl Physiol* 36:618–620, 1974.
10. Cumming GR, Alexander WD: The calibration of bicycle ergometers. *Can J Physiol Pharmacol* 46:917–918, 1968.
11. Seldinger SI: Catheter replacement of the needle in percutaneous arteriography: A new technique. *Acta Radiol (Stockh)* 39:368–376, 1953.
12. Sorbini CA, Grassi V, Solinas E, et al.: Arterial oxygen tension in relation to age in healthy subjects. *Respiration* 25:3–13, 1968.
13. Harris EA, Seelye ER, Whitlock RML: Revised standards for normal resting dead-space volume and venous admixture in men and women. *Clin Sci Mol Med* 55:125–128, 1978.
14. Wasserman K, Whipp BJ, Koyal SN, et al.: Anaerobic threshold and respiratory gas exchange during exercise. *J Appl Physiol* 35:236–243, 1973.
15. Wasserman K, Van Kessel AL, Burton GG: Interaction of physiological mechanisms during exercise. *J Appl Physiol* 22:71–85, 1967.
16. Bradley CA, Harris EA, Seelye ER, et al.: Gas exchange during exercise in healthy people: I. The physiological dead-space volume. *Clin Sci Mol Med* 51:323–333, 1976.
17. Givoni B, Goldman RF: Predicting metabolic energy cost. *J Appl Physiol* 30:429–433, 1971.
18. Workman JM, Armstrong BW: Oxygen cost of treadmill walking. *J Appl Physiol* 18:798–803, 1963.
19. Bruce RA, Kusumi F, Hosmer D: Maximal oxygen intake and nomographic assessment of functional aerobic impairment in cardiovascular disease. *Am Heart J* 85:546–562, 1973.
20. Hansen JE, Vogel JA, Stelter GP, et al.: Oxygen uptake in man during exhaustive work at sea level and high altitude. *J Appl Physiol* 23:511–522, 1967.

CHAPTER 23

Regulation of Ventilation

JAMES E. HANSEN, M.D.

Accurate assessment of ventilatory regulation requires consideration of a variety of complex factors. In addition to the voluntary and emotional influences on ventilation, breathing is modified by stimulation of the mechanical receptors in the chest wall, stretch and irritant receptors in the airways, and juxtapulmonary capillary (J) receptors in the lung parenchyma, all of which send impulses to the medullary respiratory center. Respiration is stimulated by reduced arterial pH (pHa) and arterial oxygen tension (PaO_2) in the peripheral chemoreceptors (primarily the carotid bodies) and also by decreased pH in the tissue extracellular fluid in the medullary chemoreceptors (as influenced by $PaCO_2$ and cerebrospinal fluid HCO_3^-). The resulting central drive must be transmitted through the intercostal and phrenic nerves to the ventilatory musculature of the neck, chest, and abdomen. Ventilation of the lung is affected not only by anatomical defects or neuromuscular diseases of the thorax and abdomen, but also by upper airway disorders and obstructive or restrictive diseases of the lung. There are several excellent reviews of the regulation of ventilation and suggestions for instrumentation (1-5).

Ventilatory drive is commonly evaluated with blood gases and physiologic tests, with historical and physical information as aids for test interpretation. Exercise testing (Chapter 22) allows assessment of the ventilatory response to exercise. The carotid body contribution to the ventilatory response during steady-state exercise is measured by the magnitude of the decrease in ventilation that occurs a few seconds after hyperoxic breathing. Hypercapnic response is a measure of the change in ventilatory output associated with increases in inspired CO_2 concentration when oxygenation is adequate. Hypoxic response is a measure of the change in ventilatory output associated with decreases in inspired O_2 concentration while end tidal CO_2 is stabilized at one or more levels. Among the

ISBN 0-12-788125-5

methods used to access neural output, measurements of the negative pressure generated by the muscles of inspiration when inspiratory flow is not allowed to begin (''occlusion pressures'') are superior to the more traditional measurements of minute ventilation, which may be limited by obstructive or restrictive pulmonary diseases.

Although formerly used principally in research, the assessment of ventilatory drive is increasingly used clinically for the evaluation of patients with unexplained depression of respiration (e.g., hypoxia and or hypercapnia), for evaluating the response to hypoxia or hyperoxia (e.g., high altitudes or oxygen supplementation), and for evaluating patients with disordered respiration during sleep. As disorders of ventilatory regulation and their therapy become better understood, the clinical application of this testing will increase.

This chapter will discuss the measurement of breath-holding time, the performance of several rebreathing tests, and the ventilatory and inspiratory occlusion pressure responses to hypercapnia without hypoxia and hypoxia with eucapnia.

EQUIPMENT

The rebreathing and inspiratory occlusion tests require equipment similar to that diagrammed in Fig. 1.

If the flow, CO_2, O_2, and pressure signals are sent via an analog to digital converter to a computer, the collection, analysis, and plotting of data are simplified: The integrating and differentiating channels are not needed and switching of recorder paper speeds is minimized. The Lloyd valve is used because of its small dead space (64 ml) and configuration. A transparent cylinder, approximately 17 cm in length and 5 cm in diameter, to enclose the CO_2 absorber, can be fabricated using a large stopper at each end. A compressor with needle valve provides variable flow (up to 30 liter/min) through the CO_2 absorber circuit. The apparatus is filled with fresh cylinder gases through the inlet. During hypoxic testing, oxygen can be introduced through the inlet by adding a flow meter and valve.

The Starling resistor noiselessly occludes the inspiratory side of the rebreathing circuit. It is fabricated of plastic or metal tubing 3 cm in internal diameter and 8 cm long and equipped with a side tap, a rubber condom with the end cut off, two rubber bands, connecting plastic tubing, and a 100-ml syringe. If inspiratory occlusion tests are not performed, the Starling resistor and transducer for mouth pressure are unnecessary. A screen to block operator movements from the view of the patient is useful. To measure the rapidly changing pressure during inspiratory occlusion, a recorder paper speed of 50 mm/sec is desirable. Oxyhemoglobin saturation in arterial blood (SaO_2) can be measured easily and accurately with a suitable ear oximeter (6).

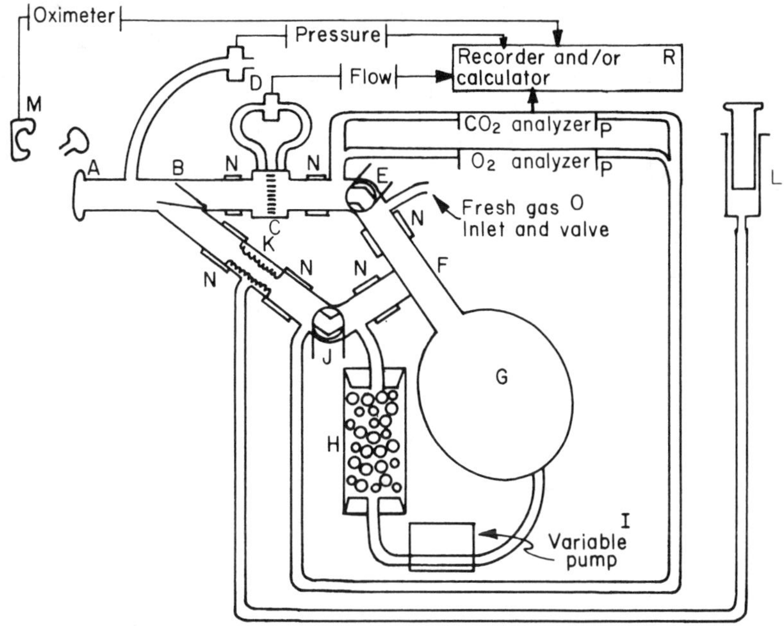

Fig. 1 *Equipment for rebreathing. (A) Mouthpiece and noseclip or mask; (B) Lloyd valve with tap at mouthpiece for tube to transducer for mouth pressure;* (C) *#3 pneumotachograph (heated); (D) transducers for mouth pressure and expiratory flow: (E) three-way Y valve with taps to O_2 and CO_2 analyzer; (F) plastic or metal T-piece; (G) 7-liter anesthesia bag; (H) plastic cylinder filled with CO_2 absorber; (I) pump with needle valve to vary flow (0–30 liters/min); (J) three-way Y valve with taps from (1) CO_2 absorber and bag and (2) CO_2 and O_2 analyzers; (K) Starling resistor (plastic or metal tube 3.3 cm in diameter with side tap and thin rubber tubing; (L) 100-ml glass syringe; (M) ear oximeter; (N) six short connecting pieces of 3.3 cm in diameter rubber connecting tubing; (O) fresh gas inlet and valve; (P) O_2 and CO_2 analyzers; (R) recorder and computer. Plastic connecting tubing is used as diagrammed.*

QUALITY CONTROL

The mouth pressure transducer should be linear from 0 to −30 cm of water as tested against a water manometer. To check for leaks in the circuit, pump a 1–4-liter calibration syringe several times at the mouthpiece with the circuit valves turned for recirculation. The volume signal (integrated flow) should be within 10% of the correct value at both high and low flow rates. When high oxygen concentration is used in the hypercapnic response test, the pneumotachograph conversion factor needs to be decreased to 90% of room air values due to the high viscosity of oxygen (see Chapter 12). The O_2 and CO_2 analyzer should be calibrated as in Chapter 22 (Exercise Testing). The scale of the recorder needs to be set to display the CO_2 signal from 0% to 10% and the O_2 signal from 21% to 5%. The ear oximeter measurement should occasionally be compared with arterial blood samples. The Starling resistor valve should close and open silently and completely. As with many other tests of pulmonary function, one of the best quality control procedures is the periodic performance of tests in normal subjects, comparing results either with previous testing or published normal values.

PREPARATION OF SUBJECT

An American Thoracic Society workshop on assessment of respiratory control in humans (1) established the following recommendations:

> The ventilatory responses to hypoxia and hypercapnia even in normal individuals vary considerably. To prevent extraneous influences from further increasing this variability, the following is recommended. 1) Studies should be performed in the fasting state with the bladder empty. 2) The subject should be comfortable and should rest for at least 30 minutes before the test. 3) The room should be quiet. 4) Body temperature should be determined. 5) Tests may be performed in either the sitting or semi-supine position. 6) Preliminary evidence suggests that normal subjects may have greater (presumably exaggerated) hypoxic responses when using nose clip and mouthpiece than when using masks. 7) Tests should be performed in duplicate with at least 10 minutes of rest between tests.
>
> Ventilatory responses to hypoxia and hypercapnia are potentially hazardous. The clinical condition of the patient should be considered when evaluating the potential hazardous effects of the test procedure, and the usual precautions for safety of the patient used in any stress test should be taken.

In addition, the subject's eyes should be closed. As a minimum, the subject should be unable to see the various meters, monitors, and manipulators.

Because the procedures and calculations for each of the various tests of ventilatory regulation differ, each will be discussed individually in the following sections.

BREATH-HOLDING TIME

Procedure

With nose clamped, the subject exhales to residual volume, inhales to total lung capacity (TLC), and holds his breath as long as is comfortably possible. If the volume of the valve and distance from A to I (Fig. 1) are low, analyses of the expired gases can be made to estimate end-tidal CO_2 concentrations ($P_{ET}CO_2$).

Calculations

Breath-holding time equals the average time in seconds from the cessation of inspiration to TLC to the first expiration. The test is repeated until the subject achieves reproducible breath-holding times or $P_{ET}CO_2$s.

Normal Predicted Values

Mithoefer (7), summarized 278 observations from nine series in the literature; for breath holding at TLC, the mean time was 78 seconds. (Room air was inspired without prior hyperventilation.)

Expected Reproducibility

Davidson et al. (8), studied six normal subjects, and found at TLC a mean ± SEM breath-holding time of 75 ±3 seconds at sea level; subjects were trained until the expired $P_{ET}CO_2$ was reproducible within 2 mm Hg. Such reproducibility cannot often be obtained when testing patients in clinical labs.

HYPERCAPNIC RESPONSE

Procedure

The following methodology is as described by Read (9): The anesthesia bag is filled with a volume equal to the subject's vital capacity plus 1 liter with a mixture containing 7% CO_2 and 93% O_2 (the latter to eliminate hypoxic drive). The valves E and J (see Fig. 1) are turned so the patient breathes room air and expires into the room. Expired flow and $P_{ET}CO_2$ are recorded. After a period of stability, valves E and J are turned (J during a forced maximal expiration, and E during the next inspiration) so that the subject now breathes into and out of the anesthesia bag. The test is continued until the patient terminates the test because of dyspnea, until the $P_{ET}CO_2$ equals 9%, or until 4 minutes have elapsed.

Calculations

The ventilation in liters per minute (BTPS), either breath-by-breath or averaged over 5–10 breaths, is plotted on the Y axis and the mean $P_{ET}CO_2$ in millimeters Hg on the X axis for the same periods. The slope [the change in minute ventilation ($\Delta\dot{V}_E$) divided by the change in $P_{ET}CO_2$] is determined for all of the periods, preferably by linear least squares regression and analysis, eliminating the first 30 seconds of rebreathing.

Normal Predicted Values

There is large variability between normal subjects. Expressed as $\Delta\dot{V}_E$ in liters per minute BTPS/$\Delta P_{ET}CO_2$ in millimeters Hg, Read (9) found in 21 normal adults a mean ± standard deviation (SD) of 2.65 ± 1.21 with a range of 1.16–6.18. Irsigler (10) found in 126 adults a mean ± SD of 2.6 ± 1.2 with a range of 0.47–6.22; 79% of the subjects ranged between 1.5 and 5.0. Kronenberg et al. (11) found, in nine men ages 22–30, a mean of 2.4 for $PaO_2 > 200$ (high inspired O_2).

Hypercapnic response has been shown to correlate with weight and especially height, and vital capacity (12). Therefore, these measurements should always be reported concurrently.

Expected Reproducibility

Irsigler (10) measured and plotted $\dot{V}_E$ in liters per minute BTPS versus $P_{ET}CO_2$ in mm Hg in 111 students on 2 occasions 15 minutes apart. The mean ± standard error of the estimate (SEE) slope of the first test was 2.60 ± 0.11, and of the seond test was 2.46 ± 0.10. The mean ± SEE intercept on the CO_2 axis (at 0 $\dot{V}_E$) was 32.42 ± 0.67 mm Hg for the first test and 31.17 ± 0.71 mm Hg for the second test. Thus, although the slopes did not differ significantly, the intercepts did. When 10 of thc samc subjects were retested 9–24 months later, the difference in slopes from earlier values varied from 0.04 to 3.57 liter/min/mm Hg and the differences in X axis intercepts from 0 to 7.6 mm Hg.

HYPOXIC RESPONSE

Procedure

The following procedures are according to the methodology of Rebuck and Campbell (13). The anesthesia bag is filled with a volume equal to the patient's vital capacity plus 1 liter with a mixture containing approximately 7% CO_2, 70% N_2, and the balance O_2. Valves E and J are turned so the patient is inspiring from and expiring into the room. Expired volume, $P_{ET}O_2$, $P_{ET}CO_2$, and ear oximeter O_2 saturation values are sent to the recorder. When the $P_{ET}CO_2$ values stabilize, valve J is turned during a normal expiration and valve E during the next inspiration so that the patient now rebreathes from the bag. The subject then takes three deep breaths to facilitate mixing. After these three breaths, the CO_2 signal is noted. The operator attempts to maintain the CO_2 at this level by manually decreasing the CO_2 scrubber flow if $P_{ET}CO_2$ declines. Rebreathing is continued until the $P_{ET}O_2$ declines to 45 mm Hg, the saturation declines to 75%, or the subject evidences distress. If ventilation increases too rapidly as saturation declines below 85%, the addition of oxygen through inlet O at a rate of 125–200 ml/min will reduce the rate of change.

Calculations

The mean $P_{ET}CO_2$ is noted. The ventilation in liters per minute BTPS, either breath-by-breath or averaged over 5–10 breaths, is plotted on the Y axis and the mean SaO_2 in percent on the X axis for the same periods. The slope (change in $\dot{V}_E$ per 1% desaturation) is determined, preferably by linear least squares regression analysis.

Normal Predicted Values

There is large variability in hypoxic response during eucapnia in normal subjects. Expressed as increase in $\dot{V}_E$ in liters per minute BTPS per 1% desaturation, Rebuck and Campbell (13) found in nine normal subjects a mean ±SD of 1.65 ± 1.20 with a range of 0.26–4.12 at an average $P_{ET}CO_2$ of 51.2 ± 3.7 mm Hg. In 11 normal subjects, Rebuck and Woodley (14) found a mean ± SD of 0.56 ± 0.42 liters per minute BTPS per 1% desaturation with a range of 0.16–1.76 at average $P_{ET}CO_2$ of 39 ± 1.4 mm Hg and a mean ± SD of 2.20 ± 1.07 liters per minute per 1% desaturation (a range of 1.21–4.90) at average $P_{ET}CO_2$ of 51.7 ± 2.1 mm Hg, (The latter $P_{ET}CO_2$ was considered to be equivalent to the estimated mixed venous CO_2.) The difference in slopes shows that hypoxic response depends markedly on the level of $P_{ET}CO_2$ selected. Approximately 10% of the population has a flat response to hypoxia (J. Severinghaus, personal communication, May 1980).

Expected Reproducibility

Rebuck and Campbell (13) repeatedly measured and calculated the increase in $\dot{V}_E$ in liters per minute BTPS versus change in SaO_2 in five subjects from day to day. Variance within the individuals was 0.76 whereas that among cohorts was 7.75.

INSPIRATORY OCCLUSION PRESSURE AT 100 MSEC OR MAXIMAL CHANGE IN PRESSURE

Procedure

When breathing room air or while the hypercapnic or hypoxic response is being tested, the mouth pressure at 100 msec (P_{100}) or the maximum rate of inspiratory pressure change [(dP/dt)max] can be measured. To measure P_{100} brief inspiratory occlusions should be randomly performed, always preceded by three or more tidal ventilations (15). Out of view of the patient, the operator compresses a syringe during expiration to close the Starling resistor and occlude the inspiratory channel, and then decompresses the syringe as soon as possible after the inspiratory attempt begins. The recorder speed should be 50 mm/sec during the subject's inspiratory attempt.

Alternatively, one measures the mouth pressure and its differential, the change in pressure, in the 10–50 msec before the inspiratory valve opens. This takes advantage of the inherent "stickiness" or resistance in the valve and can be measured at a slow recorder speed for every breath without requiring a Starling resistor or other operator maneuvers (16). It is difficult to make P_{100} measurements every 30 seconds; measurements every minute are more practical. For consistency, P_{100} readings must be measured at the same time after inspiratory effort begins, e.g., 100 ± 10 msec.

Calculations

The P_{100}s of single partially occluded breaths or the average (dP/dt)max of several breaths are measured directly from the recording and plotted on the vertical axis. On the horizontal axis can be graphed either (1) mean $\dot{V}_E$ expressed in liters per minute BTPS, calculated from three or more breaths preceeding inspiratory occlusion, (2) $P_{ET}CO_2$, or (3) SaO_2.

Normal Predicted Values

Kryger et al. (17) in five normal subjects found a mean P_{100} of 2.6 cm H_2O (with a range of 1.5–5.0 at a $PACO_2$ of 39–42 mm Hg). With progressive hypercapnia, Cherniack et al. (18) found a mean increase ± SEE of 0.60 ± 0.11 cm H_2O/mm Hg PCO_2 in the range of $PACO_2$ 45–55. Gelb et al. (19) in 15 normal subjects during increasing hypercapnia found a mean ± SD increase of 0.52 ± 0.19 cm H_2O/mm Hg PCO_2.

In 32 normal adult colleagues during quiet breathing, Matthews and Howell (16) found (dP/dt)max to vary from 12.5 to 25 cm H_2O/sec. During progressive hypercapnia, the increase in (dP/dt)max ranged from 0.6 to 4.6 cm H_2O/sec/mm Hg CO_2 while $P_{ET}CO_2$ rose from 50 to 60 mm Hg. In 47 studies on the 32 subjects, the correlation between the ventilatory slope (liters/min/mm Hg CO_2) and the (dP/dt)max response slope was excellent (r = 0.84).

Expected Reproducibility

Whitelaw et al. (15) demonstrated a series of five consecutive inspiratory occlusion pressure tracings from a subject during constant hypercapnia ($P_{ET}CO_2$ = 56). The mean ± SD P_{100} was 13.2 ± 0.76 cm H_2O. Cherniack et al. (18) studied normal subjects during progressive hypercapnia and found a linear correlation between P_{100} and $\dot{V}_E$ exceeding 0.80 in 34 of 35 trials. Shekleton et al. (20) measured the negative inspiratory occlusion pressures in centimeters H_2O at 150 msec (P_{150}) and $\dot{V}_E$ in liters per minute during hypercapnia ($PACO_2$ in millimeters Hg) in seven normal subjects. Three of the subjects were studied four times, and the following ranges were observed in the three individuals: The ΔP_{150}/$\Delta PACO_2$ varied from 0.42 to 0.86, 0.31 to 0.53, and 0.98 to 1.25 cm H_2O/mm

Hg. The $\dot{V}_E/\Delta PACO_2$ varied from 1.72 to 4.34, 1.96 to 2.83, and 2.84 to 4.76 liters/mm Hg.

Matthews and Howell (16) found that individual resting breath-to-breath (dP/dt)max varied up to 20%. In three subjects, each studied four times during incremental hypercapnia, the (dP/dt)max/$PACO_2$ ranged from 82% to 123% of each individual mean.

TROUBLESHOOTING

If the O_2 or CO_2 analyzers are erratic or do not record room air values when sampling room air, the sampling tubes or heads may have become clogged or wet. Water or saliva on the pneumotachograph will cause erroneous flow and volume measures. The Starling resistor should be checked for leaks by attempting to breathe through it during occlusion. It must be closed before inspiration begins and should be opened completely as soon as possible after inspiratory effort begins in order to minimize interruption to ventilation.

CONTROVERSIAL ISSUES

Safety of Rebreathing Measures

The only side effect to the CO_2 response test is the frequent occurrence of headaches. With hypoxic testing, there is the risk of hypoxic damage or syncope, but no reports of damage attributable to testing have been reported.

Gas Concentrations

Some investigators initiate hypercapnic response tests using 0% inspired CO_2 rather than CO_2 near mixed venous levels. Using an initial low P_ICO_2, there is a delay in increase in $\dot{V}_E$ until $P_{ET}CO_2$ gradually increases to mixed venous levels. One group considering this problem (21) has recommended the use of the inspired CO_2 at mixed venous levels (approximately 7% CO_2). In patients with CO_2 retention, the use of a P_ICO_2 about 4 mm Hg above the measured or estimated mixed venous PCO_2 eliminates the delay.

In assessing hypoxic response, some investigators stabilize $P_{ET}CO_2$ at resting end-tidal values rather than near mixed venous values. Thus, it is important to record the level or levels of eucapnia used during hypoxic response testing.

Alternative Equipment

The use of bag-in-box methods for measuring tidal volume are uncomplicated and obviate the necessity to recalibrate the pneumotachograph for varying compositions, thus providing more accurate integration of flow into volume. However, room air control measurements are not possible with these methods. Systems that control the inflow of N_2, CO_2, or O_2 are more complex than rebreathing systems, but they do allow closer control of the rate of change in inspired gas tensions. A more gradual decrease in inspired O_2 concentration during hypoxic testing can also be achieved with the equipment suggested in this chapter simply by using a larger rebreathing bag.

Other Methods of Assessing the Regulation of Ventilation

Serial blood gas and pH measurements obviously give a great deal of information about the regulation of ventilation. Classical steady-state methods are more time-consuming and tiring and do not appear to add significant additional information. The equipment and method described by Severinghaus et al. (22), allow rapid step changes in the patient's PO_2 while PCO_2 is stabilized, and offer the advantage of a brief stable period of hypoxia.

Other methods of assessing the regulation of ventilation include electromyographic measurements of the diaphragm, the measurement of isometric inspiratory loads, and the use of doxapram (which stimulates the carotid body) (4). None of these methods has yet been widely used clinically.

Calculating and Expressing Values

In plotting and calculating hypercapnic response, the slope of the $\Delta\dot{V}_E/\Delta PCO_2$ line is often denoted as S with the zero-ventilation intercept being denoted as B (23). Hypoxic response is usually expressed as $\dot{V}_E/1\%$ desaturation, but it can be expressed in other ways (23, 24). These, however, require considerably more complex calculations and several steady-state measurements. The $\dot{V}40$ (liters per minute per square meter) is the increment in ventilation, standardized to normal body size, produced by decreasing PaO_2 from hyperoxic levels to 40 mm Hg at the resting $PaCO_2$. If $\dot{V}_E$ is plotted against PAO_2 at a constant $PACO_2$, $\dot{V}_E$ normally increases steeply as PAO_2 declines. The hyperbolic curve can be characterized by the parameter A, which is the increase in ventilation for a decrease in PaO_2 to 33 mm Hg, assuming that ventilation becomes infinite when PaO_2 equals 32 mm Hg.

REFERENCES

1. Assessment of respiratory control in humans; editorial and workshop. *Am Rev Respir Dis* 115:1-5, 177-181, 363-365, 541-544, 713, 715-716, 883-887, 1977.

2. Berger AJ, Mitchell RA, Severinghaus JW: Regulation of respiration. *N Engl J Med*. 297:92-97, 138-143, 194-201, 1977.
3. Control of breathing: Assessment in intact man. *Proc R Soc Med* 68:237-245, 1975.
4. Laurenco RV (ed): Clinical methods for the study of regulation of ventilation. *Chest* 70 (suppl): 109-195, 1976.
5. Pavlin EG, Hornbein TF: The control of breathing; Basic of RD. *Am Thoracic Soc*. November 1978.
6. Saunders NA, Powles ACP, Rebuck AS: Ear oximetry: Accuracy and practicability in the assessment of arterial oxygenation. *Am Rev Respir Dis* 113:745-749, 1976.
7. Mithoefer JC: Breathholding, in Fenn WO, Rahn H (eds): *Handbook of Physiology*. Washington DC, Am Physiol Soc, 1965, chap 38; pp 1011-1025.
8. Davidson JT, Whipp BJ, Wasserman K, et al.: Role of the carotid bodies in breathholding. *N Engl J Med* 290:819-822, 1974.
9. Read DJC: A clinical method for assessing the ventilatory response to carbon dixoide. Australas Ann Med. 16:20-32, 1967.
10. Irsigler GB: Carbon dioxide lines in young adults: The limits of the normal response. *Am Rev Respir Dis* 114:529-536, 1976.
11. Kronenberg R, Hamilton FN, Gabel R, et al.: Comparison of three methods for quantitating respiratory response to hypoxia in man. *Respir Physiol* 16:109-125, 1972.
12. Patrick JM, Cotes JE: Letter: Hypoxic and hypercapnic ventilatory drives in man. *J Appl Physiol* 40:1012, 1976.
13. Rebuck AS, Campbell EJM: A clinical method for assessing the ventilatory response to hypoxia. *Am Rev Respir Dis* 109:345-350, 1974.
14. Rebuck AS, Woodley WE: Ventilatory effects of hypoxia and their dependence on PCO_2. *J Appl Physiol* 38:16-19, 1975.
15. Whitelaw WA, Derenne J, Milic-Emili J: Occlusion pressure as a measure of respiratory center output in conscious man. *Respir Physiol* 23:181-199, 1975.
16. Matthews AW, Howell JBL: The rate of isometric inspiratory pressure development as a measure of responsiveness to carbon dioxide in man. *Clin Sci Mol Med* 49:57-68, 1975.
17. Kryger MH, Yacoub O, Dosman J, et al.: Effect of meperidine on occlusion pressure responses to hypercapnia and hypoxia with and without external inspiratory resistance. *Am Rev Respir Dis* 114:333-340, 1976.
18. Cherniack NS, Lederer DH, Altose MD, et al.: Occlusion pressure as a technique in evaluating respiratory control. *Chest* 70 (suppl): 137-141, 1976.
19. Gelb AF, Klein E, Schiffman P, et al.: Ventilatory response and drive in acute and chronic obstructive pulmonary disease. *Am Rev Respir Dis* 116:9-16, 1977.
20. Shekleton M, Lopata M, Evanich J, et al.: Effect of elastic loading on mouth occlusion pressure during CO_2 rebreathing in man. *Am Rev Respir Dis* 114:341-346, 1976.
21. Cherniack N, Dempsey J, Fencl V, et al.: Conference Report. Workshop on assessment of respiratory control in humans: I. Methods of measurement of ventilatory responses to hypoxia and hypercapnia. *Am Rev Respir Dis* 115:177-181, 1977.
22. Severinghaus J, Ozanne G, Massuda Y: Measurement of the ventilatory response to hypoxia. *Chest* 70 (suppl): 121-124, 1976.
23. Severinghaus JW: Proposed standard determination of ventilatory responses to hypoxia and hypercapnia in man. *Chest* 70 (suppl): 129-131, 1976.
24. Weil JV, Byrne-Quinn E, Sodal IE, et al.: Hypoxic ventilatory drive in normal man. *J Clin Invest* 49:1061-1072, 1970.

CHAPTER 24

Bedside Testing and Intensive Care Monitoring of Pulmonary Function

ROBERT J. FALLAT, M.D.
JOHN C. MCQUITTY, M.D.

Monitoring in intensive care medicine has increased considerably during the past decade but respiratory monitoring has lagged behind cardiovascular monitoring. There is a need for pulmonary monitoring in acute care situations since many episodes of sudden death or cardiac arrest may have a respiratory origin. Shock, coma of various etiologies, pneumonia, congestive heart failure, obstructive airways disease, and postoperative states make up the bulk of admissions to intensive care units; all of these conditions may be associated with respiratory failure. Therefore, pulmonary monitoring in the intensive care unit may be critical in preventing respiratory failure and is of demonstrated usefulness for the management of patients already requiring ventilatory support.

Bedside pulmonary testing includes assessment of pulmonary mechanics (measurements of pressure, flow–volume relationships), and gas exchange (inspired and expired oxygen and carbon dioxide and noninvasive monitoring of blood gases). Each of these two catagories of testing are discussed separately in the following sections. Chapter 25 reviews the important area of hemodynamic monitoring.

PULMONARY MECHANICS

The major aim of pulmonary function testing in the critical care unit is to determine the adequacy of ventilation by monitoring respiratory rate and tidal volume (V_T) and assessing the patient's respiratory status. Monitoring of respiratory rate and tidal volume is routinely done in patients receiving mechanical ventilation, but is still in a developmental state for spontaneously breathing patients.

PULMONARY FUNCTION TESTING
GUIDELINES AND CONTROVERSIES

ISBN 0-12-788125-5

EQUIPMENT

Volume Pressure and Flow Measurements

Devices for measuring volume may be divided into three major categories: volume displacement spirometers, pneumotachographs, and chest wall or body devices.

The most commonly used instruments for volume monitoring are volume displacement devices. A dry expanding bellows, such as the Bennett spirometer, can be used to monitor the expired volume from any ventilator. Volume can also be measured with devices such as Wright and Drager respirometers, which operate by the rotation of a vane. Since none of these devices lend themselves easily to electronic output and automation, they are used primarily for manual monitoring and alarm purposes.

A second method of volume measurement involves the integration of flow measurements from pneumotachographic type devices (see Chapter 9). Pneumotachographs are usually small and relatively lightweight, and because they offer little resistance to air flow they may be inserted into ventilator circuits to provide an electrical output for continuous automated monitoring. Pneumotachographs are of three different types. The type most widely used are those that measure flow on the basis of a pressure drop. Of these, the most commonly used is the Fleisch pneumotachograph; it consists of corrugated metal columns that provide a fixed resistance with laminar flow. Screens are also used for producing resistance as is the case with the Siemens ventilator. More recently, a plastic flap has been used as a resistance device in order to obviate the change in calibration that occurs as secretions accumulate (1). For optimal performance, it is essential that the linear range of the pneumotachograph selected be appropriate for the low flow rates that may be encountered in the intensive care setting, especially when monitoring infants and children.

The hot wire anemometer is another type of pneumotachograph that measures gas flow by the change in the electrical current needed to maintain the temperature of the wire. These are usually limited to unidirectional measurements and are seriously affected by temperature and humidity changes, and particularly by secretions that accumulate during prolonged monitoring. Therefore, these hot wire anemometers have generally been used downstream from the patient to monitor only inspiratory or expiratory volume.

The third type of flow-measuring pneumotachograph is the ultrasonic pneumotachograph. It has the potential to measure flow without the necessity of mechanical structures in the airstream, but problems with accuracy have limited the widespread use of this type of device to date. However, it does hold considerable promise for the future.

A third general method of volume measurement uses the change in the electrical impedence of the chest between electrodes, or the change in inductance between coils placed over the chest and abdomen. These methods may prove to be of value in continuous monitoring of tidal volume and respiratory rate in spontaneously breathing patients since they require no connection to the mouth or airway. They can give accurate measurements of V_T in controlled laboratory settings but their clinical use has been limited to monitoring respiratory rate.

Intra-airway pressures may be measured manually from the aneroid gauges that are present on every ventilator; these are sufficiently accurate for a direct simple assessment of ventilator function and patient mechanics.

In automated systems, airway pressure (P_{aw}) is measured with strain gauge transducers. There are a variety of reliable, stable gauges available that provide a linear electrical output spanning the range of 0–200 cm H_2O with an accuracy of $\pm 0.5\%$ full scale. If an esophageal balloon is used to measure intrathoracic pressures, a differential pressure transducer will be needed; negative intrapleural pressure must be measured *relative to* mouth pressure.

Quality Control

Unlike diagnostic spirometry, where the needs for accuracy are more readily definable, the accuracy of instrumentation and frequency of quality control that are required for bedside monitoring of volumes and flows will vary according to the specific clinical applications. Measurements of volume by bellows displacement and pressure by anaeroid gauges on ventilators are generally quite reliable for routine clinical purposes but should be checked for accuracy during routine servicing of the ventilator system at weekly or monthly intervals. Volume should be calibrated using a standard 1-liter syringe; for pressure, a mercury manometer is convenient.

Volume Calibration

Rotating vane respirometers, wet- and dry-gas meters, and pneumotachographs need to be calibrated more frequently and at differing flow rates because of their susceptability to errors at low and high flows. Pneumotachographs must be calibrated at frequent intervals (at least once daily or more often) according to the conditions of use because of their susceptability to errors. Calibration is usually most easily accomplished using a large 1–3-liter hand-driven calibrating syringe, but one should remember that temperature and humidity factors will be different when measurements are made on patients. (See Chapters 4 and 9.)

In the acute care setting, errors due to temperature and humidity variations may be considerable because of the use of heated humidifiers and because patients may be febrile or hypothermic. Pneumotachographs are also dependent on gas viscosity and, therefore, on gas concentration. For example, there is about a

16% change in calibration when 100% O_2 is substituted for air. Because of this sensitivity of pneumotachographs to temperature, humidity, and gas composition, calibration should be done reproducing clinical conditions whenever the need for accuracy justifies the extra work involved.

Flow Calibration

Flow may be calibrated with a rotameter. Calibrated rotameters are available in different flow ranges to give the desired resolution. Their accuracy should always be checked initially; this is most easily accomplished from volume measurements at stable flow rates using a Tissot spirometer. In most monitoring systems (and in all pneumotachograph systems), the primary signal is related to flow, which is then integrated to obtain volume. Volume measurements should be accurate to within $\pm 3\%$ or ± 50 ml when tested at the extremes of flow rates expected; e.g., 0.1 l/sec and 2.0 l/sec. This can most easily be assessed by emptying a 1-liter syringe through the system slowly (10 sec) and very quickly (0.5 sec). Flow rates should be measured with an accuracy of ± 0.1 liter/sec and should be linear over a range of 0 liter/sec to at least 2.5 liter/sec for accurate monitoring of ventilator patients. Note that patients with severe lung disease, such as those with adult respiratory distress syndrome, may have expired flow rates more than 5 liter/sec when on a ventilator.

Pressure Calibration

Calibration of pressure gauges can readily be done using a mercury manometer and a Y-connector attached to the ventilator tubing. Accuracy and precision of airway or intrathoracic pressure measurements should be ± 2 cm H_2O.

CALCULATIONS

Figure 1 shows characteristic flow, volume, and pressure curves of a patient on a ventilator. Maximum inspiratory airway pressure (P_{aw} max), static or plateau pressures (P_{st}), and positive end expiratory pressures (PEEP) may all readily be measured manually using the pressure gauges on the ventilator. These pressures in combination with tidal volume (V_T) may be used to calculate compliance of the lung and chest wall. Two parameters are most commonly measured—static compliance (C_{st}) and dynamic characteristic (C_{dyn}):

$$C_{st} = V_T/(P_{st} - \text{PEEP}) \qquad \text{(Eq. 1)}$$

$$C_{dyn} = V_T/(P_{aw}\ \text{max} - \text{PEEP}) \qquad \text{(Eq. 2)}$$

It should be understood that these compliance measurements may differ significantly from measurements of *lung* compliance measured using the esophageal

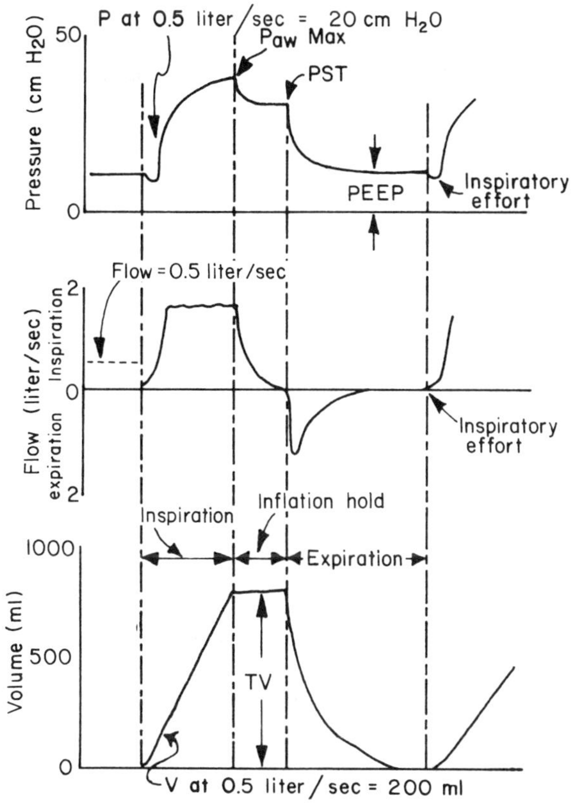

Fig. 1 *Airway pressure is measured in the airway close to the patient's endotracheal tube. A small inspiratory effort is seen which initiates inspiratory flow. The flow is of the square wave type, very quickly reaching a plateau. There is a period of inflationary hold and flow falls to zero, but the lungs are maintained inflated: during this time a static airway pressure (P_{st}) is obtained prior to exhalation. Pressure returns to some predetermined positive end-expiratory pressure (PEEP) level. Flows are not readily obtained except from flow measuring devices such as the pneumotachograph. Pressure readings may be readily obtained from the pressure gauge on the ventilator. Tidal volume (V_T) can also be measured from a spirometer placed in the exhalation line.*

balloon (or some other estimate of pleural pressure) because of the inclusion of the compliance of the chest wall. Any active contracture of respiratory musculature (chest wall and diaphragm) may affect these measurements. Meaningful and reproducible measurement of lung mechanics on ventilator patients without utilizing an esophageal ballon requires the patient to be passive (neither pulling against nor "fighting" the ventilator) during the measurement. A short period of negative pressure which initiates inspiration, as shown in Fig. 1, can be present without seriously affecting the results.

Dynamic compliance as measured in the intensive care unit (ICU) setting is not identical to the compliance as defined by Mead, since in the former setting, the $P_{aw}max$ measured under conditions of flow includes resistance elements; these elements are subtracted electronically with the classic (Mead) technique. The difference between $P_{aw}max$ and P_{st} may be viewed as a measure of airway resistance (R_{aw}):

$$R_{aw} = (P_{aw}max - P_{st})/\text{Flow} \qquad \text{(Eq. 3)}$$

where flow is end-inspiratory flow at the time of the $P_{aw}max$ measurement. In Fig. 1

$$P_{aw}max = 37.5$$

$$P_{st} = 30$$

and

$$\text{Flow} = 1.5$$

$$R_{aw} = (37.5 - 30)/1.5 = 5 \text{ cm } H_2O/\text{liter/sec}$$

Alternatively, R_{aw} can be calculated at any other point during inspiration using the flow at that point and the pressure corrected for the component due to the static compliance factor. A flow of 0.5 liter/sec is commonly used for R_{aw} measurement, e.g., from Fig. 1, at a flow of 0.5 liter/sec, and volume of 200 ml where:

$$P_{st} = 30 \text{ cm } H_2O$$

$$\text{PEEP} = 10 \text{ cm } H_2O$$

and

$$V_T = 800 \text{ ml}$$

$$C_{st} = 800/(30 - 10) = 40 \text{ ml/cm } H_2O$$

Assuming a constant C_{st}, the pressure due to compliance (P_c) at $V = 200$ is

$$P_c = V/C_{st} = 200/40 = 5 \text{ cm } H_2O$$

R_{aw} at 0.5 liter/sec then is

$$R_{aw} = (P \text{ at } 0.5 - \text{PEEP} - P_c)/\text{Flow}$$
$$= (20 - 10 - 5)/0.5 = 5/0.5 = 10 \text{ cm } H_2O/\text{liter/sec}$$

Note that the R_{aw} at 0.5 liter/sec is twice that calculated at end inspiration from Eq. 3. Such large and variable R_{aw} measurements can be expected in ventilator patients because of the large flow-dependent resistances found in the endotracheal tube and the expansion of airways that occurs during inflation.

PROCEDURES

Measurement of compliance (C) is most commonly done manually from point readings of pressure from a gauge or from analog recorder signals and V_T measurements. At least three breaths should be measured when the patient is quiet and being ventilated passively. Changes in ventilator settings should not be made for at least 1 minute and preferably not for 15 minutes prior to measurement. Changes in inspired gas concentration, particularly increases in O_2, may result in progressive changes in lung mechanics, but most pressure and volume characteristics stabilize within 5 minutes after a step change. Comparison of compliance measurements made at differing levels of PEEP or V_T is now commonly made to optimize the ventilator settings as suggested by Suter et al. (2). Such studies can be done 1-2 minutes after the PEEP or V_T change but should be repeated to ensure stability and reproducibility.

Volume history is well recognized as having a significant effect on compliance measurements. Hyperinflation to P_{aw}max of 40 cm H_2O for three breaths should be done 1-5 minutes before making a series of compliance measurements. Such hyperinflation may be omitted when one is attempting to determine the change in compliance that may be occurring as a result of some step change in the ventilator setting, for instance, a change in PEEP when determining the optimum PEEP level.

Dynamic compliance and R_{aw} will obviously be dependent on the flow rates. However, static compliance will also be effected by flow rates since some high resistance lung elements will not be inflated with higher flow rates. Therefore, the ventilator flow settings should be noted and not indiscriminantly changed when a series of compliance measurements are being done to determine optimum ventilator settings.

Automated methods of compliance measurements have been described (3). Manual procedures should still be done, perhaps once every 8 hours, even when automated methods are used, to check for reliability. The automated measurements should agree with simultaneous manual measurements to within 10%.

The measurement of static or plateau pressure is most prone to difficulties. If the ventilator has an inflationary hold this may be used for 0.5-2.0 seconds. A stable pressure (P), as shown in Fig. 1, should be obtained; occlusion of the expiration line for longer periods may be necessary to obtain a stable plateau. More often, there is a continuous decline in P_{st} due to leaks, and accurate or reproduceable results are not possible until the leaks are corrected. An alternate method of obtaining P_{st} is to use a very slow inspiratory flow; P_{aw}max may then approximate P_{st}. But this method is frequently associated with active inspiratory effort by the patient, which would cause imprecise results.

Normal Values

Normal values for pulmonary mechanics obtained from conscious subjects on ventilators are not available. Rahn et al. (4) measured relaxation pressure volume data in ten spontaneously breathing, conscious, relaxed, supine subjects and found a mean value of 130 ml/cm H_2O at 20 cm H_2O pressure. Nims et al. (5) found a lower mean value, 111 ml/cm H_2O, in twelve conscious relaxed subjects. They further found that when six anesthetized subjects were studied after paralysis with succinyl choline or after hyperventilation (i.e., when more complete relaxation of the chest wall muscles was attained) the compliance fell to 62 ml/cm H_2O. They hypothesized that the decrease resulted from the decreased compliance of the chest wall due to loss of tone of the inspiratory intercostal muscles. Since the chest wall muscles of a patient being ventilated continuously in the clinical setting are probably more relaxed than those of the spontaneously breathing subject, the predicted values reported by Nims et al. are probably most applicable to intensive care patients. The compliance will be dependent upon the size of the lungs and chest. The six subjects studied by Nims were females averaging 36 years of age and 157 cm in height with a mean predicted functional residual capacity (FRC) of 2.6 liters. The compliance can be normalized by dividing it by FRC; it is then called the specific compliance. Using an average compliance of about 90 ml/cm H_2O:

Specific $C_{st} = 90/2.6 = 35$ ml/cm H_2O/liter.

Expansion volume in ventilator tubing should be subtracted when comparing clinical measurements. More details about this are described in the troubleshooting section.

In the ICU setting, most adult patients will have a C_{st} in the range of 50–100 ml/cm H_2O. When C_{st} is less than 25 ml/cm H_2O, one can expect difficulty in weaning. When C_{st} is over 100 ml/cm H_2O, one should suspect either emphysema or erroneous measurements (most likely due to leaks in the system). The range of normal values for dynamic characteristic is wide, since the measurements vary with the flow rate and the size of the endotracheal tube used. Since P_{aw}max is generally about 10–20% higher than P_{st}, C_{dyn} would be proportionately lower than C_{st}.

Expected Reproducibility

Since volume and pressure measurements under optimal calibration conditions are each expected to be accurate to ±3%, the largest compliance error due to instrumentation should be ±6%. But because of the inherent physiologic and biologic variability of the compliance measurements, no better than 10% reproducibility should be expected and a 20–30% difference between breaths is possible. Under optimal conditions, in a paralyzed or a well-sedated patient with low airway pressures and no leaks, ±5% may be achieved.

TROUBLESHOOTING

Volume Measurements

With the volume displacement devices such as the Wright and the Drager respirometers, one must be careful about the extremes of flow measurements. At the very low flows (below 0.2 liter/sec), the vanes in these devices may not rotate and will, therefore, underestimate volume. On the other hand, very high flow rates may cause overshoot due to momentum and result in erroneously high volume determinations. Detection of leaks is always important in doing spirometric determinations but is critical in a bedside or acute care setting when endotracheal tubes, and perhaps open tracheostomies, are used.

The point at which volume measurements are made will effect the result. When measured directly at the tracheal tube, both inspiration and expiration can be assessed. If the expansion volume of the inspiratory tubing is measured downstream as part of the expired volume, leaks in the system will be missed.

Compliance

Validity of compliance measurements depends on several factors. Leaks in the system will make the volume and pressure measurements (particularly the static pressures) quite erroneous. Any voluntary muscular action on the part of the patient (either actively inspiring or "fighting" the respirator) will produce very erratic and meaningless pressure and compliance measurements, unless an esophageal balloon, which allows the pressure effects of the chest wall to be separated from the elastic recoil of the lung, is used. Multiple determinations of the compliance of the lung and the chest wall (made over several breaths) are needed for accuracy and reliability.

Another complicating factor in compliance measurements is the expansion volume in the ventilator tubing, which is added to the expired volume even though it has never entered the patient's lung and is, therefore, additional dead space ventilation. A rough rule of thumb which may be used to estimate the expansion volume is 3 ml/cm H_2O airway pressure, but this will vary, depending upon the tubing and ventilator used. In patients with very stiff lungs, such as occurs in acute respiratory distress syndrome (ARDS) where airway pressures are high and V_T low, there can be considerable error in compliance calculated from downstream exhaled volume due to inclusion of the tubing expansion volume in the measurement. When research accuracy is desired, this volume should be measured by simply occluding the out-flow from the ventilator and simulating the pressures used on the patient. The air released during the expiratory cycle, then, is the expansion volume.

GAS EXCHANGE

Arterial blood gas measurements are the most common way of monitoring acutely ill patients (see Chapter 21). However, when a patient is on a ventilator, the measurement of airway oxygen and CO_2 concentrations offers a noninvasive means of monitoring gas exchange. Although the need for monitoring airway gas concentrations is somewhat controversial, the use of such measurements may obviate the need for some blood gases and thereby justify the medical costs involved.

Monitoring the inspired oxygen concentrations is desirable, if not necessary, in the patient who is hypoxemic. Oxygen monitoring capabilities are built into most ventilators but generally depend upon a volume displacement from the oxygen source rather than a direct oxygen detector. Inexpensive oxygen monitors can be placed in line with the ventilator and used as alarms to detect clinically significant changes in oxygen concentration.

Monitoring of carbon dioxide seems particularly desirable in patients on ventilators because ventilatory requirements can vary considerably with subtle changes in a patient's condition. Most hospitals depend on arterial blood-gas monitoring to detect such alterations but, clearly, such invasive and intermittent monitoring is less than optimal. The technology now exists to monitor CO_2 accurately and continuously at the bedside, but clinical studies are still needed to verify the usefulness of CO_2 monitoring in routine, nonresearch settings.

The measurement of airway O_2 and CO_2 allows calculation of the alveolar-arterial gradient $P(A-a)O_2$. For oxygen, this gradient should be less than 30 torr when breathing room air, and less than 50 torr when breathing higher inspired oxygen concentrations. The effects of age and inspired O_2 on the $P(A-a)O_2$ gradient are described by Harris et al. (6). Arterial O_2 should always be related to the inspired-oxygen concentration to make a valid assessment of lung function. It should be emphasized that end tidal O_2 and CO_2 may not *accurately* measure the alveolar concentrations in the sick ICU patient, but often serve as *useful* clinical approximations.

Alveolar-arterial carbon dioxide gradients have not been as readily accepted or utilized in the clinical setting. It is well established that the gradient between end tidal $CO_2(P_{ET}CO_2)$ and arterial $CO_2(PaCO_2)$ is small (i.e., less than 2-3 torr) in normal subjects, but may increase considerably in diseased patients. What has not been established is the stability of the $P_{ET}CO_2$-$PaCO_2$ gradient and, therefore, the usefulness of the $P_{ET}CO_2$ measurement for monitoring arterial CO_2 tension noninvasively. A change in the $P_{ET}CO_2$-$PaCO_2$ gradient may not accurately represent the arterial PCO_2 change, but will still have physiologic and diagnostic usefulness. A rise in the $P_{ET}CO_2$-$PaCO_2$ gradient indicates an increase in wasted ventilation, which may be an indication of emboli or other ventilation-perfusion abnormalities. Prospective clinical studies are needed to verify the applicability of such measurements in routine clinical use. For more detailed information on the multiple potential uses of CO_2 monitoring and on problems associated with such uses, the reader is referred to Fallat and Osborn (7).

Equipment

O_2 Measurement

Oxygen monitors have been available in the form of a number of inexpensive devices that employ standard polarographic detectors such as those used in blood-gas machines. Recently, mass spectrometers have been advocated for continuous monitoring of multiple gases from several patients. Less commonly, low or high temperature fuel cells or paramagnetic detectors are used. Of all these devices, only the high temperature fuel cell and the mass spectrometer are sufficiently rapid to allow instantaneous monitoring of oxygen; the other devices have time constants of several seconds and therefore must depend either on batch processing or on giving mean values of airway gases over a period of several seconds. By incorporating a series of electronic circuits that follow the sensor's time response and then predict a result in a 100–200 msec response time, a polarographic sensor has been developed with an effective response time of 200 msec, which can thus be used for instantaneous O_2 monitoring. However, the instantaneous measurement of airway O_2 is not necessary for most monitoring purposes; instead, the less expensive, slow-reacting O_2 monitors are generally used. These are set to sound an alarm if the airway O_2 falls outside of a 5–10% desired range. Since inspired and expired O_2 concentrations differ by 1–3%, and inspired O_2 may vary over a wide range depending upon the mode of ventilation, accuracy of better than 5% in slow reacting systems is unnecessary.

CO_2 Measurements

Carbon dioxide monitoring has been available for many years using infrared detectors. These give instantaneous readings with a 90% response time of less than 100 msec. The application of these devices for long-term monitoring in intensive care units has not received widespread use because of the difficulty in maintaining calibration. When care is taken to avoid accumulation of moisture by use of heaters or flushing with dry gas, accurate measurements are possible. This difficulty has been avoided by developing a miniaturized infrared system that looks at the airway gas through a window.

In recent years there has been increasing interest in the use of mass spectrometers for monitoring gases. A mass spectrometer, which costs in excess of $25,000, has the capability of measuring multiple expired gases using minimal sampling volumes. Reliability has been increased and the technology now exists to monitor several patients with a single instrument, thereby potentially justifying the expense. The response time is fast enough to obtain continous on-line analysis of O_2, CO_2, N_2, CO, and many anesthetic gases. As many as five or six gases may be measured simultaneously. Small-bore, high-vacuum lines may be used over distances in excess of 30 m without significant loss of the waveform, allowing multiple beds to be monitored at a distance. The number of units monitored is limited primarily by the duration and frequency of the monitoring needed for each unit.

Quality Control

Calibration

If measurements of airway gas concentrations are to be useful, calibrations must be done at least daily and preferably at more frequent intervals, particularly prior to a series of measurements. Calibrations can readily be carried out using room air and one test gas of 40–50% O_2 and 3–5% CO_2. Accuracy and precision of both oxygen and CO_2 concentrations will depend upon the instrument used and its purpose. Automated calibrations are possible.

Some of the devices are alinear over a wide range of gas concentrations. Calibrations should be done in the range of use. If a wide range is necessary, as is frequently the case in O_2 measurement, the alinearity must be measured or corrected (8). Mixing chambers are available for providing a wide range of known gas concentrations. Alternatively, several tanks with gas mixtures determined by Scholander or chromatographic techniques may be used.

With continuous gas sampling, most of the gas measurements are done at a site several feet away from the sampling port; care must be taken to ensure that the waveform has not been distorted by mixing in the tube. With standard ⅛-inch tubing, fast flow rates of 0.5 liter/min are necessary to obtain accurate waveforms at distances of 2–3 m. With mass spectrometers, much lower flows are possible when very small diameter tubing is used under vacuum conditions; this allows lines up to 30 m with minimal loss of waveform (9).

Procedure

The procedures used for measuring gas concentrations will depend upon the choice of instrumentation. If the response time is slow, then a batch or mixed sample must be obtained. Instruments with a fast response may use continuous sampling techniques. Batch or mixed samples of the expired gas can be collected in large bags (Douglas or weather balloons) and both minute volume and gas concentrations can be accurately obtained. Alternatively, a baffle or mixing box can be placed in the low-pressure exhalation line (10). When any step change in ventilator or gas concentrations is made, sufficient time must be allowed for washout of the ventilator circuit and baffle box, but this will be rapid relative to the time constant of the change occurring in the patient.

When fast responding instruments are available (Infrared CO_2, mass spectrometer, or high-temperature fuel cell) sampling can be done at the patients' airway and both inspiratory and expiratory gas analysis is possible. A major problem with rapid gas analysis, however, is the difficulty of matching the gas concentration with the gas flow, which is usually measured with a pneumotachograph. The difficulties involved are too extensive to cover here but the reader is referred to Osborn (3) and Osborn et al. (11).

The sampling times and procedures required will vary depending upon specific clinical needs. O_2 changes should be capable of being detected within 1–2 minutes. Changes in alveolar–arterial gradients and end-tidal PCO_2 are adequately monitored every 5 or 10 minutes. This allows a single instrument such as the mass spectrometer, to monitor several beds with 30–60 seconds of sampling for each bed.

Calculations

Many variables may be calculated from continuous or batch measurements of airway O_2 and CO_2. These measurements may be combined with flow and volume measurements to obtain values for O_2 consumption, CO_2 production, respiratory quotient, and ventilatory equivalent. When combined with arterial blood gas data, alveolar–arterial gradients and wasted ventilation may be calculated. When batch methods are used, these calculations will be similar to those presented in the chapter on exercise (Chapter 22). In automated systems, these derived variables may be obtained on a breath-by-breath basis as described by Beaver et al. (12). In the acute care setting, similar measurements have been described by Osborn (3, 11). When high concentrations of O_2 are used, variables calculated using values for O_2 consumption are of dubious accuracy.

Troubleshooting

The major problem in continuous monitoring of airway gas tension is the stability of the measurement devices. The mass spectrometers are reliable but when problems occur, engineering expertise may be needed to detect and correct them. The infrared CO_2 monitoring device exhibits gross errors when moisture enters the system. For this reason, systems have had to be developed to prevent the build-up of moisture in the infrared analyzers. This is best done by frequent flushing with a dry gas. The accurate estimate of arterial CO_2 from end tidal CO_2 measurements depends on sufficient tidal volume to clear the dead space up to the gas measurement device. If tidal volumes are too low and the dead space is not cleared, the airway CO_2 seen will be low in relation to the arterial CO_2, which may be rising. Such a situation may commonly occur, e.g., during a weaning process or whenever the respiratory rates are high and tidal volumes are low.

Noninvasive Monitoring of Blood Gases

Ear Oximetry There are many situations when continuous monitoring of pO_2 and pCO_2 would be valuable but, because of the risks, discomforts and delays in intra-arterial blood sampling, it is not done. (e.g., during bronchoscopy, during treadmill exercise studies, or during manipulation of ventilators). Ear oximetry, a rapid, noninvasive method to measure oxygen saturation, has been available for some time. The principles of optical transmission devices were described in the early 1930s and an ear oximeter was described by Millikan in 1942 (13). Instruments developed in this era had the significant limitations of extensive calibration requirements and bulky size, and they yielded relative and not absolute values of oxygen saturation. In the past few years, these problems have been overcome with new ear oximeters that use microcomputer circuitry; these units provide the capabilities of continuous assessment of oxygen saturation with sufficient accuracy for many clinical applications.

The principal advance that allows the current instrument manufactured by Hewlett-Packard, Inc. to provide accurate measurement is the use of multiple wavelengths, each specific for one optical absorption factor. A filter wheel rotating at 1300 rpm is used to transmit light of eight different wavelengths between 650 and 1050 nm. Thus, 20 measurements per second are obtained at each wavelength to compare to a second reference beam. The microcomputer is asked to solve eight simultaneous absorbance equations. The constants for these equations have been determined empirically from a "select group of volunteers" as described by a Hewlett-Packard (Waltham, Massachusetts) brochure on the model 47201a. This oximeter is relatively bulky and heats the ear lobe to 41° C to maintain arterialization of blood, but can be worn without serious discomfort for several hours. The accuracy of this unit is quite good above 60% saturation ranging from ±2.6% at 60–70% saturation to ±1.7% at 90–100% saturation. When oximetry saturation values were compared with simultaneous arterial samples in one study, they correlated with an r of 0.99 (14). Another study reported an r of 0.98 with 95% confidence limits for accuracy of ±4% (15). Drift is stated to be less than 0.255%/hour. The response time is exponential with a normal time constant of 3 seconds (15).

Several factors may lead to inaccuracies. Bilirubin elevation and use of cardiogreen dye interfere with readings and introduce errors. Ear perfusion must exceed metabolic demand in order for arterialization of the blood to occur. If the cardiac output is markedly diminished, saturation will decline due to poor perfusion rather than inadequate arterial oxygenation. Elevated levels of carboxyhemoglobin may result in spuriously elevated readings of oxyhemoglobin (15). Despite these limitations, ear oximetry is demonstrating increasing usefulness particularly in noninvasive testing and monitoring.

Cutaneous Electrodes Another approach to noninvasive estimates of arterial O_2 (and CO_2) levels is through the use of cutaneous electrodes. By heating the skin under an enclosed surface, it is possible to estimate the partial pressures of O_2 and CO_2 using standard polarographic electrodes. Such measurements were first made in 1951 by Baumberger and Goodfriend (16). Huch and Huch (17) later refined the polarographic methods to make clinical applications possible. Others have explored using mass spectrometry to measure the transcutaneous gases, but only units using the polarographic methods have been made commercially available. Such units contain a heating element and a polarographic cell similar to the Clark electrode of blood-gas analyzers. A platinum cathode and silver anode are used in combination with a liquid electrolyte, and these are covered with a membrane. When the sensor is applied to the skin, the current flow is close to zero; the current flow increases when the heating element within the electrode heats the skin and vasodilates the capillary bed below the skin surface. It has been found that the ideal skin temperature is 43–45°C, at which point the PaO_2 and transcutaneous PO_2 ($TCPO_2$) correlate well and the skin is not seriously burned.

Several factors affect the accuracy and sensitivity of cutaneous electrodes (18). As with ear oximetry, the phenomenon of depletion is important in this case; the perfusion of the skin below the chamber must greatly exceed the cellular metabolism in order to provide enough O_2 for consumption by the electrode. In order to achieve good perfusion, skin and sensor temperatures must be raised and then carefully controlled, since temperature is an obvious critical factor in determining partial pressures of gases. Errors will be introduced if blood flow is insufficient to the region due to central or peripheral vascular conditions. Also, the development of gas gradients because of impaired diffusion of gases through the thickened dermis becomes a factor that limits accuracy, except in infants.

Currently, the most accepted use of transcutaneous electrodes is for monitoring infants, particularly neonates (see Chapter 26). In such patients the correlation of $TCPO_2$ with PaO_2 has been good ($r = 0.96$) with the exception of patients with compromised hemodynamic function and hypotension (18). In adults, $TCPO_2$-PaO_2 correlation coefficients of 0.918 and 0.947 have been reported for two different electrode systems (19). Another study of adults noted that $TCPO_2$s were generally lower than PaO_2s with a mean gradient of about 10 torr (range +20 to −40) (17). Although these electrode systems may be useful for a variety of research applications, the problems with accuracy currently limit their use in individual adult patients. They do hold considerable potential for monitoring purposes, although definitive data establishing their usefulness for such applications is not currently available.

Cutaneous monitoring may also be done using either a modified Severinghaus PCO_2 electrode, a mass spectrometer, or an infrared optical absorption sensor. Each of these remains in the developmental phase but commercial units of the electrode and infrared types can be expected in the near future. For the adult patient, these electrodes may be more reliable than the O_2 sensors, since the required flux of CO_2 through the skin is not as great as that needed for O_2.

Maintenance and Quality Control Electrode maintenance should include the following: Clean the electrode and change the membrane according to manufacturer's recommended procedures. Check for wrinkles, air bubbles, and debris under the membrane. The optimal frequency of performing the above procedures should be determined according to the amount of usage of the machine. Have a second electrode available as a back-up.

The electrode can be applied to the skin without special preparation; multiple skin sites (thorax, abdomen, thigh, flank, and back) are useful. A tight seal to the skin is accomplished by a double-sided adhesive ring. To avoid burning the skin, the sensor should have its position changed every 4 hours and the sensor temperature should be checked frequently when in operation. It is important to use the proper amount of contact solution between the electrode and the skin. If too little solution is used, there may be air trapped under the electrode and there may not be sufficient heat transfer from the electrode to the skin to ensure adequate perfusion. Also, the electrode should be stabilized so that minimal pressure and torque are applied; if these conditions occur, erroneous values may be observed. Pressure on the electrode will generally cause erroneously low $TCPO_2$ values and low relative heat power consumption. The site chosen for placement can have a large influence on the accuracy of the resultant $TCPO_2$. It has been our experience that the abdomen or subclavicular regions are the best sites for optimal results. The area should be relatively flat and well perfused. Sites to avoid are bony areas, sites directly over large veins, and extremities.

Calibrating transcutaneous PO_2 monitors usually requires a check of the electrical zero (most instruments can be checked for electrical zero by disconnecting the electrode from the instrument), and adjustment of the true zero setting. Setting the true zero for PO_2 can be done with a solution that has been chemically depleted of O_2 ("zero solution"). Some instrument electrodes can be damaged by use of a zero solution; specific manufacturer's recommendations should always be carefully followed. True zero conditions can also be established with a gas such as 100% nitrogen, which should be humidified. Note that the response time to true zero can be a good indicator of in vitro electrode response. If this method is used, be sure to standardize conditions under which it is performed. The step change signal size and strip chart recorder speed should be standardized when using 100% N_2 for in vitro electrode response time. The calibration of the span or high O_2 can be done with either a tonometered solution, or room air (ambient or saturated with water vapor). Either method is acceptable as long as the relevant variables are taken into account. Some of these variables include electrode temperature, barometric pressure, type of tonometered solution, and the water vapor content of the gas.

The midrange check is used to estimate the amplitude of the signal coming from the electrode itself, which should be reproducible. It is accomplished by turning the calibration knob to its minimum setting and noting the digital readout while the electrode is in a standard condition (such as room air and calibration chamber). The number that is obtained can then be compared to previously obtained results. If the midrange readout is considerably above values obtained previously (when the electrode was known to be functioning properly), it can be assumed that the electrode is in need of cleaning. Since all transcutaneous PO_2 monitors available to date use a Clark electrode, the reason for an increase in the midrange value is usually silver or silver chloride depositing on the cathode or anode, respectively. These deposits can be removed using the manufacturer's recommended procedure for cleaning and buffing the electrode.

For each patient, initial in vivo correlation of transcutaneous electrode measurements with arterial samples should be obtained whenever possible. In newborn infants, correlation samples are often obtained through umbilical arterial catheters, because the levels of PAO_2 and PaO_2 are extremely responsive to the infant being handled, and it is often difficult to correlate TCO_2 with PAO_2 drawn from an arterial puncture. (Infiltrating xylocaine prior to arterial puncture helps to alleviate this problem.) It should be noted that if the patient has a possibility of intracardiac shunting (such as is found in patent ductus), correlation between arterial PO_2 and $TCPO_2$ may be poor. This disparity is readily explained in those cases where the transcutaneous electrode is in a preductal area (i.e., right subclavicular area) while the arterial blood is obtained from a postductal artery (i.e., umbilical artery).

REFERENCES

1. Osborn JJ: A flowmeter for respiratory monitoring. *Crit Care Med* 6:349–351, 1978.
2. Suter PM, Fairly HB, Isenberg MD: Optimum end-expiratory pressure in patients with acute pulmonary failure. *N Engl J Med* 292:284–289, 1975.
3. Osborn JJ: Cardiopulmonary monitoring in the respiratory intensive care unit. *Med Instrum* 11:278–282, 1977.

4. Rahn J, Otis AB, Chawick LE, et al.: The pressure-volume diagram of the thorax and lung. *Am J Physiol* 146:161–178, 1946.
5. Nims RG, Connor EH, Comroe JH: Compliance of the human thorax in anesthetized patients. *J Clin Invest* 34:744–750, 1955.
6. Harris EA, Kenyon AM, Nisbet AD, et al.: The normal alveolar-arterial oxygen-tension gradient in man. *Clin Sci Mol Med* 46:89–104, 1974.
7. Fallat RJ, Osborn JJ: Patient monitoring techniques, in Burton GG, Gee GN, Hodgkin JE (eds): *Respiratory Care: A Guide to Clinical Practice*. Philadelphia, J. P. Lippincott Inc, 1977, pp 950–965.
8. Gabel RA: Calibration of nonlinear gas analyzers using exponential washout and polynomial curve fitting. *J Appl Physiol* 34:400–401, 1973.
9. Fowler KT: The respiratory mass spectrometer. *Phys Med Biol* 14:185–199, 1969.
10. Jones NL, Campbell EJM, Edwards RH, et al.: *Clinical Exercise Testing*. Philadelphia, WB Saunders Co, 1975.
11. Osborn JJ, Beaumont JO, Raison JCA, et al.: Computation for quantitative on-line measurements in intensive care ward, in Stacy RN, Waxman BD (eds): *Computers in Biomedical Research*. New York, Academic Press Inc, 1969.
12. Beaver WL, Wasserman K, Whipp BJ: On-line computer analysis and breath by breath graphical display of exercise function tests. *J Appl Physiol* 34:128–132, 1973.
13. Drabkin DL: Measurement of O_2 saturation of blood by direct spectrophotometric determination, in Comroe JH (ed): *Methods of Medical Research*. Chicago, Year Book Publishers, 1950, vol 2, pp 145–154.
14. Flick MR, Block AJ: Continuous in-vivo monitoring of arterial oxygenation in chronic obstructive lung disease. *Ann Intern Med* 86:725–730, 1977.
15. Douglas NJ, Brash HM, Wraith PK, et al.: Accuracy, sensitivity to carboxyhemoglobin, and speed of response of the Hewlett-Packard 47201A ear oximeter. *Am Rev Respir Dis* 119:311–313, 1979.
16. Baumberger JP, Goodfriend RB: Determination of arterial oxygen tension in man by equilibration through intact skin. *Fed Proc* 10:10, 1951.
17. Huch A, Huch R: Transcutaneous, noninvasive monitoring of PO_2. *Hosp Pract* 11:43–52, June 1976.
18. Proceedings of the "Workshop on methodologic aspects of transcutaneous blood gas analysis, Severinghaus J (ed). *Acta Anaesthesiol Scand*, suppl 68, 1978, pp 76–82.
19. Schonfeld T, Sargent CW, Bautista D, et al.: Transcutaneous oxygen monitoring during exercise stress testing. *Am Rev Respir Dis* 121:457–462, 1980.

CHAPTER 25

Hemodynamic Monitoring

ROBERT J. FALLAT, M.D.

In the acute care setting where pulmonary problems are critical, arterial blood-gas determinations are frequently needed; as a result, arterial catheterization is frequently used. These catheters can also be used for continuous monitoring of blood pressure and pulse rate. Jugular vein, subclavian veins, or brachial veins have long been used in the critical care setting not only for infusion of drugs but also for monitoring of central venous pressure, a useful determinant for fluid and diuretic administration. In many situations, however, there is an uncoupling of right and left heart pressures. Acute myocardial disease may be indicated by the finding of high left-sided pressures with perhaps low or normal right-sided pressures; conversely, when pulmonary hypertension exists, right-sided pressure [central venous pressure (CVP)] might be high, whereas left-sided filling pressures may be inadequate. In each of these cases, the use of flotation catheters in the pulmonary artery has become essential for diagnosis and monitoring.

The insertion of monitoring catheters and the interpretation of pressure waveforms during advancement of the catheter is most commonly a physician's responsibility; relevant literature on these techniques is available. Although the details of these procedures may seem inappropriate for this text, we have included these recommendations and suggestions in the following sections, because proper technique is essential for successful monitoring measurements. Technical personnel who have a clear understanding of what these procedures involve can contribute significantly to the quality and efficiency of hemodynamic monitoring.

PULMONARY FUNCTION TESTING
GUIDELINES AND CONTROVERSIES

ISBN 0-12-788125-5

CENTRAL VENOUS CATHETERIZATION

Standard intravenous catheters can be used. Generally, one chooses a larger size catheter, at least 18-gauge, in order to have good pressure transmission and ease of infusion. The antecubital fossae veins are commonly used, preferably the medial basilic vein. The catheter should be inserted into the superior vena cava or right atrium. Difficulty may be encountered passing through the shoulder region. Alternatively, one may use the external or internal jugular veins in the neck, but bleeding control is more difficult there. Finally, the use of subclavian veins is possible, but increases the risk of pneumothorax. Measurement of the CVP is most directly done via a manometer connected to a stopcock, but a venous pressure strain gauge transducer may also be used.

RIGHT HEART AND PULMONARY ARTERY CATHETERIZATION

Recently, flow-directed, balloon-tipped catheters have been introduced for directly measuring right-sided pulmonary artery (PA) pressures in the intensive care unit. Several catheters of various sizes are currently available, some of which are capable of measuring cardiac output using thermal dilution techniques. Insertion of these catheters is now most commonly done by the percutaneous technique, using the internal jugular vein. An 18-gauge needle is used to introduce a guide wire, followed by an 8-French (F) ''introducer'' catheter. The large size is needed to admit the 7-F pulmonary artery catheter usually used. However, with such large catheters, there is an increased risk of bleeding. Surgical cutdown to the brachial vein may be done instead of the percutaneous procedure, particularly when a bleeding tendency exists. Cournand-type catheters can be used percutaneously, but these do not have a balloon tip for flotation insertion and generally are limited to use under fluoroscopy in catheterization laboratories.

EQUIPMENT

A cutdown tray is needed for the cutdown technique. For the percutaneous technique, an introducer, a Cournand needle, and a guide wire are needed. For both techniques the following are needed: sterile gowns, gloves, drapes, towels, preparation solution and dressings, 1% Lidocaine, a surgical light, a sterile bowl with 1000 units of heparin in 250 ml of sterile intravenous normal saline, strain gauge, pressure transmission set, and bolus of Lidocaine.

A pressurized bag containing sterile heparinized solution (1500 units of heparin per 500 ml of 5% dextrose in 0.9 NaCl) is connected to the distal port lumen for continuous slow flushing (3 ml/hr) to prevent clotting. If a triple-lumen catheter is used, the proximal port should also have a slow continuous infusion, or else the lumen may occlude with clots.

Monitoring Catheters

There are five types of pulmonary artery monitoring catheters that are effective for obtaining right atrial pressure, pulmonary artery pressure, and pulmonary wedge pressure. These same catheters also permit sampling of mixed venous blood and injection or infusion of solutions.

The *double-lumen catheter* is the basic catheter of the flow-directed monitoring series. Two lumens extend the length of the soft, pliable body. The small lumen (external end is red) serves to inflate and deflate the balloon, and the large lumen (external end is yellow), terminating at the tip of the catheter, is used to obtain pressures, to obtain mixed venous blood samples, and to infuse heparinized flush solutions.

The *triple-lumen catheter* has the additional capability of measuring the CVP, since the opening of the third lumen lies in the area of the right atrium (the external end of the proximal lumen is blue).

The *thermodilution catheter* is a quadruple-lumen line, with each lumen labeled for function. The distal lumen terminates at the tip of the catheter; the proximal lumen is in the area of the right atrium and is used for injecting cold solution and measuring right atrial (RA) pressures. The red lumen is for balloon inflation and deflation, and a final lumen is for computer connection to the thermistor, which measures the blood temperature changes for thermodilution cardiac output. Other monitoring catheters have been modified for pediatric use and for continuous readout of oxyhemoglobin saturation by fiberoptic catheters.

PROCEDURES

Calibration of Oscilloscope and Transducer

Calibration of pressure transducers is best accomplished using a mercury or anaeroid barometer connected in a "Y" to the strain gauge. After zeroing the signal on the oscilloscope or recorder, a known pressure is exerted on the mercury manometer; the amount should be in the range desired for the particular catheter being used (approximately 10 torr for CVP, 30 torr for pulmonary artery, and 100 torr for an arterial line). It is important that the system used is free of leaks, so that a steady calibrating pressure is maintained while the appropriate gain setting is made on the recorder or oscilloscope. Note particularly that the transducer must be kept at a zero reference level, which is usually considered to be at the midpoint of the patient's chest when he is in an absolutely supine position.

Procedure for Catheter Insertion

Explain the procedure to the patient (and family), and verify that a well-functioning intravenous line is in place. (Arrhythmias rarely occur, but infusion of antiarrythmic drugs may occasionally be necessary. A Lidocaine bolus should be immediately available). Although the catheter may be placed without fluoroscopy, a fluoroscope and technician should be available; also, it is advisable to place the patient on a fluoroscopy bed or surgilift prior to draping. (If fluoroscopy is not available, a portable chest x-ray machine should be used to verify catheter position.)

Prior to insertion, using sterile technique, grossly inspect the catheter for any defects and lubricate the external surface with the sterile solution of heparinized saline. Take care not to damage the latex balloon during catheter preparation. Note the maximal balloon inflation capacity, which is printed on the catheter shaft. Check the balloon integrity by inflating the balloon to capacity while it is immersed in a sterile solution. Air is an acceptable inflation medium, unless an atrioventricular communication is suspected; then filtered carbon dioxide is recommended. Fill the monitoring lumens with sterile fluid to minimize the chance of introducing air into the venous system.

The insertion should be the responsibility of an attending physician. Surgical hand scrubs, masks, caps, sterile gowns and gloves must be used. The site should be shaved if necessary, surgically cleansed with Betadine scrub, prepped with Betadine solution, and draped.

If a cutdown is selected, an incision is made over the desired vein. If entering percutaneously, directions provided with each percutaneous catheter introducer should be followed. Isolate the appropriate vein. After venotomy, introduce the catheter and, with continuous pressure and ECG monitoring, rapidly advance it until the tip is in the intrathoracic region. At this point, partially inflate the balloon and continue rapid advancement into the right atrium. Record all pressures while proceeding through the right heart and pulmonary artery [right atrial (RA), right ventricular (RV), pulmonary artery systolic (PAS), diastolic (PAD), and wedge (PAW)], then inflate the balloon to the recommended volume.

When the catheter crosses the tricuspid valve and enters the right ventricle, the first significant pressure change will occur (see Fig. 1), as evidenced by the pressure excursions. Note that it may be useful to obtain blood from the right atrium, right ventricle, and pulmonary artery to determine the possible presence of left to right shunts.

Continue to advance the catheter into the pulmonary artery, where the next

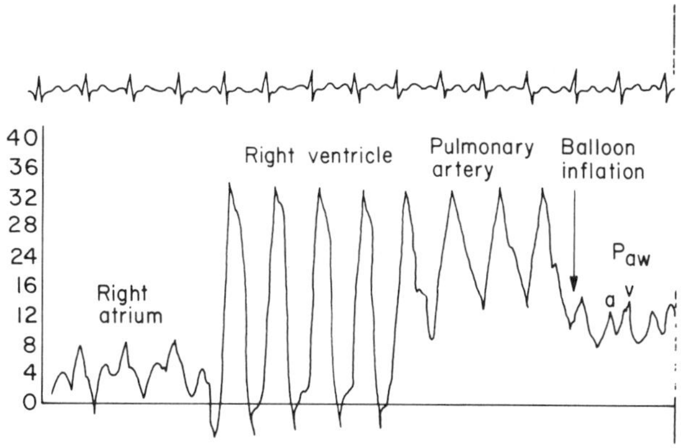

Fig. 1 *Pressure waveforms during Swan-Ganz insertion.*

readily evident pressure change occurs, an increase in diastolic pressure. Continue advancing the catheter until it is wedged in a smaller branch of the pulmonary artery. This is best accomplished by allowing the catheter, with the balloon inflated, to float into the wedge position from the main pulmonary artery. When catheter wedging occurs, it will cause a marked change in the pressure waveform, as indicated by PAW, Fig. 1. Normally, the PAW pressure is slightly less than pulmonary artery diastolic pressure.

If a pulmonary wedge pressure cannot be recorded with the balloon at maximal recommended volume, or if the balloon must be fully inflated in order to get a reading, the catheter is not far enough into the vessel. In this case, deflate the balloon, advance the catheter 1–2 cm, and again check the position by slowly inflating the balloon. On the other hand, if a reading can be obtained with the balloon minimally inflated, the catheter may be wedged too far into the vessel. In this situation, deflate the balloon and gradually pull the catheter back until the wedge pressure can be recorded with the balloon fully or almost fully inflated.

As soon as the catheter is properly positioned, record the wedge pressure, then immediately deflate the balloon. Inflation is an occlusive maneuver, and lengthy balloon inflations during wedge pressure recordings may cause pulmonary infarction. After deflation, the catheter tip will spring back to a more central position in the pulmonary artery. In this position, the pulmonary artery pressure will be continuously recorded until you are ready to record the next pulmonary wedge pressure. Once the catheter is in place, it can be withdrawn slightly, but should never be advanced, as sterility cannot be maintained.

The catheter should be sutured securely in place before application of sterile dressings.

Technique for recording Wedge Pressures

When ready to record wedge pressure, slowly inflate the balloon with a tuberculin syringe while observing the pressure waveform. Use only the minimal amount necessary to change the PA waveform to a PAW waveform. (Overdistension of the balloon may cause rupture of the balloon or the small pulmonary artery.) The 7-F catheter will hold 1.5 cc of air. Generally, not more than 1 cc is needed to inflate the balloon. (The 5-F catheter will hold 0.8–1.0 cc of air.)

To deflate the balloon, take the syringe off the line and allow the air to flow out passively. If the air does not come out (waveform still shows PAW), slowly deflate the balloon by withdrawing the air with the syringe. *Never* leave the balloon inflated, as pulmonary infarction may result. *Never* push air in and out. Flush the distal line with the intraflow heparinized solution after deflating the balloon.

If a wedge waveform persists after balloon deflation, the physician should slowly pull the catheter back until the wedge position is relieved. PAS, PAD, and PAW should be recorded with each reading. Wedge position can be verified either by noting a and v waves in appropriate position to the EKG (see Fig. 1) or by obtaining arterialized blood pO_2.

Blood Samples

Mixed-venous blood samples should be drawn with the balloon completely deflated. Samples should be drawn slowly to prevent contamination with arterialized capillary blood. Only mixed-venous samples for arterio-venous oxygen differences should be drawn from this site. All other blood samples should be drawn from another site, e.g., the arterial line. The catheter should be well flushed after withdrawing blood.

Infusions

Only heparinized normotonic solutions should be given through the distal catheter lumen. Hyperosmolar solutions and medications may clog the lumen, distort the waveforms, as well as threaten the integrity of the vessel, and they should never be given through the distal lumen. Any solutions or medications may be given through the proximal lumen, one end of which is located in the right atrium.

NORMAL VALUES

Normal values are summarized in the following table.

RAP	Right atrium pressure	3-10 mm Hg
RVP	Right ventricle pressure	
	Systolic	20-30 mm Hg
	Diastolic	3-10 mm Hg
PAS	Pulmonary artery systolic	20-30 mm Hg
PAD	Pulmonary artery diastolic	10-15 mm Hg
PAW	Pulmonary artery wedge	5-10 mm Hg
CVP	Central venous pressure	2-12 mm Hg

TROUBLESHOOTING

Thrombophlebitis at Insertion Site

To prevent thrombophlebitis, use sterile technique during insertion, lubricate the catheter before insertion, change the dressing and scrub the insertion site periodically, and NEVER advance the catheter after it is sutured in place.

Damped Waveform

To prevent a damped waveform, use a continuous pressurized heparinized drip, and flush thoroughly after blood sample drawing. Be sure the position of the catheter is optimal and aspirate any clots.

Balloon Rupture

This is prevented by slow, gentle inflation with minimal air and passive deflation as soon as the wedge reading is taken. Always check the balloon for integrity before insertion.

Special Precautions

1. At the site chosen for insertion, there should be no compromise of skin integrity, such as infection or burn.
2. As a special precaution, when a cardiac valvular abnormality is suspected or known, systemic antibiotic therapy may be considered.
3. Carbon dioxide should be used to inflate the balloon if a right-to-left intercardiac shunt or pulmonary a–v fistula is suspected. Never use air if it may enter the arterial circulation.
4. Any temperature elevation in the patient should be investigated. If septicemia or infection at the insertion site is suspected, removal of the catheter may be indicated.

Complications of pulmonary artery catheterization reported are pulmonary infarction or embolism, perforation of the pulmonary artery, conduction and rhythm disturbances, intracardiac knotting, persistent damping, and endocarditis. These complications are minimized with the use of proper technique.

Pulmonary Artery Waveforms

Familiarity with the normal and abnormal waveforms that are seen as the catheter is passed through the heart is essential (see Fig. 1). The reader is referred to Schroeder and Daily (1, pp. 76–90) as one of many articles dealing with waveforms.

Some key points to remember include

1. Frequently the a and v waves are not clearly seen in the RA or in the PAW position. The amplification may be inadequate in some types of oscilloscope.
2. The RV end-diastolic pressure is approximately the same as that of the RA (in the absence of tricuspid disease).
3. The PA systolic pressure is the same as that of the RV systolic (in the absence of pulmonary valve disease).
4. The PA diastolic pressure will be nearest to that of the PAW and should be recorded periodically in the event of balloon rupture.
5. Pressures of each vessel and chamber should be recorded during insertion.

Intra-arterial Catheterization

Although cuff pressures and current noninvasive means of automatically measuring blood pressure are available, in the case of the critically ill patient, more accurate and continuous assessment of peripheral arterial pressure is frequently essential for management. In-dwelling intra-arterial lines have become routine, not only in the management of patients with hemodynamic problems but also in patients with lung disease who are on ventilators, where frequent arterial blood-gas determinations are necessary.

Intra-arterial Catheterization Techniques

The sites of insertion of arterial catheters include the brachial artery, radial artery, and femoral artery. The femoral artery is the largest artery and usually the easiest to use in critically ill patients. Since the femoral artery is deep within the soft tissues of the groin, however, detection and control of active bleeding are more difficult. The radial artery, on the other hand, is the most superficial and the easiest to palpate, but, because of its small size, it may be difficult to cannulate with a large enough catheter to provide good continuous-pressure measurements without clotting. However, Gardner and co-workers have reported a 92% success rate in 536 radial artery catheterizations; using a continuous-flush system, only five catheters became nonfunctional after 1 to 25 days (mean, 3.4 days) (2). Because the radial artery is a more terminal artery, the adequacy of the "reserve" blood supply to the hand via the ulnar artery should be tested for by occluding both arteries, ulnar and radial, exercising the hand, then releasing pressure on only the ulnar artery. A rapid reperfusion of the hand should occur (within 5 seconds). The brachial artery is probably the best artery for catheterization for short periods of time, since it is of intermediate size and depth. However, because it is in the antecubital fossae, where frequent bending of the arm may occur, it is not as good a site as the radial or femoral artery for prolonged catheterization in critically ill patients. For more discussion of the methodology and problems encountered in intra-arterial monitoring, refer to Schroeder and Daily (1, pp. 95–103).

HEMODYNAMIC CALCULATIONS

When both pulmonary and peripheral arterial blood samples are available, a number of useful physiological variables may be calculated.

Arterial–Venous O_2 Difference

Arterial-venous O_2 difference [$C(a\text{-}v)O_2$] in vol % (ml/100ml) is derived as follows:

$$C(a\text{-}v)O_2 = CaO_2 - CvO_2$$

where CaO_2 is the arterial O_2 content in milliliters O_2/100 ml and CvO_2 is venous O_2 content in milliliters O_2/100 ml.

$$CaO_2 = 0.0031\ PaO_2 + 1.39\ (Hb)(SaO_2)$$

$$CvO_2 = 0.0031\ PvO_2 + 1.39\ (Hb)(SvO_2)$$

where Hg is grams of Hg/100 cc blood, and SaO_2 or SvO_2 is oxygen saturation of hemoglobin (in decimal form) in arterial (a) or venous (v) blood).

Cardiac Output

Cardiac output (Qt) in liters per minute is given by

$$Qt = \frac{\dot{V}_{O_2}}{10[C(a\text{-}v)O_2]}$$

where $\dot{V}_{O_2}$ is O_2 consumption (in milliliters per minute) (see Chapter 22).

Right-to-Left Shunt Fraction

Right-to-left shunt fraction (Qs/Qt) is given by

$$Qs/Qt = (CcO_2 - CaO_2)/(CcO_2 - CvO_2)$$

where Qs is blood flow through shunt and CcO_2 is the pulmonary end-capillary O_2 content.

$$CcO_2 = 0.0031\ PAO_2 + 1.39 \times (Hb)(SAO_2)$$

where PAO_2 is alveolar O_2 tension, and SAO_2 = alveolar O_2 saturation (generally 1.0).

For derivation of these equations and sample calculations, refer to Comroe et al. (3).

CONTINUOUS INTRAVASCULAR MONITORING OF BLOOD GASES

The ability to continuously monitor blood gases without blood sampling has two major clinical advantages: (1) in neonatal and small infants, it obviates the problem of depleting already small blood volume with repeated samples and (2) it provides immediate information relating to critical management decisions, such as altering ventilators or drug perfusions in acute respiratory failure (tidal volume, positive end-expiratory pressure, etc.). Several methods of continuous blood-gas monitoring have been proposed and used in physiological research. These methods include: (1) intravascular polarographic O_2 electrodes; (2) spectrophotometric O_2 saturation, using fiberoptic technology; (3) analysis of both CO_2 and O_2, either by gas chromatography or by mass spectrometry of gases obtained from intravascular catheters with semipermeable membranes. None of these methods has received wide enough usage to be considered ready for routine clinical applications. Current use of these methods is limited to specialized clinical research centers.

REFERENCES

1. Schroeder JS, Daily EK: *Techniques in Bedside Hemodynamic Monitoring*. Saint Louis, MO, CV Mosby Co, 1976.
2. Gardner RM, Schwartz R, Wong HC, et al.: Percutaneous indwelling radial-artery catheters for monitoring cardiovascular function. *N Engl J Med* 290:1227–1231, 1974.
3. Comroe J, Forster RE, Dubois AB, et al.: *The Lung*. Chicago, Yearbook Medical Publishers, 1962.

CHAPTER 26

Pulmonary Function Testing of Children

JOHN C. MCQUITTY, M.D.
NORMAN J. LEWISTON, M.D.

To achieve reliable pulmonary function measurements in the young child requires careful planning of the laboratory milieu. Physically, the room should be designed for the child's comfort and decorated pleasantly. If possible, all invasive or painful procedures should be done elsewhere and by other personnel, and all equipment associated with such procedures should be kept out of sight. Patience and skill are necessary to elicit the child's maximum cooperation, and personnel should be selected for these qualities. Extra time must be allowed for the preliminary coaching of the pediatric patient (1); in some cases an introductory visit to the laboratory is helpful. It is better to have no data than erroneous data, and it may be better to defer the test if the technician senses that inordinate patient fear or discomfort could cause poor test results.

The indications for testing the pulmonary function of a child are similar to those for testing adults. These are discussed in detail in the general references (2–7) but most completely by Polgar and Promadhat (2) whose book is essential for any laboratory that deals with children. The indications are (1) diagnosis of lung disease, (2) categorization of lung disease, (3) assessment of severity of lung disease, (4) evaluation of therapy, (5) prognostication of the course of disease, (6) prognostication of ventilatory response to general anesthesia and surgery (8), (7) determination of limitations to the tolerance of physical exertion, and (8) objective documentation of patient responses to therapeutic management.

This chapter does not reiterate techniques of pulmonary function testing described elsewhere in this book, but instead, describes those technical variations unique to testing a small child. Certain tests useful in the adult population, such as diffusion capacity, measurement of resistance and compliance, detection of closing volume, and the distribution of ventilation are done so infrequently in children that standard techniques have not been developed. It is recommended

ISBN 0-12-788125-5

that these tests be performed by specially trained personnel in tertiary care centers. A number of measurements of pulmonary function in the neonate also have been described in the literature but currently are considered to be research procedures. Thus, the main thrust of this chapter will be the discussion of special problems and normal data in the analysis of arterial blood, measurement of exhaled flow and lung volumes, and exercise testing of the small child.

ARTERIAL BLOOD-GAS ANALYSIS

The first problem encountered in blood-gas analyses in children is sample size. The total blood volume in infants is approximately 85 ml/kg of body weight. Unless sample size can be minimized, a small, sick infant quickly develops anemia from repeated blood samplings. The sample of arterial blood for gas and pH analysis should therefore be minimal and in most cases no greater than 0.5 ml. The volume of the sampling syringe should not be greater than twice the sample volume (9) and the volume of heparin introduced should be no greater than 10% of the sample size or arterial CO_2 ($PaCO_2$) and pH will be adversely affected. There is an increased incidence of osteomyelitis, nerve palsy, and bleeding associated with brachial and femoral artery punctures, and these arteries should not be used routinely to obtain samples (10). The sites of choice for obtaining samples in children are the radial and temporal arteries, and, in newborn infants, the umbilical artery. Before the radial artery is punctured, patency of ulnar artery flow should be assessed by compressing both the radial and ulnar artery and looking for a radial palmar flush when the ulnar artery is released (Allen Test). Most children will hyperventilate during arterial puncture, whether or not they are crying, and it has been shown that small infants with lung disease can change their PaO_2 dramatically by crying or holding their breath. There is considerable debate over the choice of technique for arterial puncture and also over the use of local anesthetics prior to puncture; some authorities believe better results are obtained by using a heparin-washed 25-gauge scalp vein needle to puncture the artery. If this technique is used, special care must be taken to allow the first drop or two of heparin to fall out of scalp vein tubing onto a piece of gauze before attaching the infusion set to the syringe for sample collection.

The small blood volume in infants limits the number of arterial samples that can be drawn. In addition, the size of suitable arteries presents technical problems in arterial sampling in many infants. For these two reasons, "arterialized" capillary sampling is often resorted to for estimating arterial pH, PCO_2, and O_2 tension (PO_2). Studies that have assessed the accuracy of capillary sampling (from comparisons with simultaneously drawn samples of arterial blood) have concluded that arterialized samples are suitable for assessing arterial pH (11–17). Most (11–15) but not all (16) studies concluded that capillary samples are also suitable for assessing arterial PCO_2. However, the adequacy of these samples for estimating arterial PO_2 is somewhat controversial. A number of studies have observed a marked underestimation of arterial PO_2 from "arterialized" capillary samples when arterial PO_2 values are greater than 60 mm Hg (15–17); Other have found that capillary samples were accurate even when arterial PO_2s were above 60 mm Hg (11–13). All three of the latter reports studied adults or children older than 1 year. The fact that some studies *have* reported good agreement between capillary and arterial measurements of PO_2 suggests that (at least in children and adults) differences in "arterialization" procedures, sample transfer, or the blood gas analyzer used for measurements may limit the adequacy of capillary samples for assessing arterial PO_2. The GAP conference on standardization of lung function testing in children concluded that "arterialized" capillary samples do not accurately reflect arterial PO_2 in the following three circumstances (9):

1. in the first few days of life, particularly when arterial PO_2 is greater than 60;
2. in patients of any age with shock; and
3. in patients with local reductions in blood flow to the sampling site.

Optimal "arterialization" of capillary blood can be accomplished by heating the puncture site to 42° C for 5 minutes (using immersion in water, a double wrapped moist cloth preheated to 42° C, or a heating pad) or using commercially available vasodilator creams (12, 13). The puncture itself must be deep enough to cause a free flow of blood and is best achieved with a 3-mm deep scalpel blade incision. In the newborn, the lateral aspect of the foot is the best puncture site. In the older child, the heel, lateral aspect of the toes, finger near the nail, or the lower end of the ear lobe may be used as sampling sites. The sample must be collected within 1 minute of the puncture from freely flowing (not squeezed) blood. Begin et al. recommended elevating the sampling site above the level of the heart to minimize venous blood admixture (11).

The depletion of the very limited blood reservoir in neonates from sampling of arterial blood and the limitations of "arterialized" capillary blood samples have stimulated interest in alternative methods of assessing PaO_2 and $PaCO_2$ in such patients. Transcutaneous measurements of PO_2 and PCO_2 show particular promise in newborns (18). However, the accuracy of the measurements is critically dependent upon the technique of electrode placement, and the absence of hypotension (18). Differences in electrode design may also be responsible for some of the differences in accuracy that have been observed (18, 19). In children, adults, and infants more than a few weeks old, transcutaneous electrodes have not proven to give satisfactory estimates of arterial gas tensions although they may have some use as trend monitors (see Chapter 25 for further discussion). Improved electrodes and more specific recommendations regarding their use are likely to be available in the near future. Ear oximetry is a useful measure of hemoglobin oxygen saturation in children more than 5 years of age. (This is also discussed in more detail in Chapter 25).

EXPIRATORY FLOW AND VOLUME MEASUREMENT

A maximal forced vital capacity (VC) maneuver is required for the accurate measurement of flow rates. Most children can accomplish this by age 6, although it may take 4 or 5 minutes to teach the child to perform accurate and reproducible VC maneuvers. If the child cannot make a sustained effort for 3 or more seconds, the results are unreliable and the child should be asked to return to the laboratory later. Children usually find it easier to perform the VC maneuver while standing. The report, however, should state how the child was tested and the degree of cooperation achieved between the child and technician. Younger children may be able to provide a "crying" VC but usually cannot generate maximal flow rates suitable for measurement. Vital capacity should be reported as the largest volume obtained whether a forced or slow maneuver was performed. Children often find it easier to perform a forced maneuver and a notation should be made of which value (forced or slow) was selected.

Lemen (3) has outlined technical requirements for machines used in pediatric testing (Table 1). The GAP conference recommended the following specification

Table 1 *Recommendation for Pediatric Pulmonary Function Equipment*[a]

Static calibration
Volume
range: 0–6 liters
discrimination: 20 ml/mm
linearity: within ±1%
Flow
range: 0–8 liters/sec
discrimination: 40 ml/sec/mm
linearity: within ±1%
Time
range: 0–8 sec
discrimination: 0.05 sec/mm
activated timer
threshold: 50 ml/sec
marker at 1.0 and 3.0 sec
Dynamic calibration
inertia and resistance: low
flat amplitude response (±5%) to 15 Hz

[a] From Lemen (3, p. 168).

for spirometers used in pediatric testing (9): Instantaneous flows should be within ±5% of the reading or ±0.1 liter/sec, whichever is greater. Volume measurements should be accurate to ±3% of reading or 30 ml, whichever is greater. Instruments used to measure flows at high lung volumes must have a flat frequency response (<5% distortion) to at least 8 Hz for flow and 5 Hz for volume.

Spirometers used in clinical laboratories should meet performance standards from at least one of the two sources cited (3, 9). As discussed in the chapter on spirometry (Chapter 7), because suitable equipment for testing the frequency response of spirometers is not readily available, buyers will usually need to rely on performance characteristics published by manufacturers when selecting equipment for purchase.

Lung volumes in children are most commonly measured by helium dilution, nitrogen washout, or plethysmography. Steady-state helium dilution by the technique of Hathirat et al. (20) is probably the easiest to perform. With this method, (1) the initial volume and helium concentration of the spirometer system and (2) the equilibration concentration of helium in the spirometer-patient system (after rebreathing) are used to calculate the child's lung volumes. ($C_1V_1 = C_2V_2$). If the volume of the spirometer system is large relative to the child's lung volume, then small percentage errors in the circuit volume can lead to large absolute volume errors in the child's measured volume. Therefore, we recommend that the dead space of the spirometer system be reduced as much as possible.

For measurement of volume or flow in children, the capability to double or quadruple the usual sensitivity of electronic measuring devices is desirable.

Normal Values

There are numerous reference studies for predicting normal pediatric values. As they are probably the most frequently used, we have presented the equations of Polgar and Promadhat (2), which were calculated from composite data from a number of studies published prior to 1971 (see Table 2). Subsequent comparison of many of these equations with those developed from more recent publications indicated that both sets of equations are nearly identical (21). We suggest that each laboratory test a group of normal children and compare them with the standards selected for use in that laboratory. Most of the standards currently available are based on data collected from Caucasian children, and they may not be applicable to other racial groups (22). There are also several discrepancies existing between reference standards for the oldest (tallest) group of children and independently produced results on adults. In most of the populations of children studied, the number of subjects are not evenly distributed by age. There are fewer data points for the youngest (smallest) and oldest (tallest) group. We do not know how to link this oldest group of children with normal adults, because normal adult data was obtained from only a few young subjects. Data needs to be

Table 2 *Summary Equations and Variability from Polgar and Promadhat*[a]

Function[b]	Equations of summary curves[c]	Average coefficient of variation[d]	Reproducibility (% of mean)[e]	Day-to-day variation %
VC (in ml)				
males	$VC = 4.4 \times 10^{-3} \times H^{2.67}$, or $\log VC = -2.3554 + 2.6727 \times \log(H)$	13	1.4–2.9	4.9
females	$VC = 3.3 \times 10^{-3} \times H^{2.72}$, or $\log VC = -2.4756 + 2.7194 \times \log(H)$			3.9
FRC (in ml)				
males	$FRC = 0.75 \times 10^{-3} \times H^{2.92}$, or $\log FRC = -3.1274 + 2.9173 \times \log(H)$	18	4	3.7
females	$FRC = 1.78 \times 10^{-3} \times H^{2.74}$, or $\log FRC = -2.8622 + 2.795 \times \log(H)$			5.8
RV (in ml)				
males and females	$RV = 4.41 \times 10^{-3} \times H^{2.41}$, or $\log RV = -2.355 + 2.4101 \times \log(H)$,	22.8	8	27.0
	or $RV = -919.2123 + 11.419 \times H$			22.0
TLC (in ml)				
males	$TLC = 5.6 \times 10^{-3} \times H^{2.67}$, or $\log TLC = -2.2469 + 2.669 \times \log(H)$	11.6		5.7
females	$TLC = 4.0 \times 10^{-3} \times Ht^{2.73}$, or $\log TLC = -2.3880 + 2.7302 \times \log(H)$			4.5
MVV (in liters/min)				
males and females	$MVV = -99.507 + 1.276\ H$	21.0	6	—
C_L (in ml/cm H_2O)				
males	$C_L = 17.0945 + 0.0459 \times FRC$ (ml)	22.0	9	—
FEV_1 (in ml)				
males and females	$FEV_1 = 2.1 \times 10^{-3} \times H^{2.8}$, or $\log FEV_1 = -2.6781 + 2.7986 \times \log(H)$	8.8	4	—
MIFR (in liter/sec)				
males and females	$MIFR = -5.26 + 0.06 \times H$	23	—	—

Table 2 *Summary Equations and Variability from Polgar and Promadhat[a]—Continued*

Function[b]	Equations of summary curves[c]	Average coefficient of variation[d]	Reproducibility (% of mean)[e]	Day-to-day variation %
$FEF_{25-75\%}$ (in liters/min)				
males and females	$FEF_{25-75\%} = -207.70 + 2.621 \times H$	32.9	—	—
PEFR (in liters/min)				
males and females	$PEFR = -425.5714 + 5.2428 \times H$	13	—	—

[a] From Polgar and Promadhat (2, p 254).

[b] VC is vital capacity; RV, residual volume; TLC, total lung capacity; MVV, maximum voluntary ventilation; C_L, lung compliance; FEV_1, forced expiratory volume at 1 second; MIFR, maximal inspiratory flow rate; $FEF_{25-75\%}$, mean forced expiratory flow during middle half of forced vital capacity; PEFR, peak expiratory flow rate.

[c] In all equations, height (H) is measured in centimeters.

[d] The average of coefficients of variation $\left(\frac{SD}{mean}\right) \times 100$ for observations within the population samples for the studies reviewed by Polgar.

[e] SD of duplicate measurements expressed as $\frac{SD}{mean} \times 100$.

collected on a large number of normals in their adolescent years. Until such information is available, we recommend that children's standards be followed up to age 16 and adult standards be used after that age. This cut-off for pediatric standards is somewhat arbitrary but clinically realistic and appropriate. At present there is no practical way to reliably test children between the newborn period and 6 years of age, and data for normal lung function in these ages is incomplete. Milner has published normal data for peak flows using the Wright Peak Flow Meter; included in this study were a small number of children as young as 3½ years of age (23). Among the publications that include normal values for flow-volume loop parameters are those of Knudson (24) and Schoenberg (25).

Exercise Testing

There are two types of exercise testing appropriate to the pediatric age group. The first type, classic exercise testing, measures the ability of the cardiopulmonary system to oxygenate pulmonary arterial blood during periods of increased oxygen uptake. The second type tests for the presence of exercise-induced bronchospasm (26). The two test protocols are quite different and the type of test desired should be clearly specified by the referring physician.

Classic exercise testing in the child (6) is performed very much as in the adult (see Chapter 22). A cycle ergometer is easier, safer, and better accepted by children than a treadmill. However, treadmill exercise elicits exercise-induced bronchospasm better. The incidence of complications of exercise testing is much lower in children than in adults. However, it is still important to perform a careful history, physical examination, and chest X-ray prior to the actual testing. The patient should be carefully monitored during the test by an individual trained in cardiopulmonary resuscitation, and an emergency cart and defibrillator should be available in the unlikely event that a severe cardiac dysrhythmia occurs. Special caution is necessary when exercising children with hyperreactive airway disease if the baseline FEV_1 is less than 60% of the predicted value (9), since severe bronchospasm and poor gas exchange may occur.

The detection of exercise-induced bronchospasm is useful in children with asthma, since the phenomenon can often be prevented by the use of a sympathomimetic drug, a theophylline preparation, or by cromolyn sodium. Testing is done in the following way:

Some type of exhaled flow is measured as a baseline, preferably FEV_1, but peak expiratory flow (PEF) rate is also acceptable. The individual is then exercised by free running, treadmill, or cycle ergometer for 8 minutes or until the heart rate reaches 80% of the maximal rate (predicted by age). Exercise is terminated and expiratory flow is measured at 3-minute intervals for 15 minutes and then at 5-minute intervals for a total of 45 minutes. Flow rate values are plotted as a function of time. A drop of 15% in expiratory flow rate from the baseline is considered evidence of exercise-induced bronchospasm although decreases of 50% are not uncommon. If acute bronchospasm is precipitated by the testing, it should be treated promptly.

Normal values for exercise testing are found in a number of publications; the best pediatric values are presented by Godfrey (6).

OTHER MEASUREMENTS

The need for special tests, such as respiratory resistance, airway resistance, and diffusing capacity, may arise occasionally. Because of the expensive equipment and trained personnel necessary for optimal performance of these tests, it is usually advisable to refer the patient to a laboratory that does a large volume of such testing as is often found in tertiary pediatric pulmonary centers.

The measurement of *respiratory* resistance by oscillation techniques assesses the total impedance of the lungs and chest wall as well as the airways. This resistance varies with factors such as the volume at which the measurement is made and the frequency of the oscillating current. Thus, it is suggested that the lung volume at which the resistance is calculated be measured, and that the oscillation frequency be specified.

In measuring airway resistance by plethysmography, if a correction factor is used to correct for the displacement volume of a subject, before reporting results on small children, it is advisable to check the validity of the correction formula by calibrating the box pressure (or volume) signal with a small subject within the box. In the young sick child, adequate panting may be difficult to achieve. With plethysmographs that are suitable for such measurements, such patients may be studied during tidal breathing. During the panting maneuver, some small children do not produce flows of 0.5 or even 0.25 liters/sec. To measure resistances in such cases we suggest calculating resistance from the straight line which most nearly fits the more linear portion of the curve crossing the zero flow line.

Measurements of diffusing capacity also often present unique problems in pediatric patients. Some young children may find it difficult to hold their breaths properly for the single breath test; in such cases steady-state measurements may be preferable. However, the paucity of normal predictive data for steady-state measurements in the pediatric age range limits the usefulness of this methodology. Until adequate normal values are available, laboratories making these measurements need to develop their own normal predictive values. When studying smaller children with the single-breath technique, the washout volume and volume of expired air collected for analysis frequently must be smaller than that used routinely in adult patients.

REFERENCES

1. Brough FK, Schmidt CD, Dickman M: Effect of two instructional procedures on the performance of the spirometry test in children five through seven years of age. *Am Rev Respir Dis* 106:604-606, 1972.
2. Polgar G, Promadhat V: *Pulmonary Function Testing in Children: Techniques and Standards*. Philadelphia, WB Saunders Co, 1971.
3. Lemen RJ: Pulmonary function testing in the office and clinic, in Kendig EL, Chernick LC (eds): *Disorders of the Respiratory Tract in Children*, ed 3. Philadelphia, WB Saunders Co, 1977, pp 166-176.
4. McBride JT, Wolh MEB: Pulmonary function tests. *Pediatr Clin North Am* 26:537-551, 1979.
5. Waring WW, Jeansonne LD: *Practical Manual of Pediatrics*. Saint Louis, MO, CV Mosby Co, 1975, pp 73-78, 292-303.
6. Godfrey S: *Exercise Testing in Children*. Philadelphia, WB Saunders Co, 1974.
7. Doershuk CF, Orenstein DM: Pulmonary function and exercise testing, in Lough MD, Doershuk CF, Stern RC (eds): *Pediatric Respiratory Therapy*. Chicago, Yearbook, 1979.
8. Froese AB: Pre-operative evaluation of pulmonary function. *Pediatr Clin North Am* 26:645-659, 1979.
9. Taussig LM, Chernick V, Wood R, et al.: Standardization of lung function testing in children. *J Pediatr* 97:668-678, 1980.
10. Pape KE, Armstrong DL, Fitzhardinge PM: Peripheral median nerve damage secondary to brachial arterial blood gas sampling. *J Pediatr* 93:852-856, 1978.
11. Begin R, Racine T, Roy JC: Value of capillary blood gas analyses in the management of acute respiratory distress. *Am Rev Respir Dis* 112:879-881, 1975.
12. Davis RH, Beran AV, Galant SP: Capillary pH and blood gas determinations in asthmatic children. *J Allergy Clin Immunol* 56:33-38, 1975.
13. Godfrey S, Wozniak ER, Courtenay-Evans RJ, et al.: Ear lobe blood samples for blood gas analysis at rest and during exercise. *Br J Dis Chest* 65:58-64, 1971.

14. Gandy G, Grann L, Cunningham N, et al.: The validity of pH and PCO_2 measurements in capillary samples in sick and healthy newborn infants. *Pediatrics* 34:192–197, 1964.
15. Glasgow JFT, Flynn DM, Swyer PR: A comparison of descending aortic and "arterialized" capillary blood in the sick newborn. *Can Med Assoc J* 106:660–662, 1972.
16. Hunt CE: Capillary blood sampling in the infant: Usefulness and limitations of two methods of sampling, compared with arterial blood. *Pediatrics* 51:501–506, 1973.
17. Van Kessel AL: The blood gas laboratory, an update: 1979. *Lab Med* 10:419–429, 1979.
18. Peabody JL, Gregory GA, Willis MM, et al.: Transcutaneous oxygen tension in sick infants. *Am Rev Respir Dis* 118:83–87, 1978.
19. Whitehead MD, Halsall D, Pollitzer MJ, et al.: Transcutaneous estimation of arterial PO_2 and PCO_2 in newborn infants with a single electrochemical sensor. *Lancet* 1:1111–1114, 1980.
20. Hathirat S, Renzetti AD, Mitchell M: Measurement of the total lung capacity by helium dilution in a constant volume system. *Am Rev Respir Dis* 102:760–770, 1970.
21. Polgar G, Weng TR: The functional development of the respiratory system. *Am Rev Respir Dis* 120:625–695, 1979.
22. Binder RE, Mitchell CA, Schoenberg JB, et al.: Lung function among black and white children. *Am Rev Respir Dis* 114:955–959, 1976.
23. Milner AD, Ingram D: Peak expiratory flow rates in children under five years of age. *Arch Dis Child* 45:780–782, 1970.
24. Knudson RJ, Slatin RC, Lebowitz MD, et al.: The maximal expiratory flow-volume curve. *Am Rev Respir Dis* 113: 587–600, 1976.
25. Schoenberg JB, Beck GJ, Bouhuys A: Growth and decay of pulmonary function in healthy blacks and whites. *Respir Physiol* 33:367–393, 1978.
26. Jones RS, Buston MH, Wharton MJ: The effect of exercise on ventilatory function in the child with asthma. *Br J Dis Chest* 56:78–86, 1962.

CHAPTER 27

Selection of a Computer for the Pulmonary Laboratory

JAMES K. LARSON, P.E.

The most significant change in pulmonary laboratory technology in the last decade has been the increasing use of computers. The selection of a satisfactory computer system is a task that requires careful thought and consideration of a number of factors. These factors range from the obvious such as cost, to the less obvious such as printer noise, to the seemingly obvious such as data storage capabilities. Proper attention to these many competing factors will lead to the selection of a system that will perform well for many years and significantly increase the efficiency of a lab; otherwise, the lab may be saddled with an expensive piece of furniture. It is the purpose of this section to advance the understanding of the factors involved in the selection process.

Before delving deeper into the components of complex computer systems, it is very important to emphasize that, because of the costs (in terms of both time and money) of custom programing, a packaged preprogramed system is usually most suitable for the majority of pulmonary labs. Unless the services of an experienced programer are available and ample time is allowed for the completion of the programing, the purchase of an unprogramed system often means many months or even years of delays before the system is operating to its full potential.

Two very common terms used in discussing computer systems are "hardware" and "software." Hardware is the physical equipment: the computer, the printer, the disk drives, the terminal, etc. Software refers to the programs that make all the hardware actually do something besides gather dust. The importance of the software cannot be overemphasized, for without it the finest hardware available will do nothing.

Two other terms that need definition are "bit" and "byte." A bit is simply a single digit in the binary number system, specifically, a 1 or 0. A byte is eight bits. Bits and bytes are used in several contexts to describe computers and

PULMONARY FUNCTION TESTING
GUIDELINES AND CONTROVERSIES

ISBN 0-12-788125-5

peripherals. The number of bits that a given computer can handle simultaneously gives an indication of the speed and complexity of the instructions it can execute. For example, an 8-bit computer will not have the performance of a 32-bit computer. This is significant if more than one task is to be performed at one time. For example, if two tests are being done simultaneously, a small machine (8-bit) might not perform satisfactorily. On the other hand, 32-bit machines are expensive and may offer little measurable advantage over a 16-bit machine. More specific recommendations will follow. Bits are also used to measure the accuracy of analog to digital and digital to analog converters (refer to section on peripherals). Note that a 12-bit converter may be used with a 32-bit or 8-bit computer; that is, the bit size of one does not dictate the bit size of the other. Bytes are often used to refer to the storage capability of the computer memory or mass storage device. Each byte may be thought of as one character, so that a report that has 1500 characters will require about 1500 bytes of storage. The terms ''M,'' or ''mega,'' and ''K,'' or ''kilo,'' are often used to mean 1,000,000 and 1,000 bytes, respectively.

There are many tasks around the lab for which the computer is especially suited and which justify the purchase of a system. The computer is outstanding at doing calculations and preparing reports. These are the most common lab applications. Recently, many computers have become available that can process data simultaneously with testing (via an analog to digital interference) and do the necessary calculations without further input from the person conducting the test. In addition to reducing the chances of errors during manual entry of data and markedly reducing calculation time, this allows an immediate review of the test results. The computer can also do many calculations that would be prohibitively tedious if done by hand.

Further tasks suitable for a computer system include its use as a record keeper. Via magnetic disks and/or magnetic tape, the computer can maintain and rapidly access a large file of patient records. The system can maintain departmental personnel records, calculate payrolls, keep supply inventories, and monitor quality control programs. Using a video terminal (also known as a cathode-ray tube or CRT), the task of word processing (archaically called typing) may be simplified considerably. Using a word processor, a document is viewed on the video screen as it is being typed. Corrections may be made easily, without correction fluid, and only the finished document need be printed.

Obviously, the applications for a computer are multitudinous and conceptually limited only by the imagination. I say conceptually limited, because, in practice, the computer does only what it is programmed to do. Software, then, is the key to having a system that can do any or all of the functions previously listed.

In establishing criteria for system selection, the first thing to consider is exactly what tasks the system *must* do. These would be the primary requirements. Next, what further tasks would you *like* it to do? These would be the secondary requirements, and should be considered on a cost/benefit basis. Keep in mind that having a system that is *capable* of doing a certain task is not the same as having one that *will* do it. The point here is that if you do not have the software to do the task, the system will not do it, even though it may be capable of doing the task.

This fact leads to two further observations. First, your system will do exactly what it is programed to do, no less and no more. Therefore, it is important to test any programs that may be purchased with the system to ensure that they work as intended. Second, just because your system will not presently do a given task does not mean that it cannot, given the right program. This implies that the hardware purchased today should be purchased with an eye to what further tasks might be desired tomorrow.

SELECTION CONSIDERATIONS

Any section on computer system selection should include mention of a very important and often overlooked type of computer: the microprocessor. The microprocessor is a single electronic component that can be designed right into a piece of test equipment and will perform many of the functions of a large computer. In the last few years, several types of test equipment—including spirometers, helium dilution spirometer systems, and blood-gas analyzers—have appeared with microprocessors built into them. The microprocessors sequence test procedures, calculate results, and may control a small printer to generate a report of the test. These systems cannot generally be reprogramed by the user and are often restricted as to the types of tests they can perform, but as their prices continue to drop, they offer an attractive alternative for small labs unable to afford larger computer systems. In buying microprocessor-based test equipment, you should insist on seeing results of comparison tests done using standard laboratory apparatus and techniques. It is also a good idea to test the device in your own lab to assess its usefulness.

The remainder of this section is addressed mainly to those interested in larger systems capable of performing more sophisticated tests than a microprocessor system; however, it should be useful to anyone considering any computer-based system.

Basically, there are two ways to buy a computer system. You can buy a special-purpose system, which is generally sold as a package including software and often including physiological test equipment as well (e.g., a spirometer). This type of package will generally be designed to perform only a few specific tasks (e.g., data collection and calculation). It may or may not be possible to program such a system to do other tasks. The other alternative is to buy a general-purpose system, which is perhaps more difficult, since it requires the purchaser to choose every element of the package from the computer to the printer to the software. This approach allows the maximal flexibility, however, and, if done with the assistance of someone experienced in computer selection, often results in a very satisfactory system, especially if several tasks are to be performed on one system and existing physiological test equipment is to be used. If possible, any consultant employed should have experience in pulmonary labs, so that the system recommended will fit smoothly into the lab routine. When choosing larger and more sophisticated systems, a consultant is essential, unless the system is an exact duplicate (including software) of an existing system that the buyer knows meets all needs of a pulmonary lab.

One important question to be addressed is whether or not you will have programing capability within the lab. That is, will you have personnel that will program your system or will you need to rely on outside sources for software? This question must be considered early in your selection process, since it will determine whether to buy a special-purpose system (which is preprogrammed), to hire a consultant to do your programming, or to figure on doing your own programming after you get the system (see the section on languages and programs). Often, a combination of the previously mentioned options will prove the most satisfactory. For example, a spirometry and pulmonary function testing (PFT) program might be written by a consultant, a word-processing program purchased from a software vendor, and a record-keeping program written at a later date by someone in the lab.

Another key question is what size computer to buy. ''Size'' as used to describe computers can have several meanings. It may refer to physical size, main memory size, mass storage capability, or data word size. Realizing that there is no single answer for all cases, most labs will need a 16-bit minicomputer with 64K to 256K bytes of main memory and 1M to 5M bytes of disk storage. (This applies to general-purpose systems; special-purpose systems will use suitable computers chosen by the system vendor.) A reputable salesman or consultant can help greatly in this area, but if his recommendation is significantly different from the one just mentioned, be wary and ask for a thorough explanation. In 1981, a system of this type could be purchased for $15,000 to $40,000, including a printer and terminal. The actual cost will depend on exactly what peripherals (see the section on peripherals) and software are desired. It is important to note that good software is not cheap and can easily make up one-third to one-half of the system cost, especially if it is custom written. It is a good idea to talk with other labs about their systems, and it is sometimes possible to simply copy an existing system. Note that copying the hardware of an existing system still requires you to give careful consideration to the source of adequate software, since it may be illegal to copy existing software if it is copyrighted. Again, if a large, sophisticated system is being purchased, the services of an experienced consultant are recommended.

In order to store programs and data effectively, some sort of mass storage device(s) is required. These may be divided into two main types: magnetic disk drives and magnetic tape drives. Disks are the most flexible and are available as either hard or floppy disks. Floppy disks are inexpensive and easy to handle, but they are slower and not as durable as hard disks. Floppies are great for program interchange, data filing, and similar tasks in which they are not used on a continuous, daily basis. Hard disks offer more storage (5 to 50 times as much) and stand up well under continuous use. Hard disks are either fixed or removable. Removable disks offer some of the advantages of floppies, but are much more expensive and require careful handling. Most clinical labs will find a floppy disk system satisfactory. Magnetic tape drives using reels of tape are expensive ($15,000 versus $5000 for a disk drive) but can cheaply store large amounts of data. If a major record-keeping effort is anticipated (such as university-type epidemiological studies), a tape drive should be considered. Recently, tape drives costing $5000 to $7500 have been advertised; if these prove reliable in service, they should be cost-effective in those labs needing tape storage. Another type of tape drive is the cassette drive. It stores less data than reel types but is much less costly. It might be considered as a substitute for floppies, but this is generally not recommended, because programs and data are accessed very slowly on cassette systems and much more user attention and interaction is required to make proper use of the system.

PRECAUTIONARY NOTES

In concluding this section on computer selection, let us mention a few commonly overlooked aspects of computer selection (see section on languages and programs, also). Software packages must be carefully designed and thought out if they are to function satisfactorily. A package for a clinical lab should fit in with the flow of patients and sequence of tests in the lab. On-line test procedures should be in accordance with standard recommended methodology. Report formats should be easy to read and understand. In a busy lab, simultaneous tests on two or more patients may be required. The software must be designed to perform all these tasks efficiently and reliably. There must be enough terminals to allow lab work to flow smoothly. These terminals should be fast, quiet, and easy to use. If a special-purpose system is purchased, it should be flexible enough to allow some reprograming and should allow the user to expand system capabilities if he wishes to at a later date. Sufficient space must be available in the lab for the system. For large systems, it is best if the computer can be kept in a separate room with enough storage space for such things as data disks, tape reels, and documentation. Special temperature or humidity limits may be required and should be considered. Look for hidden costs, such as cables for data collection, spare hard disk packs, a storage cabinet, etc. Include these in your budget. Choose an analog to digital converter (see the section on peripherals) that will give the degree of accuracy you require. Do not overlook the cost of a service contract to maintain your computer. Deal with an established, experienced vendor, since this is the best way to get a reliable system. *A key step is a detailed consultation with an objective expert in the state of the art of computer technology.* He should review the entire system to be ordered, including any software. Try to find a consultant that is familiar with a pulmonary lab. If he or she is not, then the recommended system may not be satisfactory in the lab and may cost considerably more than necessary.

TALKING TO YOUR SYSTEM: PERIPHERALS

Peripherals are those devices which allow one to communicate with one's computer and allow it to communicate with other devices (such as a spirometer or printer). The most important peripherals include printers, terminals, analog to digital and digital to analog interfaces, plotters, digitizer tablets, and light pens. Each of these has certain purposes, characteristics, advantages, and pitfalls, which will be discussed in the following. Discussion centers on the hardware aspects of what they can do. Keep in mind, however, that it is the software that determines what the hardware will do and that a device such as a plotter or a graphics terminal is useless without the specific software necessary to drive it. This software is often available at reasonable additional cost, but the cautions set forth in the section on languages and programs must be observed.

The first peripherals we consider are those devices that actually give you a piece of paper: printers. A printer is essential in almost any lab system, since a printed report (called "hard copy") is generally required. The width of the paper used is important, since you will generally want to use standard 8 ½" x 11" sheets. You may choose either impact or thermal printers: impact printers actually hit the paper (like a typewriter), whereas thermal printers use heat to mark specially treated paper. Thermal printers are quieter, but require special paper, which has a tendency to fade and is relatively expensive compared to regular paper. Impact printers use regular paper but are noisier, are often more expensive, and may require more maintenance. Impact printers are available in two basic types, letter-quality and dot matrix, depending on the way the letters are formed. Letter-quality printers generate letters that look like they were made with a typewriter and allow typefaces to be changed in the manner of an IBM typewriter. They are expensive ($3000) and relatively slow (30 characters per second). Buy one if you will be using the computer to do a lot of word processing (letter writing) or want publication-quality printing. The other type of impact printer is the dot matrix, and, as the name implies, it uses a matrix of tiny dots to form the letters. The printing looks like a computer did it, but it is easy to read, fast (up to 180 characters per second), and less expensive ($1000) then a better-quality printer. If noise is a problem with an impact printer, an acoustic enclosure may be purchased for a few hundred dollars.

The next important peripheral is the terminal. Terminals are those devices that allow you to tell the computer what to do, usually via a keyboard. They also have a display to let you see what you said and to let the computer talk back. This display is usually either a hard copy or a CRT. Hard-copy terminals are essentially a printer with a keyboard, and all the comments made concerning printers apply. The CRT terminal has a screen much like a television, on which letters and numbers typed on the keyboard or by the computer appear. This is by far the easiest and most satisfactory type of terminal to use, since it is quiet and allows users to see what they are doing easily without having to struggle with a roll of paper. Also, in most systems, a CRT will be much faster than a hard-copy terminal (3 to 30 times as fast, typically). A hard-copy terminal should be chosen over a CRT only if a low purchase price is an overwhelming consideration, since a separate printer would not be required. CRTs are basically one of two types: alphanumeric, which essentially display only letters and numbers, and graphics type, which can display continuous curves, line diagrams, etc., like an X–Y recorder. Alphanumeric types are cheaper ($700 to $1200), but the graphics type is needed to accurately display spirometry or body box loops. Graphics type terminals are available with built-in hard-copy devices that will accurately print the screen image on light-sensitive paper ($4000). Another type of terminal that has recently become available is the color terminal. These may be had with or without graphics capability, and are often useful in an intensive care environment where a lot of patient information must be reviewed quickly. Color can emphasize important information. Color terminals cost from $2000 to $8000.

Analog to digital and digital to analog converters (known as ADCs and DACs, respectively) allow the computer to process electronic signals sent from or to other devices (such as a spirometer). Analog signals are those signals that vary continuously, e.g., from 0 to 5 V. Digital signals are those signals that are discrete in nature, such as 0 or 5 V only. Digital signals are used inside the computer to represent numbers for calculation, whereas analog signals are the type commonly output from most test devices and used for controls, such as controlling ergometer work load during exercise testing. The need for conversion from one mode to the other is obvious if the computer is to directly communicate with test devices. One important consideration in selecting ADCs or DACs is their resolution. Resolution is expressed in bits. For example, an 8-bit ADC can resolve one part in 256 (2^8), whereas a 12-bit ADC can resolve one part in 4096. Practically, this means that a vital capacity output that varies from 0 to 6 liters will be divided into 256 discrete steps by an 8-bit ADC (23cc/step). If this is not precise enough, then a 10- or 12-bit ADC must be used. See Chapter 8 for a detailed discussion of the impact of resolution and sampling rate on spirometric measurements.

When evaluating ADCs or DACs, consider their effects on the results of calculations to be done. If very precise results are required, then be sure that the data gathered will be accurate enough. In addition to the resolution, the effects of sample rate on the accuracy of data collected must also be considered. This rate is an important parameter in selecting ADCs and DACs. If a high rate is required, then a real time clock will probably be required as well. The clock will provide a high speed and stable time reference for sampling. If it is anticipated that a need for simultaneous analog to digital tasks will exist (for example, simultaneous spirometry and exercise testing), then your system may require more than one analog to digital converter. Additional clocks may also be needed. Another feature that often comes with ADCs and DACs is an event trigger. This is just a switch that allows the start of an event to be signaled (such as the start of a forced expiratory volume maneuver), or it can mark the occurrence of a certain event (such as a timing pulse). Carrying the idea of computer-controlled switches further, switch units are also available that enable the computer to directly switch other equipment on and off.

Plotters are available for computer systems, ranging from simple X–Y units to multicolor units costing many thousands of dollars. What type you need (if any) depends on your requirements. For most clinical purposes, you will not need high resolution, and can just use a special program that will plot results using symbols (e.g., "x" or "+") in a satisfactory manner. Another inexpensive alternative is to use a DAC output to control a standard laboratory X–Y recorder. Since it is possible to send data to it at a controlled rate, the results of high-speed events may be satisfactorily plotted on a low-speed plotter (e.g., body box loops). One of the preceding techniques is usually adequate for most pulmonary lab applications. If you need more rapid or convenient operation and finer resolution, then a computer-controlled unit is a good investment ($2000 to $6000). If you must plot complex data, then a multicolor unit might be considered ($8000).

Digitizer tablets and light pens may be thought of as reverse plotters, taking data gathered as curves and translating them into a form that the computer can work with. Of the two, the tablet is more precise, being suitable for such applications as determination of lung volumes from chest radiographs. The digitizer tablet is essentially a metal board on which the item to be traced is placed. A special stylus is then traced over the desired curve, and the digitizer converts the curve into digital data for the computer to use. Digitizer tablets are available in various sizes, and the comments about resolution apply here. The light pen works in a similar manner, but uses the CRT screen as a tablet. It is not usually as accurate. Light pens may be useful for program control, but are seldom necessary for most pulmonary lab applications.

LANGUAGES AND PROGRAMS

If you plan to write or buy any programs, you must give some consideration to languages. A language is a system of symbols and syntax that allows a programer to instruct the computer to perform a certain task. The computer must be told what to do in a very precise and unambiguous manner. This is the purpose of a language. The commoner languages in use today for lab applications are Fortran, Basic, and Pascal. Fortran is the oldest and probably the commonest. There are many programs already available in Fortran that may be useful in the lab. Basic is perhaps the easiest to learn and use, but is much slower at certain tasks than Fortran or Pascal and may be unsatisfactory for tasks such as controlling an ADC. Pascal is a relatively new language that combines the power and speed of Fortran with the ease of use of Basic. It has the disadvantages that there are few existing programs written in it, and that many programers are not familiar with it. The choice of languages is largely a matter of personal preference, but if major programing is contemplated, Fortran or Pascal is probably indicated.

In writing programs, or having them written, two major concerns should be uppermost. First, will the program do the job? This capability can only be evaluated by testing the program in the lab environment, and is most likely to be realized if the programer has a thorough understanding of exactly what the program is required to do. These requirements must be determined by the lab and should be set forth clearly before any programing is started or any contract for programing is let. Second, can another programer easily understand and modify it? This second requirement is met by documentation. Documentation is the explanation of the program—not just what it does but, more importantly, how it is done. This involves not only an explanation of calculation methods, including references, and a copy of the program as it was entered into the computer by the programer (the "source" program), but also an explanation of how different parts of the program interact. This is vital if the program ever needs to be changed (which it almost certainly will). It is interesting to know that, to a large extent, Pascal takes care of this need because of the way it is structured as a language—another point in its favor. A print-out of the program should be kept in a safe place. A back-up copy of the program should be kept on a disk or tape file and stored.

Writing your own programs is not a task to be undertaken lightly. A programer capable of writing a satisfactory package for a laboratory will need to have considerable experience. One or two classes at night school is usually not sufficient. It is often possible to train someone in the lab to program well, but this will require a sizable investment in time. Programming, even for the experienced, is a task that can consume a considerable amount of time; it is not usually satisfactory to ''borrow'' a programer from another department ''for a few days.'' If complete program development for a pulmonary lab is to be done satisfactorily, it usually requires a major commitment of time by a person with adequate training in the field. This does not mean that a person with a small amount of training will not be able to program effectively; it only means that it is neither wise nor fair to count on such a person to do the bulk of your programing unless they are given additional training and sufficient time for the task.

When purchasing a software package, whether it is for running an entire laboratory or just for driving a new plotter, several important considerations must be kept in mind if the package is to work satisfactorily. The package must be compatible with your system. That is, if your system is a Data General, then the software must run on a Data General. Another important consideration is the form that the software is available in. If it is on magnetic tape and you do not have a tape drive, then you must have it translated onto a medium that you do have (such as a floppy disk). This translation can often be done by a computer vendor, but will cost additional money. Obviously, you should not count on being able to do this until you verify that there is someone who can do it for the particular system you have. If the package is complex, a certain amount of training of lab personnel may be required. This training should be included as part of the program package. The software vendor should provide ''support'' for his package. Support is the continuing maintenance and updating of the package to cure any bugs or errors that might be discovered. Support often means providing the latest version whenever updates occur, for a nominal charge.

FUTURE TECHNOLOGICAL ADVANCES

The minicomputer field is without a doubt one of the fastest changing technological areas, making it difficult to accurately predict what is coming in the next few years. But the important question is not so much what is coming as what impact will it have. In the next few years, look for more capable computer systems at about the same prices. The cost of the computer will go down, but the prices for peripherals and software will continue to climb, keeping the overall price about constant. Certain costs will probably continue to fall and are important to anyone planning to expand an existing system. Specifically, the cost of main memory is considerably lower than it was just a few years ago. The cost of hard disks, particularly the so-called Winchester disk, is going down steadily. Magnetic tape drives have recently dropped considerably in price. Tape drives and hard disks will soon be available on systems at much lower prices than previously. The bottom line is that if you buy a system that meets your current needs, is made by a major manufacturer, and allows you to expand its capabilities readily, then it will provide satisfactory service to your lab for many years to come. New developments are not likely to make a satisfactorily performing system obsolete.

CHAPTER 28

Guide to Manufacturers of Pulmonary Function Testing Equipment and Supplies

CATHY FONZI, RCPT
CRAIG PEDERSON, RCPT

This guide is included in this text because similar information is not readily available elsewhere. No attempt was made to include or exclude listings based on the quality of the products. Any omissions that may have occurred were inadvertent. Inclusion in this guide does not represent endorsement by the California Thoracic Society or the authors of the text.

MANUFACTURERS BY EQUIPMENT

Blood-Gas Analyzers

AVL Scientific Corp.
Corning Medical
Instrumentation Laboratories
The London Co. (Radiometer)
Technicon Instruments Corp.

Body Plethysmographs

Cardio-Pulmonary Instruments
Collins, Warren E., Inc.
Erich Jaeger, Inc.
Gould Godart
Medi Craft Instruments, Inc.
Ohio Medical Products Div.
P.K. Morgan, Ltd.
SRL Medical, Inc.

Bronchial Provocation, Inhalation Dosimeter

Chest Corp.
Laboratory for Applied Immunology

Chromatographs

Antek Instruments, Inc.
Bendix Corp.
Bowers Instrument Co.
Camag Inc.
Clinical Analysis Products Co.

PULMONARY FUNCTION TESTING
GUIDELINES AND CONTROVERSIES

ISBN 0-12-788125-5

Hewlett-Packard Co.
Laboratory Data Control
LKB Instruments, Inc.
Micrometric Instrument Co.
QuinTron Instrument Co., Inc.

Computer Software

Chest Corp.
Digital Equipment Corp.
Equilibrated Bio-Systems, Inc.
Erich Jaeger, Inc.
Hewlett-Packard Co.
Jones Medical Instrument Co.
Medical Graphics Corp.
Personalized Software
Russell Medical Specialties
Telediagnostics Systems
Telemed Cardio-Pulmonary Systems

DL_{CO} Systems

Bio-Logic Systems, Inc.
Chest Corp.
Collins, Warren E., Inc.
Erich Jaeger, Inc.
Gould Godart
Hewlett-Packard Co.
Jones Medical Instrument Co.
Medical Graphics Corp.
Medi Craft Instruments, Inc.
Med-Science Electronics, Inc.
P.K. Morgan Ltd.
SRL Medical, Inc.

Esophageal Balloons

Young Rubber Corp.

Exercise Equipment

Alpha Technologies, Inc.
Collins, Warren E., Inc.
Erich Jaeger, Inc.
Gould Godart
Medical Graphics Corp.
P.K. Morgan, Ltd.
QuinTron Instrument Co.
Siemens Elema Ventilator Systems
SRL Medical, Inc.
Statham Instruments, Inc.

Gas Analyzers

CO_2

Applied Electrochemistry, Inc.
Beckman Instruments, Inc.
Cavitron
Erich Jaeger, Inc.
Gould Godart
Hewlett-Packard Co.
Instrumentation Laboratories
P.K. Morgan, Ltd.
Siemens Elema Ventilator Systems
Vertek

CO

Beckman Instruments, Inc.
Chest Corp.
Collins, Warren E., Inc.
Erich Jaeger, Inc.
Gould Godart
Hewlett-Packard Co.
Jones Medical Instrument Co.
Med-Science Electronics, Inc.
P.K. Morgan, Ltd.
SRL Medical, Inc.

He

Cardio-Pulmonary Instruments
Collins, Warren E., Inc.
Erich Jaeger, Inc.
Gould Godart
Jones Medical Instruments Co.

Med-Science Electronics, Inc.
P.K. Morgan, Ltd.
QuinTron Instrument Co., Inc.

N_2

Antek Instruments, Inc.
Cardio-Pulmonary Instruments
Collins, Warren E., Inc.
Erich Jaeger, Inc.
Hewlett-Packard Co.
Med-Science Electronics, Inc.
Ohio Medical Products Div.
Vertek

O_2

Applied Electrochemistry, Inc.
Beckman Instruments, Inc.
Beckton Dickinson Medical Systems
Biomarine Industries
Del Mar Avionics
Erich Jaeger, Inc.
Gould Godart
Oxford Instrument Co., Inc.
P.K. Morgan, Ltd.
Siemens Elema Ventilator Systems
Teledyne Analytical Instruments

Mass Spectrometers

Chemtrix Inc.
CVC Products, Inc.
Finnigan Corp.
LKB Instruments, Inc.
Perkin-Elmer Medical Instruments

MIP Gauges

Applied Engineering
Boehringer Laboratories
Jones Medical Instruments Co.

Miscellaneous Laboratory Supplies

Bryans Southern Instruments, Ltd.
Dade Div., American Hospital Supply Corp.
Latex Products
Lundy Medical Products, Inc.
Marquest Medical Products, Inc. (syringes)
Popper & Sons, Inc.
Vacumed

Multiple Gas Analyzers

United Technical Corp.
(see also: chromatographs, mass spectrometers)

Oximeters

American Optical
BT, Inc.
Instrumentation Laboratories
Hewlett-Packard Co.
The London Co.

Oxygen Content

Lexington Instruments Corp.

Quality Control Products, Blood Gas

ALKO Diagnostic Corp.
Analytical Products, Inc.
Corning Medical
Dade Div., American Hospital Supply Corp.
Fisher Scientific
General Diagnostics, Div.
Instrumentation Laboratories

RNA Medical Corp.
R.S. Weber and Associates
The London Company
W.T. Farley, Inc.

Spirometers

Alpha Technologies, Inc.
Armstrong Industries, Inc.
Beckton-Dickinson Medical Systems
Breon Laboratories, Inc.
Bio-Logics Systems, Inc.
Cardio-Pulmonary Instruments
Cavitron
Chest Corp.
Collins, Warren E., Inc.
Cybermedic, Medistor Div.
Datametrics
Devilbiss Co.
Draeger Medical Lts.
Erich Jaeger, Inc.
Hewlett-Packard Co.
Jones Medical Instrument Co.
LSE Corp.
Marion Laboratories, Inc.
Medi Craft Instruments, Inc.
Med-Science Electronics, Inc.
Monaghan
Ohio Medical Products Div.
P.K. Morgan, Ltd.
Puritan Bennett
Spirotech, Inc.
SRL Medical, Inc.
Technicon Instruments Corp.
Vitalograph Medical Instrumentation

Spirometry: Calibration Devices

Charles Meriam Co., Inc.
Fisher & Porter
Hans Rudolf, Inc.
Jones Medical Instrument Co.
Medi Craft Instruments, Inc.
Vacumed Inc.
Vitalograph Medical

Tonometers

Analytical Products, Inc.
Instrumentation Laboratories
R.S. Weber and Associates

Transducers, Pressure

Datametrics Inc.
Erich Jaeger, Inc.
Hewlett-Packard Co.
P.K. Morgan, Ltd.
Statham Instruments, Inc.
Validyne Engineering Corp.

Valves

Collins, Warren E., Inc.
Erich Jaeger, Inc.
Hans Rudolf, Inc.
Medi Craft Instruments, Inc.

MANUFACTURERS BY ALPHABETICAL ORDER

A

ALKO Diagnostic Corp.
412 Washington
Holliston, MA 01746
(617) 429-4600

Alpha Technologies, Inc.
22961 Triton Way
Laguna Hills, CA 92653

Ambulatory Monitoring, Inc.
731 Saw Mill River Rd.
Ardsley, NY 10502
(914) 693-9232

American Optical, Medical Div.
Box 361, Crosby Dr.
Bedford, MA 01730
(617) 275-0500

American Optical
Scientific Instr. Div.
Eggert & Sugar Rds.
Buffalo, NY 14215
(716) 895-4000

Analytical Products, Inc.
511 Taylor Way
Belmont, CA 94002
(415) 592-1400

Antek Instruments, Inc.
6005 N. Freeway
Houston, TX 77076
(713) 691-2265.

Applied Electrochemistry, Inc.
735 N. Pastoria Ave.
Sunnyvale, CA 94086
(408) 732-7880

Applied Engineering
2038 15th St. NW
Rochester, MN 55901
(507) 288-4822

Armstrong Industries, Inc.
P.O. Box 7
3660 Commercial Ave.
Northbrook, ILL 60062
(800) 323-4220
(312) 272-5577

AVL Scientific Corp.
P.O. Box 728
Pine Brook, NJ 07058
(800) 526-2272

B

Beckman Instruments
2500 Harbor Blvd.
Fullerton, CA 92634
(714) 871-4848

Beckton Dickinson Medical Systems
Route 1
Sharon, MA 02067
(617) 784-7878

Bendix Corp., Environmental & Process
Instrument Division
P.O. Drawer 831
Lewisberg, WV 24901
(304) 647-4538

Bio-Logics Systems, Inc.
422 Wakara Way
U. of U. Research Park
Salt Lake City, Utah 84108
(801) 582-5331

Biomarine Industries
45 Great Valley Center
Malvern, PA 19355
(215) 647-7200

Boehringer Laboratories
P.O. Box 337
Wynnewood, PA 19096
(215) 642-4944

Bowers Instrument Co.
2600 Monroe St.
Wilmington, DE 19802

Breon Laboratories, Inc.
90 Park Ave.
New York, NY 10016
(212) 972-4141

Bryans Southern Instruments, Ltd.
Willow Lane, Mitcham
Surrey, CR4UL, England
Tel: 01-640-3490
Telex: 946097

BT, Inc.
5589 Arapahoe Ave.
Suite 203
P.O. Box 914
Boulder, CO 80306
(303) 447-9842

C

Camag Inc.
2855 S. 163 St.
New Berlin, WI 53153
(414) 782-1220

Cardio-Pulmonary Instruments (C.P.I.)
Div. of SRL Medical, Inc.
Box 36424
6400 Westpark Dr., Suite 150
Houston, TX 77036
(713) 783-7520

Cavitron/KDC Medical Sales
A Division of Cavitron Corp.
1542 S. Embassy St.
Anaheim, CA 92802

Charles Meriam Co., Inc.
1183 N. Tustin Ave.
Anaheim, CA 92807
(714) 630-0671

Chemtrix Inc.
163 S.W. Freeman Ave.
Hillsboro, OR 97123
(503) 648-0762

Chest Corp.
31-7 Hakusan I Chome
Bunkyo-ku, Tokyo, 113 Japan
Tel: 03-812-7251
Telex: 272-3701

Clinical Analysis Prods. Co. (CAPCO)
599 N. Mathilda Ave.
Sunnyvale, CA 94086
(408) 739-7270

Collins, Warren E., Inc.
220 Wood Rd.
Braintree, MA 02184
(617) 843-0610

Concord Laboratories
21 Gregory Dr.
Fairfax, CA 94930
(415) 457-5207

Corning Medical
Medfield, MA 02052
(617) 359-7711

CVC Products, Inc.
525 Lee Rd. P.O. Box 1886
Rochester, NY 14603
(716) 458-2550

Cybermedic, Medistor Div.
P.O. Box 3468
Boulder, CO 80307
(303) 666-9253

D

Dade Division, American Hosp. Supply Corp.
P.O. Box 520672
Miami, FL 33152
(305) 592-2311

Datametrics Inc.
340 Fordham Rd.
Wilmington, MA 01887
(617) 658-5410

Del Mar Avionics
1601 Alton Ave., at Red Hill
Irvine, CA 92714
(714) 549-1500

The Devilbiss Co. (Health Care Division)
P.O. Box 552
Somerset, PA 15501
(814) 443-4881

Digital Equipment Corp.
8340 Clairemont Mesa Blvd.
San Diego, CA 92111
(714) 292-1818

Draeger Medical Lts.
(See N. Amer. Draeger)
Hertfordshire House
Wood Lane
Hemel Hempstead
Herts HP24SU
(0442) 3542

E

Equilibrated Bio-Systems, Inc.
P.O. Box 612
Syosset, NY 11791

Erich Jaeger, Inc.
P.O. Box 5465
Rockford, ILL 61125
(815) 847-9475

F

Finnigan Corp.
595 N. Pastoria Ave.
Sunnyvale, CA 94086
(408) 732-0940

Fischer and Porter
Warminster, PA 18974
(215) 674-6000

Fisher Scientific Co.
590 Lincoln St.
Waltham, MA 02154
(617) 890-4300

Fisher Scientific
Diagnostics Division
526 Route 303
Orangeburg, NY 10962
(914) 359-9200

G

Gast Manufacturing
P.O. Box 97
Benton Harbor, MI 49022
(616) 926-6171

General Electric Corp.
1211 W. 22nd St.
Oak Brook, ILL 60521
(312) 325-4217

General Diagnostics, Div.
Warner-Lambert Co.
Morris Plains, NJ 07950
(201) 540-2640

Gould Godart (see also Statham and SRL Medical)
2330 Statham Blvd.
Oxnard, CA 93030
(805) 487-8511
Telex: 65-9223

H

Hans Rudolf, Inc.
7200 Wyandotte St.
Kansas City, MO 64114
(816) 363-5522

Harris-Lake, Inc.
10910 Briggs Rd.
Cleveland, OH 44111
(216) 251-8870

Hewlett-Packard Co.
Medical Products Group
1776 Minutemen Rd.
Andover, MD 01810

Hewlett-Packard Co.
Scientific Instruments Division
1601 California Ave.
Palo Alto, CA 94304
(415) 493-1311

I

Instrumentation Laboratories
113 Hartwell Ave.
Lexington, MA 02173
(617) 861-0710

K

Kruger & Eckels, Inc.
P.O. Box 681
S. Pasadena, CA 91030
(213) 799-4200

L

Laboratory for Applied Immunology
c/o Richard R. Rosenthal, M.D.
The John Hopkins University
School of Medicine at
The Good Samaritan Hospital
5601 Loch Raven Boulevard
Baltimore, MD 21239

Laboratory Data Control
P.O. Box 10235, Interstate Ind. Pk.
Riviera Beach, FL 33404
(305) 844-5241

Latex Products
Div. of Mid-State Enterprise, Inc.
155 Van Winkle Ave.
Hawthorne, NJ 07506
(201) 427-6040

Lexington Instruments Corp.
241 Crescent St.
Waltham, MA 02154
(617) 899-0410

LKB Instruments, Inc.
12221 Parklawn Dr.
Rockville, MD 20852
(301) 881-2510

LSE Corp.
6 Gill St.
Woburn, MA 01801
(617) 935-4954

Lundy Medical Products, Inc.
1015 E. Katella
Unit C
Anaheim, CA 92805
(714) 937-1441

M

Marion Laboratories, Inc.
10236 Bunker Ridge Rd.
Kansas City, MO 64137
(800) 327-3247

Marquest Medical Products, Inc.
109 Inverness Dr. East Cl
Englewood, CO 80112
(303) 770-4835
(800) 525-7044

Medical Graphics Corp.
501 W. County Rd. E
St. Paul, MN
(612) 484-4874

Medical Instruments,
Perkin-Elmer Corp.
2771 North Garey
Pomona, CA 91767
(714) 593-3581

Medi Craft Instruments, Inc.
48 Merrick Rd.
Rockville Center, NY 11570
(516) 536-8010

Med-Science Electronics, Inc.
Science Park
600 Wheeler Rd.
Burlington, MA 01803
(617) 273-4000

Micrometrics Instrument Corp.
5680 Goshen Springs Rd.
Norcross, GA 30093
(404) 448-8282

Micro-Metric Instrument Co.
P.O. Box 22226
Cleveland, OH 44122
(216) 524-8502

MKS (Baratron)
22 Third Ave.
Burlington, MA 01803
(617) 272-9255

Monaghan
4100 East Dry Creek Rd.
Littleton, CO 80122

N

North American Draeger
148 B Quarry Rd.
P.O. Box 121
Telford, PA 18969
(215) 723-9824

Nuclear Associates, Inc.
100 Voice Rd.
Carle Place, NY 11514
(516) 741-6360

O

Ohio Medical Products Div.
3030 Airco Dr.
P.O. Box 7550
Madison, WI 53707
Telex: (910) 286-2712

Orion Research, Inc.
P.O. Box 681
S. Pasadena, CA 91030
(213) 799-4200

Oxford Instrument Co., Inc.
234 Meadow Rd.
Jackson, MI 39206
(601) 362-4411

P

Perkin-Elmer
Medical Instruments
2771 North Garey
Pomona, CA 91767
(714) 593-3581

P.K. Morgan Ltd. (in U.S.A.)
P.K. Morgan Instruments, Inc.
200 Sutton St.
Andover, MA 01845
(617) 685-8061

P.K. Morgan Ltd.
10 Manor Road, Chatham
Kent, England ME46AL
Tel: 0634-44384-47949-48627
Telegrams: Diftest, Chatham, Kent

Popper & Sons, Inc.
300 Denton Ave.
New Hyde Park, NY 11040
(516) 248-0300

Puritan Bennett
17855 E. Rowland Ave.
City of Industry, CA 91748
(213) 964-3415

Q

Quinton Instrument Co.
2121 Terry Ave.
Seattle, WN 98121
(206) 223-7373

QuinTron Instrument Co., Inc.
3712 W. Pierce
Milwaukee, WI 53215
(414) 645-1515

R

R.S. Weber And Associates
31240 La Baya Dr.
Westlake Village, CA 91361
(213) 889-4630
(805) 495-6414

Radiometer A/S
72 Emdrupvey
DK - 2400 Copenhagen
Denmark

RNA Medical Corp.
21 Cummings Park, Suite 228
Woburn, MA 01801
(617) 935-7111

Roche Medical Electronics, Inc.
Cranbury, NJ 08512
(609) 448-1200

Russell Medical Specialties
6500 Village Parkway No. 212
Dublin, CA 94566
(415) 829-1539

S

Siemens Elema Ventilator Systems
1765 Commerce Dr.
Elk Grove Village, ILL 60007
(312) 981-4940

Spirotech Inc.
4025 Pleasantdale Rd.
Atlanta, GA 30340
Suite 520
(404) 447-8881

SRL Medical, Inc.
2676 Indian Ripple Rd.
Dayton, OH 45440
(513) 426-0033

Statham Instruments, Inc.
Medical Division
2230 Statham Blvd.
Oxnard, CA 93030
(805) 487-8511

T

Technicon Instruments Corp.
Technicon Outreach Pulmonary Systems
206 Talbott Tower
Dayton, OH 45402
(513) 223-6926

Technicon Instruments Corp.
Clinical Division (Blood Gas Analyzers)
155 Benedict Ave.
Terrytown, NY 10591

Tektronic Inc.
P.O. Box 500
Beaverton, OR 97077
(503) 638-3411

Telediagnostics Systems
San Francisco, CA
(800) 227-3224

Teledyne Analytical Instruments
333 W. Mission Dr. P.O. Box 70
San Gabriel, CA 91776
(213) 283-7181 or (213) 576-1633

Telemed Cardio-Pulmonary Systems
5181 S. Third West
Salt Lake City, Utah 84107
(801) 268-3480

The London Co.
811 Sharon Dr.
Cleveland, OH 44145
(216) 871-8900

Thomas Co., Arthur H.
Vine St. at Third P.O. Box 779
Philadelphia, PA 19106
(215) 574-4500

Transmed Scientific (formerly Biocom)
860-C Capitolio Way
San Luis Obispo, CA 93401
(805) 541-1103

U

United Technical Corp.
83 Keystone Dr.
Leominster, MA 01453
(617) 537-9737

V

Vacumed Inc.
2261 Palma Dr.
Ventura, CA 93003
(805) 644-7461

Validyne Engineering Corp.
P.O. Box 9025
Northridge, CA 93128
(213) 886-8488

Vertek
364 Dorset St.
So. Burlington, Vermont 05401
(802) 863-2808

Vitalograph Medical Instrumentation
8347 Quivira Rd.
Lenexa, KN 66205
(800) 255-6626

W

W.T. Farley
23974 Craftsman Rd.
Calabasas, CA 91302
(213) 724-2118

Y

Young Rubber Corp.
P.O. Box 5147
Enterprise Ave.
Trenton, NJ 08638
(609) 392-5134

Index

D

E

I

J

L

M

R

T

V

W

X

a
b
3 c
4 d
5 e
6 f
7 g
8 h
9 i
8 0 j